MASTERING THE CLINICAL CONVERSATION

Also Available

Acceptance and Commitment Therapy:
The Process and Practice of Mindful Change, Second Edition
Steven C. Hayes, Kirk D. Strosahl, and Kelly G. Wilson

Mindfulness and Acceptance:
Expanding the Cognitive-Behavioral Tradition
Edited by Steven C. Hayes, Victoria M. Follette, and Marsha M. Linehan

Mastering the Clinical Conversation

Language as Intervention

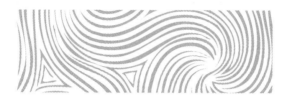

Matthieu Villatte
Jennifer L. Villatte
Steven C. Hayes

THE GUILFORD PRESS
New York   London

The authors have checked with sources believed to be reliable in their efforts to
provide information that is complete and generally in accord with the standards
of practice that are accepted at the time of publication. However, in view of the
possibility of human error or changes in behavioral, mental health, or medical
sciences, neither the authors, nor the editors and publisher, nor any other party
who has been involved in the preparation or publication of this work warrants
that the information contained herein is in every respect accurate or complete,
and they are not responsible for any errors or omissions or the results obtained
from the use of such information. Readers are encouraged to confirm the
information contained in this book with other sources.

Library of Congress Cataloging-in-Publication Data

Names: Villatte, Matthieu. | Villatte, Jennifer L. | Hayes, Steven C.
Title: Mastering the clinical conversation : language as intervention / by
  Matthieu Villatte, Jennifer L. Villatte, Steven C. Hayes.
Description: New York : The Guilford Press, [2016] | Includes bibliographical
  references and index.
Identifiers: LCCN 2015037310 | ISBN 9781462523061 (hardback) |
  ISBN 9781462542161 (paperback)
Subjects: LCSH: Psychotherapist and patient. | Psychotherapists—Language. |
  Communication in psychiatry. | Psychotherapy. | BISAC: MEDICAL /
  Psychiatry / General. | SOCIAL SCIENCE / Social Work. | PSYCHOLOGY /
  Psychotherapy / General.
Classification: LCC RC480.8 .V55 2016 | DDC 616.89/14—dc23
LC record available at http://lccn.loc.gov/2015037310

To my parents,
Michèle and Jean Villatte
—M. V.

To my partner in all things,
Matthieu
—J. L. V.

To my wife and soul mate,
Jacqueline Pistorello
—S. C. H.

About the Authors

Matthieu Villatte, PhD, is Research Scientist and Clinical Trainer at the Evidence-Based Practice Institute in Seattle. He has conducted workshops on the clinical applications of relational frame theory and contextual behavioral science in the United States, Canada, Australia, South America, and Europe. He is also an associate editor of the *Journal of Contextual Behavioral Science*. Dr. Villatte's current work focuses on the dissemination of evidence-based practices, and he has published articles and book chapters on relational frame theory, contextual behavioral science, and experiential cognitive-behavioral therapy.

Jennifer L. Villatte, PhD, is a clinical psychologist committed to advancing health equity through contextual behavioral science. She is Assistant Professor of Psychiatry and Behavioral Sciences at the University of Washington, where she partners with innovators in computer engineering, human-centered design, and data science to maximize the effectiveness and reach of behavioral interventions that enhance individual and community well-being.

Steven C. Hayes, PhD, is Nevada Foundation Professor in the Department of Psychology at the University of Nevada, Reno. He has served as president of multiple scientific and professional organizations, including the Association for Behavioral and Cognitive Therapies and the Association for Contextual Behavioral Science. His work has been recognized by the Award for Impact of Science on Application from the Society for the Advancement of Behavior Analysis and the Lifetime Achievement Award from the

Association for Behavioral and Cognitive Therapies, among other awards. The author of 41 books and over 575 scientific articles, Dr. Hayes has focused on understanding human language and cognition and applying this understanding to the alleviation of human suffering and the promotion of human welfare. His books include *Acceptance and Commitment Therapy, Second Edition: The Process and Practice of Mindful Change*, and *Mindfulness and Acceptance: Expanding the Cognitive-Behavioral Tradition*.

Preface

The human species' greatest advantage is its unique ability to wield the world's most powerful tool: language. Our capacity to learn and thrive has grown exponentially with the acquisition of language and its related mental processes. Yet this power does not come without cost. Talking, thinking, and reasoning are at the core of many, if not most, psychological problems. That is part of why we call the behavioral problems we treat "mental health" problems.

This dual nature of language creates a unique problem for psychotherapists, as language is also at the core of most psychological treatments. Many of the therapy techniques aimed at changing our words and thoughts have unintended, even paradoxical, results. Beliefs and memories tend to persist even in the face of contradictory evidence and a sincere desire to change them. Even if we can beat back troublesome thoughts, placing mental content at the forefront of the battle often reinforces its importance and influence over our lives. These battles leave both clients and therapists exhausted and discouraged. How can psychotherapists alleviate the suffering caused by language and cognition *through the use of* language and cognition? This book represents an alternate approach, where clinicians disengage from the struggle and help clients harness the power of language to promote psychological resilience and flourishing.

Many psychotherapy manuals function like recipe collections—step-by-step procedures that cooks of all skill levels can follow in order to produce a specific outcome. They are quick and easy to use, produce generally consistent results, and reduce the risk of user error by requiring relatively little input or decision making. Cookbooks have their use, but another approach is possible. Master chefs can innovate on the spot and be confident that they will achieve their desired results because their actions are based on well-tested principles. They can modify recipes and substitute ingredients based on the resources available in their current cooking environment and the personal preferences of the people they are serving. They can also adapt a recipe to their own style, emphasizing their unique strengths and creating a more personal experience for their clients.

One thing that has been missing from psychotherapy development and training is a set of solid behavioral principles that show clinicians how to masterfully wield their most essential tool—language—and turn the clinical conversation into a haven for healing. We believe the time has arrived to explore the potential of relational frame theory (RFT) to provide a way out of this seemingly unwinnable battle. Rather than waging war on language or simply ignoring that our primary weapon can cause unintentional damage, RFT provides guidelines for using language therapeutically. No need to give up the benefits of language. No need to sacrifice our clients' flourishing and vitality as collateral damage.

RFT has a notorious reputation as being hard to learn, primarily because early RFT research is characterized by the technical precision and painstaking research paradigms required to investigate novel conceptual claims and establish its relevance to basic science. The resulting data have rich and diverse implications for applied science, but understanding them requires deep familiarity with both technical terminology and complex methodology. Perhaps a greater challenge is that RFT entails an entirely new approach to thinking about language and cognition. It is an approach that runs counter to prevailing cultural norms and requires a reexamination of one's philosophical assumptions and worldview—a process that can be as unsettling as it is liberating.

We have made every effort to keep things straightforward and practical in this volume. We will focus on the implications of RFT rather than its technical aspects. Even so, there will be times when you may find yourself confused or uncertain as you begin to apply what you learn here to your case conceptualizations and treatment plans. In trainings we have conducted, however, participants tell us that even that uncertainty comes along with a sense that a new vista is opening up. You begin to see language processes in flight. With a relatively small set of language principles, we hope you will be able to adopt, adapt, and integrate evidence-based practices in a way that fits with your own theoretical ideas, is sensitive to the needs and preferences of your clients, and, most importantly, helps you accomplish your clinical goals.

WHAT YOU WILL FIND IN THIS MANUAL

This manual is organized in two major sections. The first three chapters provide a foundation in the theory and science informing the clinical approach detailed in this book. Chapter 1 introduces language as learned behavior central to all aspects of human psychology and explores how language interacts with other behavioral learning processes. This chapter explains the relationship between RFT and contextual behavioral science, and why this approach has important advantages for psychotherapists.

In Chapter 2, we consider how normal language processes are responsible for many of the problematic behaviors observed across clinical disorders. We discuss how language processes are involved in the development and maintenance of psychological problems, and how to recognize them in clinical practice.

Chapter 3 provides a framework for using RFT principles in psychotherapy. We define overarching goals that guide the clinical conersation, along with a set of language tools for accomplishing these clinical goals.

These three chapters are the most theoretical of the book. We have been careful to keep the discussion practical, with concrete examples you will find familiar from your own life and clinical practice. Every principle you will learn in these chapters will be useful in the subsequent chapters on assessment and intervention.

Chapter 4 demonstrates how to use RFT to conduct psychological assessment. The strategies we present here are intended to be broadly applicable across therapy traditions and to guide the integration of language targets and interventions in case formulation and treatment planning. This approach to assessment is designed to be inherently collaborative and validating, laying the groundwork for a strong therapeutic relationship and ensuring that both client and therapist are working toward mutually agreed-upon goals and progress markers.

The next six chapters of the book detail clinical interventions based on the experiential use of language suggested by RFT. As each principle is presented, we consider what we are trying to accomplish, why it is important, how it connects to clinical traditions generally, and how to enact it from an RFT point of view. In Chapter 5, we show how to use language to activate and shape behavior change. In Chapter 6, we examine how to apply specific symbolic relations to establish a flexible sense of self. Chapter 7 explores how language can be used to integrate clients' behavior into symbolic relations that increase motivation and provide support for meaningful actions.

Chapter 8 shows you how to craft and deliver powerful experiential metaphors that resonate with your clients' experience and maximize the possibility of clinical change. In Chapter 9, we explain how you can use RFT in formal experiential training. Finally, in Chapter 10, we apply RFT principles to the therapeutic relationship, demonstrating ways to enhance empathy, compassion, and the courage to stay present and committed to acting in your clients' best interest. At the end of this book, you will also find a quick guide to using RFT in psychotherapy, in which you can review all the skills presented in Chapters 4–7 with concrete examples, and a compilation of practical definitions of terms we are using here.

The approach we lay out here is intended to function as a guide for empowering clinical practice regardless of the brand of psychotherapy you use. We believe these principles can enhance interventions within many different evidence-based treatments. As such, this book is not meant as a collection of therapy recipes. It is not a cookbook. It is a set of principles through which you can gain mastery over the language you and your clients use in psychotherapy. We are not suggesting that you adopt a new set of techniques; we have no intention of encouraging you to abandon strategies you know to be effective. Our goal is to show that RFT principles can empower you as a therapist to be present, to listen, and to intervene in the way your training and scientific beliefs encourage—but to do so within language processes that make good sense. Our hope is that by mastering the clinical conversation, you will make an even bigger difference in the lives of those you serve.

Acknowledgments

We would like to thank our colleagues, friends, and students who provided feedback on the full manuscript or on selected chapters: Niklas Törneke, Louise McHugh, Darrah Westrup, Jennifer Plumb-Vilardaga, Pierre Cousineau, Danielle Moyer, Jillian Jacobelli, Maarten Aalberse, Yvonne Barnes-Holmes, Simon Dymond, Steven Vannoy, Stephanie Caldas, Jean-Louis Monestès, Sophie Cheval, Olivier Lefebvre, Roger Vilardaga, Carlton Coulter, Samantha and Drake Pollard, Rainer Sonntag, Jim Nageotte, and the anonymous reviewers selected by The Guilford Press. We are grateful for Kelly Koerner's generous mentorship in clinical teaching and building expert performance. We would also like to thank the numerous participants in our clinical trainings and the members of the Association for Contextual Behavioral Science who helped us refine our work throughout this challenging process of making relational frame theory accessible and useful to clinicians.

Matthieu Villatte would like to thank Jennifer and Steve for being the main sources of support and inspiration in his work since meeting them, separately, on the same day in May 2009.

Jennifer Villatte would like to thank her clinical mentors, who inspired and supported her in exploring applications of relational frame theory across a broad spectrum of evidence-based psychotherapies: Steve Hayes, William Follette, Alan Fruzzetti, Jaqueline Pistorello, Steven Vannoy, Barbara McCann, Debra Kaysen, Kate Comtois, Joan Romano, and Chris Dunn.

Steve Hayes would like to thank Jacque and little Stevie for tolerating the many hours he sat in the living room with a laptop sitting on his legs.

Contents

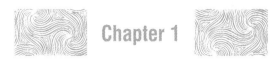

Chapter 1

The Power of Language

All psychological interventions rely on the power of language. Even those that emphasize silence, employ imagery, induce hypnosis, or conduct exercises to promote direct contact with the here and now do so by engaging language processes. Psychotherapists rarely intervene directly in their clients' lives—they create change largely through conversation. Effective therapists, by nature and by training, are skilled at using language; speaking articulately, listening with attention and understanding, and promoting psychological well-being through dialogue. Language builds alliance, provokes insight, and expresses empathy; it teaches concepts, shapes new skills, and guides therapeutic exercises. Language isn't just a vehicle for therapeutic intervention—it *is* intervention.

Not only is language an essential tool for promoting positive change in psychotherapy, it is involved in the development and maintenance of most forms of psychopathology. Language orients us to what we should be aware of, and as soon as we are aware, we begin to describe, evaluate, and analyze. Our direct experience of emotions, thoughts, memories, learning experiences, and bodily sensations become quickly interwoven with reasons and narratives that influence us as much as the experiences themselves.

The power of language to transform human experience is evident in most clinicians' caseloads. Language can transform a harmless object into a terrifying threat; imagination can become indistinguishable from reality; a memory of a long-gone trauma can open fresh wounds; anticipation of an improbable outcome can become a barrier to happiness. The ways we think and speak about our experience can take us away from the world we live in and trap us in an ever-expanding world within our own minds. Without language processes, we could not worry about catastrophic outcomes,

1

ruminate over past transgressions, or endorse delusional beliefs; we couldn't ascribe blame, defend perfectionistic standards, or doubt whether our lives have meaning or purpose. The price of language, it seems, is often our own flourishing.

Similarly, in the absence of language, it would be impossible to hope, to dream of a better life, to contemplate ideals, or to be touched by someone we've never met. Clinicians are often amazed at the resilience of the human spirit and our persistent capacity to cooperate, connect, and seek understanding. These experiences also rely on the core processes that underlie language. It is how we create and critique laws, literature, philosophies, histories, theologies, and the arts. It's no wonder that we call the fields that study these products of language "the humanities": they define us as a species.

The benefits of language are not limited to communication and understanding; language has a powerful influence on many forms of behavior. Humans alone can avoid terrible consequences by following good rules and advice. We can create useful and beautiful things, like rocket ships and cathedrals, from mathematical formulas and physical laws. We can infer the intentions and feeling states of others, allowing us to make predictions about how they will behave and adjust our behavior accordingly. After symbolically stepping into another's shoes, we may stop a bully or choose a perfect gift. We can compare, analyze, evaluate, and plan, thus solving problems more efficiently than any other species. We can even find hope and motivation to persevere in trying times by anticipating a brighter future.

Language, as we mean it in this book, is at the core of virtually all complex human abilities, including thinking, imagining, remembering, self-awareness, and perspective taking. Our relatively weak and defenseless species has been able to dominate this ancient planet after only a few thousand years of wielding this powerful tool—a tool, it seems, that is capable of creation and devastation in equal measure. Accordingly, language has long been a phenomenon of great interest within psychology and other fields concerned with improving the human condition.

TRADITIONAL APPROACHES TO LANGUAGE IN PSYCHOTHERAPY

Every mature psychotherapy system touches on the role of language, symbols, and meaning. Psychoanalytic traditions sought to resolve clinical conflicts by understanding the symbolism and covert meaning of common events through techniques such as dream analysis and free association. Humanistic therapists aim to actualize human potential by undermining comparative and evaluative language processes through unconditional regard and empathy. Cognitive therapists modify their clients' dysfunctional schemas and troublesome beliefs through Socratic dialogue and restructuring the way clients think and speak about their experiences. While holistic and present-focused approaches, including Gestalt and mindfulness-based therapies, have warned against excessive verbal analysis and emphasized the importance of awareness and direct experience, they guide this very exploration in part through verbal means. Of all the major psychological traditions, only behaviorism showed a somewhat limited interest in psychotherapy based on language and symbolic meaning. Though B. F. Skinner claimed that radical behaviorism was "the very field of purpose and intention" (1974, p. 61), his analysis of verbal behavior led to a limited range of practical applications with verbally able clients. Many doubted that a science founded on empirical studies with nonhuman animals could provide insight into the most complex human behaviors.

So far, the different approaches to language and symbolic meaning have tended to divide traditions, not unite them, and none of these approaches has led to a generally applicable understanding of the role of language in psychotherapy itself. They have usually focused on the implications of how specific symbolic or cognitive content impacts clients rather than on providing a guide for the use of language as an active ingredient in psychotherapy. Like the air we breathe, language is as useful as it is pervasive, but we rarely notice it unless something goes awry—when we can't find the right words, communication breaks down, or misunderstanding ensues. What has been missing is a theory of language that shows us how to use this tool intentionally inside a variety of psychotherapy systems and treatment protocols. What has been missing is a behavioral science of language that can promote vitality and minimize harmful responses to psychological pain.

We seek an analysis and conceptual toolkit that can cast a useful light on clinical problems and guide and empower practitioners from all therapeutic traditions. That is the focus of the present volume.

A CONTEXTUAL BEHAVIORAL APPROACH TO LANGUAGE

This manual presents a theory of language that illuminates the complexity of human behavior and provides a pragmatic toolkit that can strengthen therapeutic practices from all traditions. This approach comes from a surprising source: a branch of behavioral psychology known as *contextual behavioral science* (CBS; Hayes, Barnes-Holmes, & Wilson, 2012; Zettle, Hayes, Barnes-Homes, & Biglan, 2016). It is surprising because behaviorism is the one psychological approach that almost foundered on the rocks of language and cognition. Language was the phenomenon that seemed beyond the limits of behavioral thinking; a distinctly human ability that a naturalistic, holistic approach to psychology could never explain. Or so it was thought.

Contextual behavioral science is not your grandfather's behaviorism, however. It seeks nothing less than to alleviate human suffering and advance human flourishing by developing basic scientific accounts of complex behaviors. It is a system of philosophical assumptions, scientific values, and methodological commitments that informs all aspects of theory development, empirical investigation, and translation of knowledge to practical applications. The approach to language you will discover in this book can be useful to therapists and broadly applicable across therapy traditions precisely *because* it is rooted in a contextual behavioral approach.

At the core of CBS is a holistic and pragmatic worldview known as *functional contextualism*, which consists of the philosophical assumptions and criteria for truth that are used to create, assess, and evaluate theories and evidence. In functional contextualism, the standard against which progressivity is measured is effectiveness—*How well does this theory help me meet my goals?* In contextual behavioral science, that goal is to alleviate suffering and enhance well-being. We encourage readers to experiment with the functional contextual criterion of effectiveness when evaluating the concepts and techniques in this book—Does this help me understand my client better? Does it improve the therapeutic relationship? Does it make my interventions more effective? Then check to see if it was useful to choose effectiveness as your benchmark for what is "good" or "true."

Within contextual behavioral science, *behavior is defined as the action of a whole organism within a particular context*. Accordingly, anything a whole human does is a behavior, including thinking, remembering, attending, feeling, and perceiving. Many readers will be used to distinguishing behavior from thought (or behavior from emotion) and find this use of the word awkward, or even wrong. As functional contextualists, we choose to use this definition because it helps us meet our clinical goals by allowing us to apply a relatively concise set of behavioral principles to a wide range of clinically important phenomena. The pragmatism in this principle-driven approach affords therapists the flexibility to respond to the diversity of human experience and countless unique combinations of client, setting, and situational factors, while remaining grounded in psychological science.

You'll notice that this definition of behavior does not separate the action of an organism from the environment in which it occurs. This is because CBS is situated within the larger field of evolution science, which considers behavior in terms of variation and selective retention, and because of its pragmatic goal: the only way to determine if a behavior is effective is to see how it works in a given context. *Context is the setting in which a behavior occurs; it contains everything that influences when, how, and why it happens.* Context refers to both historical and situational sources of influence on the organism's behavior, including biological, social, and cultural variables, development and learning history, and the organism's current internal (e.g., cognitive, affective) and external environment. Behaviors are influenced by multiple elements of the context, but it is possible to weaken or strengthen the influence of particular variables, thus, altering behavior.

Altering elements of the therapeutic context, including language, can generate substantial changes in aspects of the client's experience that psychotherapists can't access directly, such as physiological, cognitive, affective, and motivational states. This puts the power to change firmly within the hands of therapists and clients because both can observe and operate the mechanism that drives therapeutic change. It also leads to interventions that are quite efficient, impacting a wide range of treatment goals by simultaneously targeting core behavioral processes and functions rather than specific forms of thoughts, feelings, and actions.

The overarching aims of this book are to help therapists and their clients to (1) identify the contextual features that influence behavior and (2) use the power of language to alter the context in ways that support adaptive responses. Our approach is based on a contextual behavioral theory of language and cognition called relational frame theory (RFT; Hayes, Barnes-Holmes, & Roche, 2001) and its dynamic program of research, which, though relatively new, includes over 150 empirical publications in the areas of psychopathology, theory of mind, implicit cognition, intelligence, rule following, problem solving, sense of self, and scores of other clinically relevant topics (Dymond & Roche, 2013). Its principles have been successfully applied in the areas of education, developmental disabilities, health and safety behaviors, performance enhancement, relationship intimacy, organizational management, and community and cultural change. Acceptance and commitment therapy (ACT; Hayes, Strosahl, & Wilson, 1999, 2012) was the first psychotherapy explicitly linked to RFT and is an empirically supported treatment for a diverse range of problems in living (see the lists of evidence-based programs maintained by the American Psychological Association's Division 12 and the U.S. Substance Abuse and Mental Health Services Administration). The present volume is not an ACT manual, however. It is not meant to describe another or better way to do ACT, nor to suggest that you need to become an ACT therapist in order to apply RFT in your clinical practice. It is not meant to replace ACT or, indeed, any other treatment. Instead, this book is an attempt to explore and explicate principles that apply to a common core mechanism of *all* psychotherapies—language.

LANGUAGE IS A LEARNED BEHAVIOR

Building and Responding to Symbolic Relations

Modern human beings have been around for under 200,000 years (McDougall, Brown, & Fleagle, 2005), but most of the psychological processes that impact us are much, much older. Operant and classical conditioning are learning processes that appear to be over 500 million years old (Ginsberg

& Jablonka, 2010); habituation is even older. Language, however, could be as young as 100,000 years old (Nichols, 1992). Even if language extends back to the time that hominids branched off from chimpanzees, as some have argued, it is a relatively recent development; five million years is an eye-blink when considered on an evolutionary time scale.

Sometime in the last few hundred-thousand years, modern human beings began to create symbolic relationships that allowed them to mentally put things together and pull things apart; to recognize similarities and detect differences; to create analogies and predict outcomes. From humble beginnings in simple acts of naming emerged a collection of amazing and uniquely human capacities—to analyze and plan, to assign and compare values, to imagine futures that have never been experienced, to be self-aware, and to adopt others' point of view. These behaviors are referred to in other traditions as symbolic behaviors, higher order cognitive processes, or executive functions. We call them language.

In everyday use, language generally refers to the capacity to communicate, but in this book we mean much more than that. For now, we can define language as *the learned behavior of building and responding to relations among objects and events based in part on socially established cues.* That last phrase simply means that these relations are not based solely on the intrinsic[1] characteristics of the things being related. If we told you "This is Alfred," you would learn that those two things (the person and the name) are the same and this knowledge would influence how you respond to them. You may look at the person when you hear the name, for example. Yet there is nothing inherently equivalent about the person and the name; the relation is symbolic, based on that little word "is." The cue (i.e., *is*) telling you how to respond to the person and the name is based on social convention. Thus, the meaning of this cue has to be learned and depends on who is speaking and listening. On the one hand, "is" has a particular meaning for English speakers, and you wouldn't learn a thing about the person and the name if you haven't learned English. On the other hand, there is nothing unique about "is." You can still learn the relationship between the person and the name if we give you a completely different set of socially established cues ("C'est Alfred"), assuming you have learned French, of course. This is what we mean when we refer to socially established cues as *symbols*, and relationships based on these arbitrarily applicable cues as *symbolic relations.* With this understanding, we can simplify our definition: *language is the learned behavior of building and responding to symbolic relations.*

---

[1]By intrinsic, we don't mean independent of our perception, but independent of our symbolic interpretation. Thus, in the context of this definition, the color of a rose we see red is intrinsic because it doesn't depend on language, but it still depends on our perception (some animals, or humans with impaired vision, might see it differently).

This behavior of building and responding to symbolic relations is special because it transforms the way we experience our world, imbuing objects and events with meaning and altering their impact on our thoughts, feelings, and actions. So, language is not a thing that we possess; it is a skill that we learn and can apply to a range of situations that extend far beyond communication.

From an RFT perspective, language doesn't have to comprise words; mathematics (a form of language), for example, uses numbers and icons to describe relationships. Nor do language symbols have to be written or spoken. They can be gestures, as when we put our thumbs up to communicate approval, or visual images, like a red octagon that signals drivers to stop. The symbols that make up a language are not meaningful by themselves, but rather gain meaning through their participation in sets of relations. These relational networks influence our psychological responses to the objects and events they contain, including our evaluations, preferences, motivations, urges, and physiological and emotional reactions. Therapists care about language because these symbolic relationships have a profound influence on virtually all clinically relevant behavior—a fact they can use to their client's advantage.

Although there is some debate as to whether symbolic relating is *unique* to humans, there is no doubt that it is characteristic of humans. Thus far, research suggests that humans alone are able to acquire all of the features of symbolic relationships without having to rely on intrinsic properties (e.g., an object's size, shape, or color). We can assign value and meaning that is not inherent to the thing we are describing, such as when we describe Christina Aguilera as a "bigger" celebrity than Meatloaf, though Meatloaf stands 8 inches taller and 100 pounds heavier than Aguilera. The particular symbol we use can be based on social whim. Since a symbol can change over time and across social groups, its meaning must be understood based on the context in which it occurs. If asked what the word "cool" means, a number of definitions might come to mind, but if told that Christina Aguilera is cooler than Meatloaf, you would understand that we weren't referring to her temperature.

There are other definitions of language that are valid and useful for different purposes, such as those used in the domains of linguistics, philosophy, or literature. There are also more technically precise and detailed RFT definitions of language available (e.g., Hayes et al., 2001; Törneke, 2010). We do not want to distract readers with a debate over which is the true definition or whether language is best thought of as a behavior, or a cognitive function, or something else entirely. We propose, rather, that approaching language as a learned behavior is particularly useful for psychotherapists. Our goal in the present volume is to distill this theory down to its practical essence, using terms that everybody can understand. Let's start with the first two terms in the theory's name.

Relational Framing

Relating is simply responding to one thing in terms of another, as when we understand "mother" to have a particular kind of relationship to "child" or when we evaluate something as "bigger" by relating it to something "less big." When we relate objects and events, we learn something about them. For example, if we told you that Michèle is the mother of Matthieu, you could derive other information from this relationship without us saying another word: Matthieu is the child of Michèle, Matthieu and Michèle are members of the same family, Michèle is a woman, Matthieu is younger than Michèle. You learned all of this information without being explicitly taught by combining the information entailed in these various relationships into a network of meaning and understanding. For this reason, the capacity to symbolically relate objects and events dramatically increases the efficiency with which we learn.

Many forms of learning are relational in a broad sense, but symbolic relations have several special characteristics that account for the incredible generativity of language and its powerful effect on the way we experience our world. Framing is a metaphor for this process.

Imagine you are looking at a landscape of sunshine streaming through the branches of majestic pines surrounding a clear mountain lake. If you were looking at this scene through a window frame, you might be motivated to interact with what you see and begin to prepare for a hike, a swim, or a picnic. Your attention might be drawn to features of the landscape related to those activities, like the gradient of a hiking trail, the privacy of a swimming cove, or a tree stump that would serve as the perfect picnic table. If the landscape was framed in gold and hanging in an art gallery, you might interact with it more passively, contemplating it as an object of beauty or inspiration. You may be more likely to notice the composition of the image or to appreciate the variations in color. If the scene was framed by a theater curtain and stage, you might not notice the landscape much at all, as you began to anticipate the story about to unfold against its backdrop. One scene. Three frames. A whole range of perceptions and responses. The landscape didn't change, but its influence on you did.

An example from daily life will help illustrate how our behaviors are shaped by conceptually framing objects and events according to how they relate to other things. Have you ever had to purchase something you didn't know much about—maybe a car, a computer, or a special bottle of wine? Confronted with the range of options that modern stores provide, you may have found it difficult to choose a product. Perhaps you asked for advice from the sales clerk, who may have made comparisons among your options (e.g., this computer is cheaper than that one, but it runs slower; this wine is perfect with meat, and that one would be better with dessert). As the salesclerk described, compared, and distinguished among products, he was building a network of relations (e.g., wines from Chile are cheaper than Bordeaux; the Left Bank of Bordeaux is more sophisticated than the Right Bank; 2009 was a good vintage; this bottle tastes great with meat but not with fish). This network of relations was like those picture frames: they changed the way you looked at your options. You started to eliminate some choices and became more attracted to others. Perhaps you were able to try the product yourself, in a test drive or taste test, and you began establishing new relations that were added to the network. Eventually, you made a purchase based in part on the meaning that emerged from the relational network, not solely based on your direct experience with a particular car, computer, or bottle of wine. Language framed your experience of the products and influenced the way you perceived and responded to them.

Relational frames not only influence your rational mind but your emotions and desires as well. Neuroeconomists at Caltech studied this phenomenon by organizing a double-blind wine tasting inside an fMRI scanner. Participants sampled five bottles of Cabernet Sauvignon that were distinguished solely by their selling price, ranging from $5 to $90. Unbeknownst to the participants, they were repeatedly sampling the exact same wine, which was alternately labeled as costing $10, $45, or $90. What did they discover? Participants took greater pleasure in drinking the "more expensive" wine, despite the fact that they were drinking the same stuff. Relating to the wines as "different" and "more expensive" increased both the subjective experience of pleasure and the brain activity associated with satisfaction (Plassmann, O'Doherty, Shiv, & Rangel, 2007).

Within the RFT literature, there are a variety of highly precise technical terms that address particular features of these processes. That literature is there to be explored, but our purposes here are simpler and more pragmatic. For now, the idea to remember is that language is a process of learning to relate things based on symbols, which in turn transforms the way we learn and the way we experience our world. We will explore the technical details a bit more by considering why this capacity for symbolic learning may have evolved in the first place. It was certainly not just to sell cars or improve our enjoyment of wine.

THE EVOLUTION OF LANGUAGE

Have you ever noticed how big the human brain is relative to the rest of our bodies? Humans have the highest encephalization quotient of all mammals, which poses a particular challenge for a class of animals that give birth to live young: how to get that big brain out of the birth canal. Evolutionary processes resulted in a neat solution to this problem; humans are born with a small brain that continues to grow and develop throughout childhood, adolescence, and even into early adulthood. This solution affords our species unique advantages. Human brains are fine-tuned by the environment in which they are meant to function, including the social and cultural contexts in which they develop. The downside is that human children are highly dependent on others to meet their survival needs and that caretakers themselves are more vulnerable due to this extra burden. This dependency requires that caregivers be so invested in the well-being of children that they respond to all the unpleasant sounds and smells that infants emit with the urge to approach and nurture rather than run away or attack. A strong interpersonal attachment, fostered by affiliative emotions, joint attention, perspective taking, and empathy, improves the chances of survival for both individuals, as well as others in their social group. This level of human bonding is so useful that it enables human groups to be the unit of evolutionary selection more so than the individuals within them (Nowak, Tarnita, & Wilson, 2010; Wilson & Wilson, 2007). Thus, human survival depends on a culture of cooperation and thrives on a culture of eusociality, both of which are enhanced by language processes.

RFT seems to make most sense if language and cognition are thought of as forms of cooperation that emerged initially to extend and take advantage of the intensely social nature of human groups (Hayes & Sanford, 2014). Consider one of the first instances of language we observe in children: naming. When a young child learns to say "apple" upon being presented with a particular round red object, and then to point to that particular object upon hearing someone say "apple," a relation has been established between the symbol ("apple") and the object (apple). Notice that these relationships always go in both directions: if an object is related to a symbol in a particular way, it implies a specific kind of relationship between the symbol and the object, too. Some functional properties of one object can thus be experienced in another object based on the bidirectional relationship that connects them. Once the child learns that "apple" means the same thing as apple, she will begin to respond to the symbol and the object in similar ways under certain circumstances. If she dislikes apples, she may wrinkle her nose in disgust when she hears "apple" even when she does not experience the unappetizing taste or texture of the fruit.

The bidirectionality inherent in symbolic relations is not built into normal learning processes. Pavlov's dogs salivated to the sounds of the bell—they did not prick their ears up when presented with food. Yet bidirectionality is at the core of the most characteristically human form of learning—language. How have humans come to depend on it?

It seems likely that it is because we are social, cooperative primates. To see how symbols extend cooperation, think of the roles involved. If a child sees an apple held up and hears someone say, "This is an apple" (this is the speaker role of "see apple → say 'apple'"), later she might be asked if there are apples across a canyon or around a corner (the listener role of "hear 'are there apples?' → look for apples)." The naming relation "is" likely began with simple objects and actions that took advantage of how social humans are. We can look from the point of view of the speaker or the listener. We can learn one side of the relation and *derive* the other side. The community had a powerful reason to train the derivation of mutual relations because cooperation leads to social success. And once we learned to do it, we had a template for other types of symbolic relations.

Switching roles between speaker and listener is also part of why it is so useful to communicate with symbols, now thousands of years of cultural evolution later. Through symbolic communication, we can influence the behaviors of other people (and even ourselves) simply by talking or thinking. It began with simple social exchanges, such as a child asking an adult to give her an apple even when it is out of sight, but human culture has expanded this ability to abstract thinking, storytelling, problem solving and the myriad abilities we see every day.

LANGUAGE IS A FORM OF LEARNING

Language did not spring forth fully formed; it evolved from learning processes that are at least 5,000 times older. *Yet language is a unique learning process in two important ways; it is the only learning process that itself has to be learned, and once learned, it alters all other forms of learning.* All psychotherapies promote some type of learning, whether it is called insight, skill building, cognitive restructuring, or actualizing potential. In this section we will briefly review the different learning processes that influence human psychology, as the RFT approach to language is best understood when compared and contrasted with these learning processes. For a more thorough, though highly accessible and pragmatic, primer on learning principles for clinicians, we recommend *The ABCs of Human Behavior* (Ramnerö & Törneke, 2008).

Habituation

One of the simplest types of learning is *habituation*, which is the decrease in response to a stimulus (or environmental cue) when the stimulus is presented repeatedly. Babies will startle and cry when exposed to sudden loud noises, but if the noises continue, the startle response will subside, and the child may sleep soundly in spite of the din. The central nervous system is involved in habituation in organisms that have one (Thompson, 2009), but single-celled organisms such as the amoeba or paramecium show habituation, as do single cells within multicellular organisms, like the macrophages in our immune system (Harris, 1943; Nilsonne, Appelgren, Axelsson, Fredrikson, & Lekander, 2011). This suggests that habituation is virtually as old as cellular life itself, arguably the first form of learning. Habituation is likely involved in some clinically significant phenomena, such as in arousal responses to possible dangers. Habituation is often appealed to when explaining the effects of exposure therapies, but the actual mechanisms of action are likely to be more complex since habituation readily mixes with other, newer, learning processes (Gallagher & Resick, 2012) including language processes (Kircanski, Lieberman, & Craske, 2012).

Respondent Learning

Imagine that a child steps on a cat's tail, and the cat returns the favor by scratching her leg. After this unfortunate experience, the child may become fearful and cry whenever she sees the cat. This tendency might readily generalize, and the girl may cry when *any* cat comes into view. This phenomenon is called *respondent learning* because individuals learn to *respond* to an element of the context based on its proximity to objects or events that trigger similar responses. The girl sees the cat, feels scared, and cries.

The cat's scratch is a *stimulus*—an element of the environment that stimulates a *response* from the girl. The girl's immediate response to the cat scratch required no learning; experience was not necessary to teach her to feel pain or jerk back her leg when scratched by the cat. These types of reactions are sometimes referred to as reflexive or instinctive. This is not true of the girl's responses to other stimuli that were present when the cat scratch occurred, such as the garden where the incident happened, the activity the child was engaged in at the time, or the size and color of the cat itself. None of these elements of the context would produce a reflexive response of distress. Since all these features were part of the context in which she was scratched, however, any of them could *acquire* the function of stimulating responses such as fear or crying. This is the process of respondent learning, which is also known as "associative learning" or "classical conditioning."

Several parameters influence which elements of the context will become cues for similar responses through respondent learning. Contextual features that are novel and highly salient are particularly likely to do so. If, on the one hand, the garden where she was scratched was unfamiliar to the child, it could more easily become associated with the painful stimulus and the girl might become fearful when approaching the garden in the future. If, on the other hand, the garden was a place she visited often, it would already be associated with a range of positive, neutral, and negative experiences that would compete with the cat scratch as a source of influence on the girl's behavior. It would therefore be less likely to acquire the function of triggering a fearful response if a painful event occurred there. The cat itself was a particularly salient feature of the environment—probably the thing she noticed most when the scratch occurred—and therefore is very likely to cue fearful responses in the future.

Contextual elements that share physical similarities with the cat (now a learned or *conditioned* stimulus) will also tend to produce a fearful reaction through *stimulus generalization*. For example, if the offending cat had long black fur, the child might be more likely to be afraid when seeing a cat with long gray fur than one with short orange hair. These reactions gradually dissipate as the child learns to distinguish among objects and events that initially seem similar. For example, she might become less frightened of cats with short hair of any color and not at all frightened of cats whose fur color is anything other than black.

Evolutionary processes have altered the parameters of respondent learning in some instances. For example, learning to avoid poisonous foods can occur through respondent learning even if sickness occurs many hours after eating the tainted food (Bernstein, 2000), even though classical conditioning typically works best when a response immediately follows a stimulus. Presumably, this is due to the strong impact of learning to avoid poisonous food on evolutionary fitness. Respondent learning is also easier in some cases than others, since evolution has preorganized certain contextual elements into functional categories. It is easier to learn to be afraid of a wiggling snake-like object than it is to learn to be afraid of an electrical outlet, even though in the modern world the electric outlet is far more likely to cause harm. Thus, even basic learning processes such as these are evolving as the contexts in which humans live are transformed.

Operant Learning

Additional learning processes may impact the child's responses to being scratched by a cat. For example, if she runs away from the cat, the cat disappears from her sight. The removal of the cat (reducing any chance of a cat's scratch) may function as an important consequence of running away, and avoidance or escape may be selected as the dominant response to seeing a cat. Without planning or thinking about it, the child is applying the most logical and adapted learning strategy of all animal species: avoiding threats to survival by avoiding stimuli that announce harmful consequences. This is the principle of operant conditioning, or learning by consequences.

Consequences that are not directly associated with threat may also influence the child's behavior. The child's parents may be distressed by seeing her expressions of pain and fear and may try to soothe her when she whimpers about cats. Being comforted is an advantageous consequence, and expressions of distress may occur more frequently due to the positive social consequences that follow. Learning of this kind is called operant learning because responses *operate on* the environment in order to alter consequences.

Consequences can also weaken the likelihood of behavior occurring. A behavior followed by a disadvantageous consequence will tend to decrease in frequency. For example, approaching the cat and accidentally stepping on its tail were followed by a painful consequence. Thus, approaching or walking near the cat may become much less likely.

Sometimes, a disadvantageous consequence comes in the form of the removal of something pleasant. For example, if the girl was carrying a lollypop and lost it as she was running away from the cat, this would be another reason for her not to play around the cat anymore.

A similar effect could happen if the parents notice that holding their child each time she whimpers leads to a greater fear of cats. They may decide not to soothe her when she acts this way, thus no longer providing this reinforcing consequence. This principle, called *extinction*, describes what happens when a maintaining consequence no longer occurs following operant behavior. The expressions of distress would be expected to increase briefly (extinction burst) and then decrease when the holding and soothing no longer occurred.

Both respondent and operant learning are sometimes called associative learning, but we prefer the term "contingency learning" to refer to them both. A contingency is simply an "if . . . then" relation. In respondent learning there is a stimulus–stimulus contingency, whereas in operant learning there is an antecedent–response–consequence contingency. Using the term "associative" when referring to operant and classical conditioning can become confusing when we examine language as a relatively new form of learning, as we will see later in this chapter. Associative models of meaning are as old as psychology and they have never worked out very well. Mistaking the relational learning that underlies language for that type of associative model would make it difficult to see what is new and useful in RFT.

Social Learning

Social animals, including humans, have a variety of behaviors that may be learned by exposure to other members of their social group. Some of these actions are genetically established, others are based on imitation, and still others are brought about by interactions with contingency learning. For example, young birds may need to hear their species' songs (even while in the egg) in order to produce them accurately as adults, as if a kind of template is laid down that the young birds will later use to determine if they are performing the song accurately (Catchpole & Slater, 1995). Children have some elements of gestural imitative responses at birth (e.g., tongue thrusting), but more complex forms of imitation rely on contingency learning processes (Ray & Heyes, 2011). However, social learning is not merely imitation. For example, after seeing an adult extract tasty ants from a log, a young chimpanzee may approach the log and figure out how to extract dinner by trial and error. The social nature of human beings gives many opportunities for social and cultural processes to interact with other learning processes. Language makes these types of interactions between social and learning processes even more likely in humans.

Relational Learning

The capacity to relate objects and events is acquired through operant learning and facilitated by social learning, so it should not be a surprise that most nonhuman animals can very quickly learn to relate things based on the intrinsic properties of events in the natural environment, such as their relative size, darkness, or speed (see Reese, 1968, for an early summary of this extensive learning literature). Modern evolution science is fairly clear that humans have evolved specialized abilities for relating events symbolically, and that the differences between humans and nonhumans become greater the more complex the relations involved (Penn et al., 2008). Evolutionists agree that in human symbolic behavior, "tacit systems of higher order relations" allow humans to "judge and discover novel relations within those domains" (Penn et al., 2008, p. 118).

What evolution science has not yet specified is where this "tacit system of higher order relations" came from, or what its properties are and how they are regulated. Such an understanding could inform clinical guidelines for regulating symbolic learning and using language principles to promote positive psychological functioning. That is what RFT and this volume aim to provide. The remainder of this chapter will explain how symbolic relational behavior is learned and how it becomes a learning process in its own right.

HOW LANGUAGE IS LEARNED

In the past 2 decades, RFT researchers have conducted over 150 studies that reproduce the stages of relational learning that underlie language development. RFT research is notoriously difficult to comprehend, even for those with a keen interest and familiarity with the jargon and experimental methodology. To be fair, testing RFT hypotheses often requires challenging and time-consuming preparations—such as building unique learning histories that mimic language development in the natural environment, but have never before been experienced by the participant—before the actual hypothesis can be tested. These challenges resulted in the development of methodological innovations and novel research paradigms leading to practical knowledge and applications that touch on all aspects of human behavior. It is not our intention to delve into RFT research here (see Dymond, May, Munnelly, & Hoon, 2010, and Dymond & Roche, 2013 for recent reviews and analysis). Nevertheless, our experience in teaching RFT to clinicians suggests that understanding RFT ideas is easier when you understand a little about how RFT researchers conduct their experiments. Spoiler alert: these next few pages are a bit geeky. We humbly ask you to hang in there while we explore these RFT principles, and we promise that you will be rewarded soon for your effort.

Contextual Cues Specify Relationships

How do we go from interacting directly with the world to talking and thinking about it symbolically? It begins with learning to relate things in particular ways, based on cues that are present in the learning environment. Consider the following example of a toddler playing with an educational game that consists of fitting three-dimensional figures into holes in a board according to their shape and color. The child looks at the board and sees holes shaped like triangles, circles, and squares. Each hole is framed in blue, red, or yellow. At the same time, an array of plastic figures shaped like triangles, circles, and squares in blue, red, and yellow are lying at his feet on the floor. By trial and error, the child learns to select the right figure according to the relation it shares with the holes. For example, he may first try to put a triangle in a circular hole. When he realizes that the corners on the triangle prevent the figure from fitting in the circular hole, he may pick up another figure and discover that the round figure with no corners fits perfectly. He is delighted when the figure is swallowed by the hole, and he continues to make things disappear by matching figures to holes of the same shape.

Now imagine that, as the child is learning to place the objects in the correct holes, his parents are around to help. When the child puts a red triangle in the triangle hole framed in red, his parents exclaim, "Hooray!" But if he puts a blue triangle there instead, they say, "No, that's not the right one. Look . . . which one has the same color?" Because the child doesn't have language skills yet, he doesn't understand the verbal[2] cue his parents just gave him. For this reason, the parents may take the hand of the little boy, guide him to the red triangle, and say, "See? This one is the same," and praise him as he places it in the correct hole. What happened in this situation is that the parents created a social context that allowed the child to learn the meaning of a *contextual cue*, in this case the word "same," which

---

[2] Although in the behavioral literature on language, the term "verbal" is used as a synonym to symbolic, we only use this term in this book when it refers to symbols made of words, in order to avoid confusion for readers unfamiliar with this literature. In this view, nonverbal cues can thus also be symbolic (e.g., gestures, images). We refer to nonsymbolic cues and functions as "intrinsic." However, when we use the term "verbal interactions," we refer to symbolic interactions, generally speaking (including gestures, postures, facial expressions, tone of voice, etc.) in order to match the more common use of this term.

describes the type of relationship shared by the color of the figure and the color of the hole.

Once the little boy has learned that the word "same" establishes a relation of equivalence between two things, his parents can teach him to relate other objects and events in the same way, for instance, that "cat" and the furry creature at his feet are the *same*. Many contextual cues can establish the same type of relation (e.g., "is," "like," "similar," "same") and don't need to be made of words. For example, sameness can be established through the application of symbols such as "=" or by gestures, as when pointing an index finger at one's chest while saying one's name out loud.

This example shows how language may develop initially based on operant learning of relationships, which are cued by features of the learning context. In this case, the relationship was based on intrinsic features—the shape and color of the figures and holes. Learning to detect intrinsic relations is a precursor to symbolic learning—it is not itself symbolic, nor is it unique to humans. Infants and fish and pigeons can readily learn similarities and differences among shapes or colors, but they cannot compare values that are socially determined.

Relationships Can Be Symbolic

Once learned, contextual cues that specify relationships can be applied to any object or event in our environment. For a young child who is not yet able to form symbolic relations, the words he hears are not unlike the stars in the night sky, disconnected and devoid of meaning and purpose. But once he learns to relate things as *similar* or *near to* or *brighter than*, he can connect those distant dots in myriad ways. "See those nine stars there? That one is Leo, because it looks like a lion. That's your sister's sign—she was born in August, which makes her a Leo." When someone shows him how these stars can be related to form constellations, the elements that were once isolated and didn't make any particular sense begin to fit together. If he views those stars as a constellation frequently enough, it will become difficult to see them as he once did; they can no longer be disconnected and meaningless. In 15 years, when he travels far away from his family, he will look up at those nine stars and feel close to his sister. He may even learn to use these constellations as a guide to know when and where he is on the planet. That is similar to the kind of transition that language training creates with symbolic learning.

In RFT terms, this behavior is symbolic because relational contextual cues can be applied arbitrarily—based on social convention, and not dependent on intrinsic characteristics of the things being related. We could all decide tomorrow that *apple* is now the word for a banana and *banana* is the word for an apple. This is the sense in which relational cues are social: if we all decided to change the terms for things, we could do so merely by specifying the proper relational cues. It would initially feel arbitrary, but it would soon become normative. This is exactly what happens when we decide to change the name of certain concepts because it no longer seems appropriate. For example, Third World countries are now called developing countries because it is considered more respectful (until it changes again). It can take a bit of time to change our habits, but a simple change of social convention can make this new appellation begin to occur.

Progressively, this ability allows us the enormous advantage of being able to bring anything into the present moment via language using symbols, even when it is not physically present in our environment. Indeed, imagine that as the child plays with his toys, the red triangle is hidden under the board and the parents say, "Where is the red triangle?" The child, who has now acquired rudimentary language skills and thus understands what all these words mean, recognizes that the red triangle is not present and begins looking for the triangle in hidden places. As we will see in the next chapters, this is also a powerful tool to bring elements of the client's life into the therapy room. Assessing and changing psychological problems becomes possible without having to directly intervene in the client's natural environment.

There Are a Variety of Symbolic Relationships

If things could only be related according to their similarities, the utility of language would be quite limited. Language probably started with the relation of sameness, however, because it is the simplest and the most central to cooperation. It is simply because the relationship between two things is exactly the same in both directions—when two things are equivalent, "this is like that" in exactly the same way "that is like this." This makes it easy to abstract information about one event based on its relationship with another (i.e., to bring the functions of a referent into the moment when hearing the name, such as when saying, "You will find my house easily. It's the one that looks like an old Victorian house."). That in turn was put to good use by those cooperative primates called "humans." But there is no reason for relating to end there, and it doesn't.

Building a symbolic world that adds to our directly experienced environment becomes really sophisticated when considering the variety of relations that can be established. RFT researchers have demonstrated the establishment of relations of opposition (e.g., Dymond & Barnes, 1996), comparison (e.g., Dymond & Barnes, 1995), hierarchy (e.g., Slattery & Stewart, 2014), temporality (e.g., O' Hora, Roche, Barnes-Holmes, & Smeets, 2002) or perspective (e.g., McHugh, Barnes-Holmes, & Barnes-Holmes, 2004). All these types of relations and many others are of interest when analyzing clinical issues and employing appropriate clinical techniques, which we will explore in detail in later chapters. For now, simply consider how crucial aspects of a client's life are related to each other in a quote such as the following:

"If only I were more confident, then I could initiate conversations, share my thoughts with friends . . . do all the things that make you feel intimate with someone. But I will never be happy because I'm worthless. You can't imagine what it's like for me. You are successful. I'm a failure."

Framed in this way, there is a network of relations that are self-supporting. We will restate what the client is saying and embolden relational cues that are particularly critical here:

"I will **never have** intimacy **because** intimacy **includes** things **like** initiating conversations and sharing thoughts, which are **conditional** on confidence, and **I am not** confident. Therefore, I and happy **are incompatible** because happy **is dependent** on confidence, and **I am distinctly not** confident—**I am** worthless. Further, **you** and I are in **opposition** because **you can't** see **my perspective** and the characteristics of **you** are the **opposite** of those for **me**. Therefore **you can't** know what it **is like** for **me**."

From an RFT perspective, each of these relations provides crucial information about the way the client perceives her life through the filter of language and how psychological interventions might address her difficulties.

Symbolic Relationships Make It Possible for Everything to Mean Anything

This is where we break away from nonhuman animals, the tiny breaking point where humans stepped forward just enough to enter the symbolic world; the point at which relational learning transitioned from intrinsic relations to open "frames" into which *anything* can be placed. We are now dealing with language.

This tiny step forward probably began merely with naming, likely controlled by that cue called *is* or cues carrying a similar function (e.g., pointing in the direction of an object while making a sound with the mouth), and an act of cooperative communication that was directly reinforced, much as any operant. But *is* has expanded now to include myriad learned relations, arranged into networks. This process of expansion began as operant learning, but by breaking away from intrinsic relations the transition to something truly new began. With millennia of cultural and social support, the expansion has become the core of the human mind: symbolic behavior.

Let's observe how this principle of symbolic expansion works. Think of two concrete nouns—any two different objects. Actually, do that before continuing. Think of two concrete nouns. Now, suppose your future depends on answering this next question: "How is [*say the name of the first object*] the father of [*say the name of the second object*]?" Take your time—don't just read these words. Do the task as if it was really important to find a great answer because your future depends on it.

We have done this exercise in scores of workshops, using many different relations, including really obscure ones (e.g., "reveals the essence of"). Given a few minutes, the groups always come up with answers. . . . and not just answers. They come up with really good ones! They often come up with answers that are downright insightful and that cause the entire group to see both objects in a different way because seemingly the relation between the two objects *exists intrinsically*. Did you find a good answer for your *is the father of* challenge? If the answer was especially apt, somehow it seems that the first object really *is*, in a sense, *the father of* the second.

This exercise shows well how tricky the mind can be. We can create any kind of symbolic relation among any objects and events. Then, we begin to believe these relations exist outside the mind. This illusion is part of what tripped up behavioral psychologists historically when dealing with human language. They missed the power of relational cues to create symbolic meaning and instead focused on the later process of how language helped humans deal with the natural (intrinsic) properties of things. You cannot understand human symbolic behavior this way because you miss the key issue—that breaking point—of relational cues being able to be applied to anything and thereby creating relations where none previously existed.

Contextual Cues Specify Functions

One of the traditional objections to considering symbolic meaning from a behavioral point of view can be summed up in the following question: if a symbol and an event are framed as "the same," why doesn't a person just lick the word "candy" or run from the word "tiger"? The answer is that the psychological functions (e.g., taste, fear) that transfer through symbolic relations are also controlled by contextual cues. Some of these cues are not symbolic; seeing ink on paper is likely enough to keep us from licking the word "candy." Some are themselves symbolic events, such as the word "taste" in the query "What does an apple taste like?" versus the word "look" in the query "What does an apple look like?" In these cases, the relation of "apple" and actual apples is the same, but the functional cues "taste" and "look" select specific functions that are evoked by the word, given the underlying relation of sameness. Sometimes these functional cues may be paralinguistic. For example, singing a depressing thought out loud may evoke different functions than saying it in a normal tone of voice.

Most often these contextual cues are used to select among the various possible functions of an event in a symbolic network, such as whether a pen is seen as a writing implement, hollow tube, sharp point, lever, something to extend reach, or so on. But contextual cues can also be used to diminish any behavioral impact of symbolic events. For example, chanting, meditation, word repetition, unresolvable paradox, and similar means can be thought of as episymbolic control systems, altering the behavioral impact of symbolic events very much as epigenetic processes can alter the likelihood that genes will produce proteins (Wilson, Hayes, Biglan, & Embry, 2014).

The Nature of Objects and Events Is Transformed through Relational Networks

When all of these properties come together, networks of symbolic relations alter the functions—that is, the meaning and impact—of the objects and events contained within them. In the clinical example we visited earlier, the client's language, in addition to simply describing different experiences, also implied a certain way of interacting with them. For example, saying, "If I were more confident, I could talk to others" implies more confidence was required to talk to others: it was necessary and sufficient. However, saying, "But I am worthless" implies that working on being more confident is useless. A no-win situation.

Language often changes the way we experience objects and events by orienting us to functional features that might be missed without language. Consider what happens when you taste some wine, read the description on the label, and then taste it again. If you are not an expert, you may only taste grapes and alcohol at first. However, after reading the label stating that this wine tastes like tobacco and chocolate, you may now start to experience these flavors. The description on the label establishes a relation of equivalence between the wine, tobacco and chocolate, and "tastes like" indicates the relevant functional features that are involved (e.g., the taste is similar but not the color). A combination of chemical elements leads the wine to taste the way it does, and to some degree language may be drawing out what was there to be tasted.

Much the same thing happens when a therapist asks her client, "Could you tell me what happens in your body when you feel anxious?" and the client answers, "My muscles are tense." The therapist's evocation of the client's symbolic network may help them have a better mutual understanding of the client's experience of anxiety. Rather than assuming that her client feels the same way other clients feel when they are anxious, asking this question allowed for a function of "anxious" that was more specific to her experience. The clinician might follow up with further questions such as, "Exactly where do you feel the tension?" or "If you could draw a line around the tense area, what is its shape and size?" With each question, the experience of anxiety is elaborated. It now has a quality that in turn has a place, a shape, and a size.

Some of the process described above is noting features of the internal and external environment that were there in the first place, but just as in the *is the father of* example, relational networks can also *create* new functions that only appear in hindsight to have been there. Deceptive blind tests are funny situations in which we observe the transformation of perceptual functions through the arbitrary application of contextual cues. Imagine that you have guests for dinner and pour them a glass of cheap wine while pretending that it is an excellent wine that was recommended to complement the particular dish you prepared. And you describe the wine this way: it offers a seamless, harmonious progression of fruit, chocolate, and black tea tones. Likely, many of your guests will actually experience these aromas. Of course, some may just want to be polite and pretend that they tasted what matched the description. But very often, even if you reveal the trick, some will sincerely maintain that they really tasted chocolate and black tea. Simply saying, "This wine tastes *like* chocolate" transformed the perceptual functions of the wine, regardless of its actual composition.

Relational Networks Expand Rapidly Due to Derivation

Once contextual relational cues are learned, they can be applied flexibly and in combination with other relational cues. Imagine that a parent says to his child at the zoo, "Look at the baby panther! It looks just like the mama panther, but smaller!" A relation of sameness between the panther and her baby is specified by the cue *just like*, while a relation of comparison is specified by the cue *but* smaller. As with all relations, there is a mutual relation to be derived: if the baby is *smaller*, the mother is larger.

Imagine that the little girl who runs away from cats and the little boy who saw a panther at the zoo end up in the same class at the same primary school. They become best friends and love talking for hours about the experiences of their young life. One day, the little girl asks, "What's your favorite animal?" The little boy says, "Panthers! I love panthers! I saw a panther and her baby once at the zoo!" to which the little girl replies, "What's a panther?" "It's like a big, big cat!" says the little boy. The little girl stops smiling, yells, "Cats are dangerous!" and runs away. Upon returning home, the little boy and the little girl both ask their parents, "Is it true that panthers are very dangerous?"

In this situation, it is fascinating to observe that the girl has never seen a panther and that the little boy has never been told that panthers are dangerous. Yet, they both now think they are. What led the little girl to think that panthers are dangerous started with the same principle we observed in the previous section of this chapter. When the little boy said, "It's like a big, big cat," he established a relation of comparison between cats and panthers using the contextual cues *like* and *big*. Since cats have the function of being dangerous for the little girl, the establishment of such a relation results in the transformation of function of the stimulus *panthers*. They are now dangerous too, and probably even more so since they are bigger. The boy also learned something that he was not directly told. In everyday language, we might say that he deduced that panthers are dangerous since cats are dangerous. From an RFT point of view, this reflects how derived relations expand from mutual relations (as in the learning of the word "apple") to entire networks of derived relations in which relations combine.

Looking at the way in which RFT experimental studies make sense of this process of language can be useful for understanding how to apply these basic principles in the therapy room. A typical experiment first consists of establishing a relation between two stimuli. For example, a relation of equivalence is established by training the participants to pick *aaa* among a series of stimuli (*aaa*, *bbb*, and *ccc*) each time *xxx* and the contextual cue "is like" are presented (see Figure 1.1). At some point in the experiment, instead of presenting *xxx*, the researchers present *aaa* and the contextual cue "is like," while the participant has to pick a stimulus among *xxx*, *bbb*, and *ccc* (see Figure 1.2). In other words, after being directly taught that *aaa* is like *xxx*, the participants have to answer the question "*xxx* is like _____?" This is exactly what happened in this paragraph. We told you that *aaa* is like *xxx*, but we never told you what *xxx* is like. Yet, how hard would it be to answer this question? It would probably be very easy. And yet, this very simple answer requires that you travel in the reverse direction of the relation that was directly trained.

In RFT, this principle is called *mutual entailment*; that is, a relation between a stimulus A and a stimulus B entails the reverse relation between

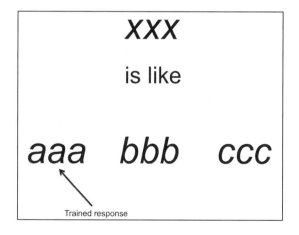

FIGURE 1.1

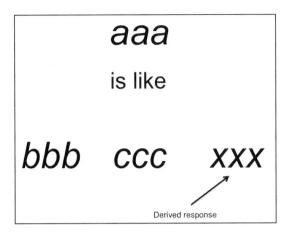

FIGURE 1.2

B and *A*. If *A* is like *B*, you can derive that *B* is like *A*. If *A* is the opposite of *B*, you can derive that *B* is the opposite of *A*. If *A* is bigger than *B*, you can derive that *B* is smaller than *A*, and so on. Thanks to this principle, children quickly learn the meaning of new words once contextual cues are established in their verbal repertoire. All they need to be told is that "*x* means *y*." Then, they can use *x* in new sentences when they want to talk about *y*. For example, if a kid asks, "What does being hungry mean?" and his father tells him, "It's when you have not eaten for a while and you feel that you need food," then the kid can say, "I am hungry," when he feels that way. The relation *being hungry = needing food* leads to derive the mutually entailed relation *needing food = being hungry*.

Let's go a little further. Now that you know that *aaa* "is like" *xxx* and vice versa through mutual entailment, imagine that we also told you that *xxx* is like *zzz*. What could you conclude about the relation between *aaa* and *zzz*? In other terms, if *A = B* and *B = C*, what is the relation between *A* and *C*? You can say that *A = C* and that *C = A* or that *aaa* is like *zzz* and *zzz* is like *aaa* thanks to the principle of derivation (see Figure 1.3). However, while deriving that *B* is like *A* after being directly taught that *A* is like *B* was based on mutual entailment, that was not the case for *A* and *C* (and vice versa) since no contextual cue ever connected these two stimuli directly. That is the same, of course, for *aaa* and *zzz*. Before we asked you what kind of relation they share, they had never even been in the same sentence together. In RFT, this type of derivation is called *combinatorial entailment*: you need to *combine* two relations to derive a third one. An easier way to think of this, instead of the technical terms of mutual and combinatorial entailment, is just to remember that symbolic relations are mutual and that they combine into networks. Teaching two relations

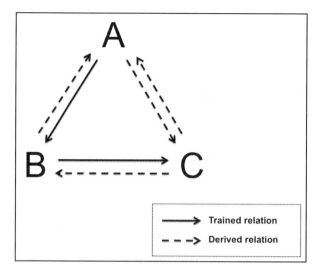

FIGURE 1.3

between three stimuli can lead to deriving four additional relations. As our colleague J. T. Blackledge says, "Buy two, get four for free!"[3]

These networks can then change the functions of things they contain. Let's go back to cats and panthers. The girl told the little boy that cats are dangerous. Before that, what he knew was that panthers are like big cats. If we translate these two sentences in RFT terms, he was told that $A = B$ (cats = dangerous) and he already knew that $C = A$ (panthers = cats). When he asked, "Is it true that panthers are very dangerous?" he derived the relation $C = B$ through combinatorial entailment. Because he also knew that along the dimension of size, $C > A$[4] (panthers are like *big* cats), he could even derive that panthers are *very* dangerous, even though he was never told so.

Language and cognition[5] in the RFT approach are based on the properties of relational framing: mutual relations combine into networks that

---

[3] Technically though, it is never totally "free," since we do have to engage in the process of derivation. But once this process is learned and well established, it becomes so rapid and natural that it can feel automatic and effortless if the relations being derived are relatively simple (we are generally much more aware of the effort required by the derivation process when we try to solve a complex problem, for example).

[4] Throughout this book, "<" means "smaller than or less than," and ">" means "bigger than or greater than."

[5] We occasionally add the term "cognition" after "language" in order to remind you that, from an RFT perspective, thinking and talking correspond to the same behavior of building and responding to symbolic relations.

then change the functions of events. All of this is controlled by the relational context and the functional context. In human beings, that is what thinking is all about.

Deriving Symbolic Relations Accounts for the Generativity of Language

The principle of derivation is a cornerstone of the RFT approach to language. It accounts for *generativity*, which is one of language's crucial properties. With language, we can produce new networks of relations, including sentences and schemas, that we have never been taught or directly exposed to. Moreover, the function of stimuli can be changed through the derivation of new relations and the presentation of the proper functional cues. Like what happened for the little girl who thinks panthers are very dangerous because of the relation they now share with cats in her mind. As we will see in the next chapters, psychological interventions can benefit from an analysis of the derivation processes operating in clients' relational networks.

Consider the following example of one of our clients, a college student who suffered from obsessive thoughts centered on the risk of being contaminated. During our first session, he told us about a TV documentary he had watched that had made things worse for him. After learning about the risks of cholera spreading through contaminated water, he felt compelled to avoid contact with water altogether. He was now stuck with a dilemma: either take a shower and risk contamination with cholera, or avoid bathing and risk contamination by germs. To resolve this crisis, he decided he would clean his entire body using only hand sanitizer. This method made him feel less anxious for a while, but quickly, water kept popping up in his relational network. He could no longer read his chemistry textbook after he saw the letters "H_2O." Because these letters referred to the chemical formula of water, he became very nervous, closed the book, and decided not to open it again. Soon, going to his chemistry class became unbearable because of the risk of being in contact, even if only psychologically, with water. In this situation, we can see that a relation between water and contamination originally established by watching a documentary led to the derivation of a new relation between chemistry class and contamination through the expansion of the client's symbolic network: a relation of condition between water and cholera, then a relation of equivalence between water and H_2O, and finally, a relation of hierarchy between H_2O and chemistry class (H_2O *is one of* the formulas used in chemistry class) led to the transformation of function of the chemistry class. Going to the chemistry class was now in a causal relation with contracting cholera, while no direct experience or direct verbal learning ever established this relation. Rather than cholera spreading through water, our client had experienced how psychological functions, such as fear, disgust, and avoidance, spread through a language network.

Although this example illustrates the excesses of human language, it also shows why language has continued to evolve culturally in the human species. Evolution works by a simple principle: variation and selective retention. Without variation, evolution is impossible. That is as true of behavioral and cultural evolution as it is of genetic evolution. Let's expand our "buy two, get four free" principle, using an example described by Deacon (1998). Suppose that we teach eight symbol → object relations. In nonhumans, if we teach them in one direction, we get them in one direction. But if we teach them to humans, each relation is mutual. We are up to 16 relations, not eight. But all of the symbols can also be related one to the other. And each object can be related to each other object. And each relation among objects can be related to each relation among objects (e.g., if two things are the same, and two other things are the same, then those two relations are also the same relation); the same goes for symbols. And each symbol can be related via combination to each object. On and on it goes. By the time you are finished, how many possible relations exist in a network with just eight symbol → object relations? Incredibly, the answer is *nearly 4,000!* Now *that's* variation!

What manages this chaos is contextual control over relating and contextual control over the change of functions. As of yet, however, human beings are not very adept at wielding such contextual control intentionally. Said more simply, we are not very good at putting our minds on a leash. We are great at generating and exploring relational networks. That is the source of our greatest achievements in science, literature, or philosophy. But that is also the source of much of our misery too, in which even taking a shower can be fearsome because of its place in an enormous relational network.

Learning to manage these relational processes is the challenge of human existence, individually and culturally. The science of RFT suggests ways that we can use language processes consciously as practitioners to do the job of psychotherapy more effectively. To that topic, we now turn.

 **CHAPTER SUMMARY**

In this chapter, we presented the basic principles of how language evolved as a unique form of learning based on building symbolic relationships among objects and events. Here are some key elements that will be useful to remember throughout the more practical sections of the book:

- We use the term "language" to refer to the learned behavior of building and responding to symbolic relations. This behavior is special because it transforms the way we experience our world, imbuing objects and events with meaning and altering their impact on our thoughts, feelings, and actions.

- Relating is simply responding to one thing in terms of another. Some animal species can learn specific relationships or how to relate things based on intrinsic characteristics, but only humans can learn how to build symbolic relationships. The capacity to relate to things symbolically dramatically increases the efficiency with which humans learn. Entire networks of derived relations can emerge from only a small number of trained relations.

- Symbolic relationships "frame" our experiences, transforming their meaning and impact. We combine the information entailed in these various relationships and derive a vast network of meaning and understanding. The ways we think, feel, and act toward things in the network are strongly influenced by their symbolic relationships with other objects and events.

- Relational learning is a behavior that results from a combination of evolution and a special kind of operant learning history. Human beings learn to relate objects and events based in part on socially established cues, rather than solely on the intrinsic properties of the things being related. Thus, language is a form of cooperation that builds on the social nature of human groups and enhances a culture of eusociality in which humans thrive.

- Although symbolic behavior is based originally on contingency learning, *it alters the impact of all forms of learning* because symbolic relationships transform the way stimuli function as antecedents and consequences.

- There are many types of symbolic relationships or "relational frames." Among them are relations of coordination, distinction, opposition, comparison, condition, hierarchy, and perspective. They are all potentially involved in the analysis and treatment of clinical issues.

- Symbolic relations are not merely words—they are deeply intertwined with virtually everything that is meaningful to human beings. Thoughts and mental images, memories, beliefs, mood and affect, self-awareness, and consciousness itself depend on symbolic relationships. Thinking in this way allows therapists to apply a parsimonious set of behavioral principles to a broad range of clinical issues in a coherent, efficient way.

- Most clinically relevant thoughts, feelings, and behaviors involve an interaction between symbolic relationships and other learned and unlearned processes. Clinicians cannot avoid language, even if it is not a central focus of their therapeutic approach. Even interventions that emphasize silence, use imagery, induce hypnosis, or conduct mindfulness exercises do so by engaging symbolic relationships.

- The capacity to derive symbolic relationships and the transformation of stimulus functions that occurs through them enables a level of behavioral variation that constitutes an enormous evolutionary advantage. Language is the source of our greatest human achievements, but it is also the source of much of our misery. On an evolutionary time scale, symbolic learning is a relatively new adaptation and we humans are still learning to harness its power without creating unintentional suffering. The conversations that happen in psychotherapy and other clinical interactions are, in part, a process of learning how to manage relational frames and the contextual cues that regulate them in the service of living well.

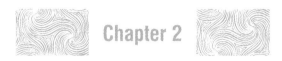

Chapter 2

Language and Psychopathology

It is a bit odd that psychological suffering is so pervasive given how successful humans have been as a species. Other species on the planet do not seem to suffer from want amidst plenty, from insecurity in the absence of danger, or from loneliness when surrounded by a caring social community. Through language, the sources of plenty, protection, and caring presence become fountainheads of struggle, angst, and isolation. Symbolic relational learning both augments and interferes with human flourishing because our strength and our struggle now share the same source.

PROBLEMS LINKED TO THE FLUENCY AND FLEXIBILITY OF RELATIONAL FRAMING

Deficits in Reasoning and Problem-Solving Skills

The RFT laboratories have shown that relational framing aptitude correlates with cognitive and social abilities in children, including effective communication (Kishita, Ohtsuki, & Stewart, 2013), the use of analogies and metaphors (Lipkens & Hayes, 2009), perspective taking and theory of mind (Barnes-Holmes, McHugh, & Barnes-Holmes, 2004), verbal intelligence (O'Hora, Pelaez, Barnes-Holmes, & Amesty, 2005), and productive and receptive language fluency (Devany, Hayes, & Nelson, 1986). These associations are based on the ability to understand and respond to specific types of symbolic relations (e.g., Weil, Hayes, & Capurro, 2011), the flexibility and fluency of these relational responses (e.g., O'Toole & Barnes-Holmes, 2009), and the degree to which they are regulated by appropriate contextual cues (e.g., Rehfeldt & Barnes-Holmes, 2009).

These are not mere correlations; improvements in symbolic relational skills lead to improvements in cognitive and social abilities. For example, training in relational skills improves IQ by 12 to 15 points in normal children and those with intellectual disabilities alike (Cassidy, Roche, & Hayes, 2011). Similarly, training in relational skills has an impact on theory of mind performance and perspective-taking ability (Weil et al., 2011). Thus, when we face deficits in human reasoning, logic, or problem solving, we are dealing with deficits in relational skills—they may not be present, they may not be sufficiently flexible and fluent, or they may not be appropriately controlled by the context.

Many psychological problems involve failures of logic, ineffective problem solving, or the inability to generate creative alternatives when faced with obstacles. Although some individuals have specific skills deficits in these areas, all humans are prone to certain cognitive biases and have difficulty reasoning quickly and accurately in complex or emotionally charged situations. Intellectual disabilities reflect problems related to reasoning and problem solving, but we commonly encounter clients without discrete intellectual disabilities who are nonetheless impulsive owing to an inability to anticipate outcomes, or who make poor choices based on an inability to generate a range of reasonable alternatives. Clients frequently commit common cognitive distortions, such as overgeneralizing or thinking in black and white when dealing with shades of gray.

Many forms of psychological intervention focus on these issues. Children are taught to avoid impulsive decisions by thinking through the long-term consequences of their actions; adults are taught to do a better job of problem solving by correctly crafting a problem, generating alternatives, and evaluating the results (e.g., Nezu, Nezu, & D'Zurilla, 2013). Cognitive errors are rooted out and examined in many forms of CBT.

Being able to reason and problem solve is essential to human functioning, and psychological problems will flow from deficits in these areas. From an RFT perspective, psychological problems relating to cognitive errors and deficits can be approached directly by an analysis of relational skills. If you can acquire relational skills that occur rapidly, with few errors, and are well regulated by context, you have established the building blocks of rationality.

Deficits in Perspective Taking and Empathy

Human beings are social animals. In order to function well, we need to understand each other, care about each other, and feel what it is like to be another person. These skills are not entirely symbolic, but they are predominantly so. Being able to see the perspective of another goes under several names in the behavioral science literature, but perhaps the best known term is "theory of mind."

Deficits in perspective taking and theory of mind (ToM) skills are enormously debilitating. Children with poor ToM skills struggle to understand the motives and actions of others, making it difficult for them to predict their social environment, to learn from stories and parables, or to find joy in relationships with other people.

In RFT, adopting the point of view of other people is a relational response that is based on perspective taking and controlled by contextual cues like I–you (interpersonal), here–there (spatial), and now–then (temporal) (for a book-length treatment, see McHugh & Stewart, 2012). These responses are called deictic framing because they are taught via demonstration. If a pen is here and a box is there, when I go there the box is here and the pen is there. As children learn deictic relational responses, they have to learn that they only make sense from a given point of view. RFT researchers have found that deictic framing emerges developmentally over time (McHugh et al., 2004), but that it can be specifically trained. There is some early evidence that when it is, perspective taking and ToM skills tend to change (Weil et al., 2011).

Without perspective-taking skills, you cannot feel empathy (Vilardaga, Estévez, Levin, & Hayes, 2012). Empathy is the change in functions that happens when we see and feel what others feel and can share to some degree their point of view. In RFT terms, the ability to feel the emotions of another is a transformation of functions that relies on the ability to view the world from another point of view. Without perspective taking and empathy, we live in a socially isolated world, unable to connect with or care about others, which is why deficits in these skills are related to such severe problems as a poor sense of self among those with autistic spectrum disorders (Rehfeldt, Dillen, Ziomek, & Kowalchuk, 2007), social anhedonia (Villatte, Monestès, McHugh, Freixa i Baqué, & Loas, 2008), or schizophrenia (Villatte, Monestès, McHugh, Freixa i Baqué, & Loas, 2010a, 2010b). RFT researchers have found that to enjoy being with others you have to have sufficient deictic framing skills to see the world through the eyes of another, you have to empathize with their emotions, and you have to be willing to experience those feelings. These three combined skills seem to provide the fundamental cognitive scaffolding for human caring (Vilardaga et al., 2012) and for undermining the tendency to objectify and dehumanize others (Levin et al., under submission).

PROBLEMS LINKED TO EXPERIENTIAL AVOIDANCE

Anything Can Become a Source of Pain

A stimulus that is not physically similar to an actual source of danger, and has likewise never been associated with it, can still acquire its aversive emotional function through language. Speaking of a past trauma can trigger the same emotions and sensations experienced in the moment it occurred, in much the same way that thinking about biting into a sour lemon can cause mouths to pucker or salivate. All the emotional, cognitive, motivational, and perceptual responses we have to an object or event can be triggered in an instant, merely by thinking or speaking about something related to it.

That process alone creates a huge challenge for human beings. It is built into the simplest act of remembering by using names and symbols, but it also means that anytime, anywhere, we can remember past painful or difficult events based on a few cues. Like any complex living creature, our histories come with us—there is no delete button—but unlike any other living creature, for us the past can become present through symbolic relationships. This human faculty can produce a kind of disconnect among emotions, situations, and actions. A nonhuman animal feels fear in situations that are similar to situations in which painful events have occurred in the past. Human beings are different. Even the word "relax" can remind a person with panic disorder of anxiety and elicit a panic attack. Anywhere we go, the possibility of pain comes with us.

This phenomenon of "cued pain" is extremely common in clinical cases. A former client who survived a childhood sexual assault hated the word "rape." She would freeze and become tearful whenever she encountered it in conversations, song lyrics, or rape prevention ads on television. This relational process made it very difficult for her to talk about that part of her life in session, and she would cry every time our conversation approached the topic. She would even hold her arms up to protect herself when she thought we might say the word. The strength and persistence of this reaction was distressing to the client, but it was also surprising. She never told anyone about the traumatic event prior to our therapy, and it had never been described as "rape." How could that word have so much power over her? From an RFT perspective, the psychological and physiological responses that result from talking about significant events makes perfect sense because symbolic relations are bidirectional. If $A = B$, then $B = A$. If an event triggers painful emotions, then stimuli in a relation of equivalence with this event will trigger painful emotions when cues are present to evoke those functions.

Notice that it is not the intrinsic nature of the stimulus but the symbolic relation it shares with the source of pain that is key. Under the influence of a contextual cue, any two stimuli can become symbolically related— even those that bear no resemblance to each other or have never occurred together. Our client relived feelings of terror when she heard loud and angry voices, even though her attacker was silent throughout the assault. Loud voices were related to terrifying threats, even though she had never been yelled at, and both set the context for fearful responses. It is likewise possible for enjoyable stimuli to become related to a source of pain, causing us to respond to pleasure as if it were painful. The kind and gentle touch of a close friend triggered anger and withdrawal in our client, who was so strongly reminded of the *lack of* kindness in her childhood that she could not contact the pleasant sensations of a loving embrace.

Not only can language remind us of past pain, it can also *amplify* pain symbolically. A study shows this process (Dougher, Hamilton, Fink, & Harrington, 2007): a relational network A–B–C was established using the kind of procedures described in the first chapter, but the relation was one of comparison (i.e., $A < B < C$). Then, using the principle of respondent learning, the researchers established an aversive function to the stimulus B by association with a slight electric shock to the participants. The emotional reactions to the presentation of each stimulus in the relational network were *lower* for A, but they were *higher* for C, even higher than those observed for B. If respondent learning per se were responsible for the transformation of function of A and C, the responses to these stimuli would have been the same as for B. Symbolic processes allow functions to be *transformed* by language. The little girl from Chapter 1 showed this: Panthers are not just cats, they are *big* cats. It is likely that the girl was even *more* afraid of panthers than she was of cats based on symbolic generalization and its amplification of pain.

This amplification commonly occurs through rumination and prediction. We are constantly reformulating the past in an attempt to control the future. But the events imagined in a feared future are often far larger and more difficult than anything that is likely to occur. We enter into an $A < B < C$ situation in which the present is bad, but the future will be even worse.

Symbolic Generalization of Avoidance

It is interesting to note that in the example of the little girl who was afraid of cats, she was not only afraid of them, but she also ran away from them. That is, she not only had strong emotional reactions to cats or symbolic stimuli related to cats, but she also actively *escaped or avoided* these stimuli. All organisms instinctively escape and learn to avoid any source of pain. From cows staying away from electric fences to humans being cautious around hot stoves, organisms avoid or escape feeling pain whenever possible. It therefore seems logical that organisms with language keep well away from any symbolic stimuli that have acquired the function of triggering painful sensations or emotions.

This prediction has been tested in a couple of RFT studies. For example, Dymond, Roche, Forsyth, Whelan, and Rhoden (2007) first trained the participants of their experiment to respond according to the relational network $A = B = C$ in which A and C are related through combinatorial entailment. Once this stage was completed, a training phase associated the stimulus A to a scary picture and sound by respondent learning. That is, each time A appeared on the computer screen, the scary picture and sound followed. After this phase, participants could avoid seeing and hearing the scary picture and sound by pressing the space bar. As expected, they quickly learned to avoid the picture and sound by pressing the space bar each time they saw *A*. In addition, the stimulus *B*, directly related to *A* during the relational learning phase, acquired the function of *A*, that is, announcing fear. Moreover, the stimulus *C*, which had never been presented with *A*, but was only indirectly related through combinatorial entailment, also acquired the same function. As a result, participants pressed the space bar each time they saw *C* on the screen. Avoidance generalized through language.

This is likely the same process that led the little girl to run away when the boy mentioned cats. Remember, the actual cat that scratched the girl acquired its scary function through respondent learning (a direct association between the cat and the scratch), and cats in general acquired their function through regular generalization (because of their similar appearance). The word "cats," however, acquired its function through its *symbolic relation* with actual cats. This also probably explains why our client suffering from obsessive–compulsive disorder stopped reading his chemistry book when he read "H_2O" (see Chapter 1). The relation of equivalence between water and H_2O transformed the function of H_2O. That is, this combination of letters and number triggered anxiety when it reminded our client that water can transmit cholera. Our client suffering from posttraumatic stress disorder displayed similar avoidant behaviors when the sexual abuse she had been victim of was mentioned. She would often stop speaking, look away, or even change the topic of discussion. She would likewise avoid any TV programs that could relate to what happened to her; possible conversations with her friends were getting narrower and narrower in an attempt to avoid hearing words related to her pain.

In all of these cases, the range of possible behaviors that these people could engage in was considerably restricted in the presence of a symbolic stimulus triggering painful emotions. While a few seconds earlier, the little girl could talk about anything and enjoy the conversation, hearing "cat" immediately reduced her potential actions. It was as if an alarm were commanding her to leave everything behind and reach the emergency doors as soon as possible. Similarly, in the presence of words related to "water" and "sexual abuse," the only actions our clients were able to do were to stop reading, stop going to class, stop talking, stop watching television, and so on.

Useful versus Problematic Avoidance

In many cases, the restriction of our behavioral repertoire in the presence of symbolic stimuli is totally appropriate. If you live in a region prone to hurricanes, weather reports advising residents to stay home during severe weather are useful. Although heeding the advice clearly narrows the range of your actions (you can no longer go wherever you want), it is certainly a wise choice. Here, symbolic control is beneficial because it allows you to avoid harm. In some cases, however, language can play tricks on us and lead us to avoid stimuli that are harmless (or even beneficial). By doing so, we can easily be led away from a more advantageous course.

Consider the following example. Imagine that you are hiking in a forest, and after a few hours you decide to go back home. Unfortunately, you get lost, and as you reach a crossroads there is no sign indicating which of three paths will lead you back to where you left your car. You pick one path at random and hope it brings you safely to your car. Let's say you choose the path on the left, but after 10 minutes, you step into a swamp and nearly drown. Fortunately, you are able to grab some tree branches and make it out. After you make it back to the crossroads you run into a fellow hiker who seems a bit lost too. Naturally, the first thing you tell him is not to take the path on the left because he is likely to end up in the swamp too.

Let's pause here a moment and analyze what just happened. Although you learned the consequence of your action through direct exposure (you followed the left path and fell in the swamp), your fellow hiker learned this consequence through language (he heard, "If you take that path, you will fall in a swamp"). Both of you will now avoid the left path, but your avoidance is the result of direct learning, whereas his avoidance is the result of relational learning (the symbolic "if–then" conditionality between the left path and falling in the swamp).

Suppose the other hiker, learning that you are looking to find your way back to your car, tells you that even though he doesn't know where to go next for his hike, he does know where the parking lot is. And, as he offers to take you there, you follow him down the center path, leaving both the right and left paths behind. Now it is your turn to learn through language, profiting from the direct experience of the other hiker. After more hours of hiking you finally reach the entrance to the forest. It is late and already getting dark. Your fellow hiker runs toward his car, excited to finally be done with his long journey, but even in the weak light it takes you only a moment to see that this is not the entrance where you left your car. He took you to the East entrance where he left his car, not the North entrance where you left yours. It turns out that to reach your car you needed to take the path on the right. Now it will take a very long walk to get back home (you'd better ask that other guy for a ride!).

This example illustrates three types of avoidance, two of which are generally useful whereas the third is commonly problematic. First, you learned to avoid danger through direct exposure to the consequences of your behavior. Falling in the swamp after taking the path on the left has taught you to avoid this path in the future. Second, by telling the hiker not to take the path on the left either, he learned to avoid danger through language. Even though he never took this path, he knows he should not take it.

Third, by hearing the hiker say that you should take the center path and not the one on the right, you learned through language to avoid something that was actually good for you and to approach something that was not helpful. This last type of avoidance is problematic because it arbitrarily takes us away from advantageous consequences.

Language Interferes with the Success of Experiential Avoidance

The symbolic generalization of avoidance provides both an advantage and a disadvantage. The advantage is that dangers and problems can be avoided without ever actually having to face them. It is not surprising that we learn a great number of useful avoidant behaviors through language because adapting our behaviors without directly experiencing negative consequences saves us time, energy, and pain. We learn not to put our fingers in electrical outlets, not to drive too fast, not to be rude to policemen, not to miss important deadlines, and so on. In contrast, language leads us to avoid artificial dangers. When we believe what we are told, or what we tell ourselves, the function of events and the way we interact with them can become strongly influenced by language rather than by the intrinsic characteristics of these events. What if this were also the case with the way we perceive our painful thoughts, emotions, and sensations? What if our tendency to avoid these psychological experiences were also the result of language processes?

We learned in the previous sections that symbolic stimuli (e.g., words) can evoke the same physiological, cognitive, and emotional reactions as the actual objects and events they refer to, owing to the mutual and networking properties of symbolic relations. When our thoughts and words reflect painful experiences, we can easily find ourselves reliving our most unpleasant moments. If you were the victim of an accident or an act of aggression, revisiting the location where it happened would likely make you feel anxious, sad, or scared; so, too, would simply thinking of the location and what happened there. How many of us have noticed our muscles tensing and our heartbeat accelerating as we think about an upcoming presentation at work or school? If you suffer from an addiction, just thinking about the substance that you are addicted to will likely make you want to use it, and so on. It is logical to avoid pain, but symbolic generalization causes us to have constant access to painful triggers and responses, which in turn leads us to focus our efforts on avoiding all symbolic forms of distress, even when they pose no danger. And how do we do that? We try to forget. We try not to think about it. We numb out. We stuff it down. We think positively. We refuse to talk about it. We pretend it isn't here.

The hard part, however, is finding a safe place where none of these symbolic stimuli will be present. Many people who suffer from alcohol addiction and want to remain sober prefer to avoid alcohol. It may be possible, for example, to choose a restaurant that doesn't have a bar or a neighborhood that doesn't have any liquor stores. It's even possible to avoid people who drink or situations where one might be offered a drink. Similarly, it may be possible for victims of violence to find a place with minimal risk of aggression, like at home with the door locked. Those who fear contamination may find a place that is perfectly clean and work tirelessly to keep it so. However, even in a locked room that is sterile and free from alcohol, it is possible to be upset by alcohol cravings, memories of aggression, or fears of contamination—because psychological functions (e.g., urges, startle, disgust) spread rapidly through symbolic relations to anything they touch, including thoughts and sensations. For example, the observation that one is in a completely sterile environment can lead to thinking about a hospital, which can lead to thoughts about disease and trigger feelings of fear and disgust. The intention of *doing this in order to avoid that* symbolically relates whatever we are doing to the target of our avoidance. A number of famous studies have demonstrated this phenomenon by asking participants not to think of a white bear (Wegner, 1989). Participants tried a variety of sensible strategies, like thinking of something else or singing loudly in one's head, but most people reported a sharp *increase* in the frequency of thoughts about white bears. Even those who were temporarily successful discovered a Catch-22: as soon as they checked to see if their strategy was working ("Am I thinking of a white bear?"), the white bear was back in their thoughts. This is how once-effective coping strategies (e.g., "I'll just distract myself or meditate until I'm no longer anxious") can get wrapped into the symbolic avoidance agenda, causing increased exposure to the very thing we're trying to escape.

RFT researchers have explored the language processes that extend the targets of avoidance in several studies. In one experiment (Hooper, Saunders, & McHugh, 2010), participants were first exposed to a typical relational training $A = B = C$. In this case, the stimuli were two nonwords and a genuine word: "Boceem = Gedeer = Bear." Then, participants were asked to not think of a bear while watching a series of stimuli appearing one by one on a computer screen. Among these stimuli were the words "Gedeer" and "Boceem," several other non-words, and the word "Bear." As you can imagine, it is difficult to not think of a bear with the word "Bear" right in front of your eyes. To help, the participants were allowed to press the space bar if they wanted to remove any stimulus from the screen. The participants logically pressed the space bar every time the word "Bear" appeared on the screen, but they also removed the word "Gedeer," which was related to "Bear" by mutual entailment, and they removed the word "Boceem" which was related to "Bear" by combinatorial entailment. They did not remove any other nonwords that were not related to "Bear." This means that the stimuli related by language alone to the target of thought avoidance also became targets of avoidance. Not only did the participants avoid "Gedeer," which was directly related to "Bear" ("Gedeer" is like "Bear"), but they also avoided "Boceem," which was only related to "Bear" through derivation ("Boceem" is like "Gedeer"). Even when a stimulus is in relation of opposition with "Bear," participants still tend to avoid it (Stewart et al., 2015). Thus, even if you try to think of something nice to avoid a painful thought, this pain will quickly catch you up anyway. In other words, once language is involved, there is no limit to how far pain can be spread. In that case, how could anyone possibly keep sources of pain to a restricted area?

Language can change the function of any event. Any event can become aversive because any event can be related symbolically to other events that are aversive. Right now it is unlikely that *neprijatelji ukrasti* means anything to you. Suppose, however, we knew that a reader of this book was trying hard to avoid memories of stealing from a friend. Just a hint of that memory sends shivers of shame through our poor reader. Let's suppose our reader enjoys playing the guitar and bike riding, and that reader comes upon the next paragraph.

Imagine playing the guitar while riding your bike. Imagine that a person named Neprijatelji plays the guitar. Oh, by the way, *neprijatelji* is also Croatian for "enemies." What is the opposite of "enemy"? Oh, by the way, the Croatian word for "steal" is *ukrasti*. *Neprijatelji ukrasti*.

We are building a network, with the perverse purpose of making it impossible for our reader to ride her bike without an uneasy sense of shame seemingly dropping out of the sky. It is not at all beyond possibility that the paragraph before this one could do exactly that for our poor reader. Language can change the function of *any* event because through derivation, language can spread changed functions through a symbolic network with virtually no end and virtually no limit. That is part of why deliberate experiential avoidance is so tricky.

When we ask our clients if their attempts to forget bad memories or not feel pain were successful, they generally tell us that they were not. Why then do we all readily persist with this strategy? Once again, language processes play an important role in this paradox.

PROBLEMS LINKED TO RULE FOLLOWING AND INEFFECTIVE PERSISTENCE

Following Rules Can Lead to Problematic Forms of Insensitivity

One of the remarkable facts of human existence is that our symbolic abilities contain a downside: when we learn what to do based on rules, it tends to undermine guidance by direct experience (i.e., contingency learning). Ironically, this insensitivity to direct experience isn't due to symbolic reasoning being unhelpful—it is precisely because they produce widespread and immediate benefits that human symbolic abilities tend to block out and overwhelm other sources of learning and human action.

Imagine you are visiting a city for the first time and want to know where the best restaurants are located. You consult a guidebook and dine at several recommended restaurants, leaving completely satisfied each time. The food is excellent, the service is fast and friendly, and the price fits your budget perfectly. The next time you are in the city you look forward to visiting your favorite restaurants where you can get friendly service and delicious food for a great value. Year after year, you visit the same spots, proud to know where the best places are.

But one day, a friend tells you that he recently visited the same city and ate at some great restaurants—none of which are on your list. Some are in a part of the city that you never visit because you were told it contained nothing very worthwhile. Your friend took the time to explore different sections of the city, check out different menus, and try a few restaurants, hoping that the food and service would be worth the price. As it turns out, over time other parts of the city have developed and so have their restaurants. Although you learned quickly and effectively where the best restaurants were, you also became insensitive to the changes of the city. Your friend's more exploratory approach rooted out restaurants with interesting menus and cheaper prices in unexpected places.

People learn much of what they do through rules, at least in part. Rules are just extensions of basic relational learning. We've already discussed how two events can be arbitrarily related regardless of their intrinsic characteristics. The same principle allows us to state rules that are independent of the actual consequences they describe. The reason is relatively simple: rules are made of a combination of symbolic relations, which can themselves be arbitrarily applied. We could tell you that reading this book is going to turn you into a great clinician or, instead, into a great cook; by putting "reading this book" into a conditional (if . . . then) relation, we have specified the consequences of an action, and that might make you more or less likely to finish reading this book. It might matter if the predicted consequences are implausible, desired, or frightening, but in each case the rule is understandable and could have an effect.

RFT researchers have been able to experimentally show how a combination of derived relations leads to the formation of rules (O'Hora, Barnes-Holmes, Roche, & Smeets, 2004). As in many RFT experiments, the first step was to build a relational network from scratch to ensure that the participants had no previous history with any of the stimuli used. The participants in this experiment had to learn what "before" and "after" meant as if they were learning it for the first time with the use of arbitrarily chosen cues (e.g., !!! for "before" and ## for "after"); and they had to learn equivalence classes for color names (e.g., ()() = yellow; ^^ = red). Participants could then press colored buttons in the right sequence after being given cues such as "()()−##−^^" (i.e., yellow–after–red).

Networks of this kind allow rules to define the consequences of a behavior without the person coming into contact with the actual consequences first. For example, a rule such as "If you feel anxious, breathe slowly and you will feel better," includes conditional relationships ("if . . . then"), equivalence relationships between "feel better" and sensations associated with a relaxed state, and so on. These relationships seem to parallel a laboratory rule such as "()()−##−^^."

When we learn through rules (in our earlier example, through a guidebook), we may learn faster, but it can come with a cost. Rule-based learning is often not as subtly fitted to the situation as actions learned through doing and getting feedback, and because the key source of behavioral regulation is a symbolic network based on a language community, rules tend to produce actions that are insensitive to changes not anticipated in the rule itself. As a result, we may persist in rule-based actions long after they are no longer adaptive.

Early research in rule-governance repeatedly reproduced this effect in the laboratory (see Hayes, 1989, for a book-length summary). In one study in which participants were asked to press a red button and a blue button (which were alternately activated) in order to earn points worth money (Hayes, Brownstein, Zettle, Rosenfarb, & Korn, 1986). When the red button worked, participants were awarded a point after an average of 10 presses; on the blue button, they were awarded a point for the first press after an average of 10 seconds. Participants were divided into two groups: one group was told that the best strategy was to press the red button fast and the blue button slowly; the other learned on their own. As you can imagine, the participants who received the tip developed a pattern that produced a lot of points much more quickly than the participants who had to figure out the best strategy on their own.

However, once both groups had learned the pattern, the conditions were secretly changed. Now a point was awarded after the blue button was pressed 10 times (on average) and only once every 10 seconds (on average) for the red button. Although participants were unaware that the conditions had changed, they could see the accumulation of points as they earned them. The participants who learned to adapt their behavior through direct experience during the first phase adapted to the new functions much more quickly than those who had received correct instructions. The rule helped them learn more quickly, but also made them relatively insensitive to the changes in their environment that were not anticipated in the rule or instruction.

In a way, this is a problem we want to have. There is an upside to insensitivity. That is in part why we teach language to our children. If we yell, "don't go into the street!" we do not want children to test the relevance of that instruction by trial and error because a single passing minivan could prove one trial too many for such a test. But language and cognition tend to wander into territory where it can be useless or even harmful if it doesn't match our direct experience. This effect is not reserved to external instructions. Sometimes generating and becoming entangled in our own rules is itself enough to create psychological mischief in areas such as social sensitivity, creativity, play, sex, and relationships. Thus, the problems we solve by establishing reason and problem solving can be accompanied by problems we create through the dominance of human language and cognition.

If we understood in more detail where the dominance of human language came from, we might be able to resolve this problem by contextual control. We could put language on a leash, getting it well established and flexible, but be able to rein it in when it was not helpful.

Different Forms of Rule Following Can Lead to Ineffective Persistence

So far we have been focused on processes involved in formulating rules, but equally important are the additional processes that lead them to be followed. We will discuss two processes in this section (others we will discuss later).

Consider the example of a parent telling a child, "Put on your coat—it is cold outside." Suppose the child puts on the coat merely because there will be hell to pay from the parent if he does not. Following a rule because there has been a history of others noting and rewarding the consistency between the action specified by the rule and the performed action is called *pliance* (a technical term deliberately chosen to remind people of the word "compliance"). Rule following starts here, and it is crucial to children's moral and social development. Profiting from an adult's experience is a huge advantage while discovering this new and dangerous world. For the sake of survival, it is important to get rule following going, without a whole lot of testing and explanation. For example, parents don't always have the time to explain to their children why they should avoid broken glass, not go into the street, or walk carefully when the floor is wet.

Much of the rule following that regulates our interactions with each other was probably initially pliance. For example, when we learned to say "please" or "thank you," we likely had little idea why we should do it except that our parents insisted, and perhaps because they withheld things until "the magic words" were said. Later on we might understand that these practices have other benefits (they enhance social connection), but initially they were established by adding social consequences for rule following. We learned simply to comply. *Systematically* disobeying a rule often corresponds to a form of pliance called "counterpliance," also maintained by social consequences for rule following per se but the form of correspondence action-rule is reversed (e.g., "I won't follow this rule because in my culture, people don't like following rules"). Said another way, compliance and rebellion both involve the domination of social reinforcers for rule following per se.

Other times we follow rules because they bring us into contact with the consequences of behavior specified in a rule. For example, a child might be told by his mother, "Put on your coat—it is cold outside," and then observe that doing so actually helps to avoid unpleasant temperatures. Following a rule because there has been a reinforcing history of contacting the consequences specified by this rule is called tracking[1] (a metaphor denoting following a symbolic path much as one would follow a map). The consequences for tracking would have been there even if the rule were not present. Wearing a coat when it is cold produces welcome warmth whether or not Mom knows that the rule was given or knows that it was followed. That is not true of pliance—you only get rewarded for "doing what you are told" if someone knows what you were told and what you did. Note that the distinction between tracking and pliance is not just whether something is socially reinforced. If we tell you how to be effective in dating, and the rules are accurate, and you can do it, you can track these rules and achieve positive social consequences. People you date will not date you because you followed the rule per se, however—they will date you because you did socially skilled things, regardless of how that happened. So, tracking can be social, but all pliance has to be because in that case it is the connection between the rule and the action that justifies reinforcement, and only people can detect such a thing.

Pliance and tracking have both advantages and disadvantages. Both can help us learn more quickly without having to first experience the actual consequences of our behavior, but when *social* consequences are added for rule following per se (as is the case in pliance), we become more easily insensitive to the *natural* consequences. For example, a child may dutifully put on his coat even when it is too warm to do so because Mom says, "Good boy!" Trying to look good, comply, or be right may overwhelm the ultimate purpose of rules, which is to be more effective. Such acquiescence can lead to the classic set of psychological problems that are based on the "shoulds," "musts," and "have tos" so clearly articulated by early leaders in CBT, such as Albert Ellis.

---

[1]Note that in Chapter 5 and later, we use the term "tracking" also for the behavior of describing functional relationships among psychological experiences (e.g., a client observes and describes the consequences of an action). We are thus using this term more broadly than in the traditional behavioral literature, but our aim is to facilitate the use of technical terms in more colloquial language. In this book, tracking thus corresponds both to describing functional relationships (i.e., formulating a rule including at least one causal connection between and action and the context) and to following a rule, under the influence of the consequences described by the rule.

Rules can be followed through tracking at first but end up encouraging pliance. Imagine if you had decided to try restaurants on your own rather than read the reviews first. It would have taken a while, but eventually you would have found the best places using this method. Then, you would have likely told yourself something along the lines of, "This one is a good one, I will have to come back again!" You may share this rule with others, proud of your discernment. Initially, what maintains following the rule may be eating good inexpensive food (tracking); following the rule might gradually be maintained not by the quality of the food but by the "rightness" of the rule giver, that is . . . you! When that happens, even if the quality of food has declined, you may keep following your rule and giving it to others. This perverse effect will likely get stronger when you share your ideas with others because observers can monitor the consistency between rules and actions even if we ourselves came up with the rules. Being "right" can in effect have you going to restaurants because you once said they were good, not because they still are. After each meal you may think, *regardless of the actual quality and price*, "This is really the best place in town, I was right to come here again!" In this case, tracking has become pliance.

This can easily happen in the therapy room. For example, suppose a client suffering from depression starts tracking the rule "If I plan and do meaningful activities even when I don't feel like it, my life will be more satisfying." Poorly crafted and timed support from the therapist could encourage the client to start to follow the rule to please the therapist more so than to increase his own life satisfaction, slowing down the development of healthy autonomy. Later in the book we will discuss how to present social support in ways that avoid this risk.

Pliance can also become tracking. For example, imagine that you had first visited the city with a friend who had done her own research on the best restaurants in town. When you arrive, she says, "Let's go to this restaurant. I know you're going to love it." You may comply with her suggestion because you think it's good manners to accept the recommendation of a thoughtful host. In this case, following her rule is pliance, not tracking. However, if you enjoy the meal you may think "I do love this restaurant. She really knows what I like." The next time you are in town, you may accept your friend's dining recommendations because you want good food, not just because it's good manners.

The shift from pliance to tracking—from complying, looking good, or being right to doing what works—is key to diminishing rule-based insensitivity. In the case of pliance, insensitivity to the environment is more likely because the issue is social support for rule following per se—the natural consequences be damned. For example, suppose a person thinks, "I have to hide that I am anxious in order to get respect," and then becomes defensive or even aggressive if someone asks him a question while he is speaking in public in order to hide his anxiety. This strategy probably does not gain a lot of respect from the audience, but if following the rule was pliance (due to a history of social demands not to display difficult feelings), it will not be sensitive to the correspondence between the predicted and the experienced consequence (checking if it actually worked).

Pliance-based insensitivity is much more likely to occur if no consequences are stated in the rule because tracking is based on specified consequences, not just adherence to the rule. That is not always the case because some tracking involves implicit consequences such as when a waiter sees us wandering with confusion near the kitchen door and says "it's down the hall and to the left" (i.e., you can find the restroom there). In general, however, a lack of specified consequences encourages pliance. For example, imagine a mother who tells her crying child to "calm down" without specifying any consequences for calming down. The mother's request leaves her reaction as the key issue in the child's decision about what to do next. The child may start to control his expression of emotion just to please his mom or to avoid criticism, even though there would have been no problematic natural consequences produced by crying.[2]

Tracking can produce insensitivity as well, but it does so in other ways. For example, a rule may be accurate in the short term but not in the long term. This is what happens when a person avoids facing an anxiety-provoking situation in order to feel better. Often, "feeling better" actually happens even though the avoidance ultimately makes the problem worse. Because short-term consequences tend to have more impact than long-term consequences, this bit of success is enough to confirm the rule and maintain the strategy of avoidance.

Tracking can also induce insensitivity when it produces specific consequences but just at a low rate compared to other strategies. For example, imagine a person who thinks the best way to develop intimate relationships is to quickly disclose very personal and negative information. On average this may be a bad strategy, but some people might respond to it by being more attentive and caring, which may maintain following the rule.

PROBLEMS LINKED TO SENSE MAKING AND COHERENCE

If language is to be useful, symbolic relations must fit together sensibly into coherent networks. Coherent networks are like superhighways, allowing us to accurately, reliably, and swiftly derive meaning through a vast system of symbolic connections. When we detect ambiguity or incoherence in a relational network, it's like hitting a roadblock that requires us to slow down, reexamine the situation, and figure out a new way forward. That is partly

---

[2]This example could be an instance of social tracking instead of pliance if the child was following a rule stating the social consequences he is actually experiencing.

how we simplify complexity and how we solve complex problems quickly through language.

Think of how a competent test-taker gets high marks on multiple-choice tests even when the material is not well known. By searching for coherent and incoherent relations among test content, implausible answers can be eliminated and remaining test items will often supply helpful information. Suppose the answer to item 10 is either "a" or "b." If "b" is the right answer to item 10, then perhaps "c" has to be the right answer for item 30; if "a" is right on 10, then "c" can't be right for 30. Back and forth the person goes until the most coherent set falls into place. Nine times out of ten, processes like this will improve the grades of test-takers who actually know little about the subject of the test but do know how to detect coherence and incoherence.

Detecting coherence and incoherence is an awesome skill—it simplifies the number of concepts we need to hold in mind and helps us respond quickly when our knowledge base is limited. We apply our core networks to ambiguous or complex situations, allowing us to give them meaning and predictability (for an RFT demonstration of that process, see Quinones & Hayes, 2014). We tend to think in ways that we have thought before; to interpret events in ways that we have done before. This is not fundamentally different from any action. The difference is that relational responses can have enormous spread. A core belief such as "people are not to be trusted" will apply to almost any social situation and the self—which is why cognitive schemas can be insidious. And if coherence per se becomes the only guide to our actions, we end up trapped in our core ideas, beliefs, or concepts (i.e., core relational networks).

Applying core networks to broad ranges of situations becomes especially risky in three ways: (1) some symbolic networks evoke actions that confirm their own coherence; (2) most actions require some contact with the contingencies in order to be learned; and (3) support for coherence might not always come in the form of effectiveness.

As an example of the first way, suppose a person who has derived or been taught the rule "people are not to be trusted" begins to protect herself by keeping people at bay, by never giving them detailed information, or by lying to them. These actions will tend to produce reactions in others (conflict, abandonment, accusations, and so on), and these actions will seemingly *prove* that "people are not to be trusted."

An example of the second way occurs when a person confronts a situation that is beyond symbolic problem solving. Many skills have to be learned by experience, and there are many ways of being in the world that are not "problem solving," in the traditional sense of the term at least. Suppose a person sees a beautiful sunset. Appreciating a sunset is not a problem-solving situation. "Nice sunset, God, but it needs a bit more blue over there" is hardly a reaction likely to support awe. In the same way, excessive or misplaced problem solving can make it hard to play a well-practiced piano piece or hit a tennis ball; it can eliminate peace of mind, or it can overwhelm our human capacity for love, appreciation, joy, and happiness.

An example of the third way is the tendency to persist in patterns even when experience shows they are unworkable, on such grounds as they should work, they work for others, they used to work, or it is not fair that they don't work. A vast amount of psychopathology fits under that broad umbrella.

An old but still interesting way of talking about this aspect of psychological problems is the idea that self-defeating behavior can become self-perpetuating—what Mowrer (1948, 1950) identified as the "neurotic paradox." From an RFT perspective, psychological problems often persist when rules overwhelm experience (e.g., following the rule "I must forget this episode of my life in order to be happy" even though it may be impossible to do so). Think of it as a clash between those 520-million-year-old processes called contingency learning, and those 100,000-to-2-million-year-old processes of symbolic influence. Speaking loosely, sometimes our minds dominate our action in an unhealthy way owing to unhealthy habits of mind (where by "mind" we mean just our collection of relational responses).

For example, the short-term success of strategies for dealing with difficult thoughts, emotions, or sensations makes them seem like the best approaches. Using television as a distraction from memories of trauma can work for a while. Excessive hand washing temporarily decreases anxiety linked to fear of contamination. Focusing attention on one part of the body in order to avoid feeling pain in another relieves suffering for a few minutes. These short successes can be powerful enough to establish "reviews" for the best strategies for avoiding pain, which then influence our future behaviors just like travel book reviews influence the way we choose restaurants. Language masks the long-term consequences of these strategies to such an extent that those consequences have little or no impact on our current behavior, so avoidance of psychological experiences persists even when it is not working in the long term.

What RFT suggests is to develop an awareness of the processes that overshadow useful contingencies and to be attentive to the contexts that promote or undermine these processes. For example, seeing the source of inappropriate problem solving as a simple extension of normal symbolic processes helps the therapist notice what in the therapy session might encourage distancing from these processes. The therapist may notice that her own tendency to try to solve the problem of the client's problem solving is yet another overextension of problem solving. That in turn leads to useful treatment alternatives, which we will address later in the book.

PROBLEMS LINKED TO MOTIVATION

Language Brings Distant and Abstract Consequences to the Present

A great deal of human behavior is motivated symbolically—this is key to our practical use of language. We can imagine positive worlds—including those that have never been—and we can track with language the consistency of our behavior with this positive vision and our progress toward these imagined outcomes. In direct contingency learning, stimulus changes that reliably track progress toward a consequence of importance also motivate action. Humans can do this with language, which provides meaning and purpose for behavior, moment by moment.

If we think of the heroic things humans have done, we see people focused on achieving or creating a better world or a better life. Fighters for social justice can imagine uplifting the downtrodden and taking steps over years and decades that have few positive consequences other than consistency with the importance of this vision (and perhaps small signs of progress in such things as recruitment of others to the cause). It is not that fighting for social justice is somehow no longer influenced by consequences—it is that the consequences are established symbolically.

One important area where this process is central is self-control. When short-term consequences exert a more powerful influence than long-term consequences, one way of reorienting the behavior is to remove the short-term consequences. This is what behavior analysts often do when they have access to the direct environment. For example, if caretakers in an institution realize that their attention is reinforcing a patient's self-harming behavior in the short term, they can switch their attention to more appropriate behaviors (e.g., asking for help). However, it is often difficult, or even impossible, to remove direct reinforcing consequences. For example, in substance addiction, decreasing withdrawals symptoms is an intrinsic reinforcing quality of using the substance. The action and its effect can't be separated from each other.

Language can help us behave according to long-term consequences. In fact, a great number of our everyday actions are symbolically linked to distant consequences through what we say and think. When the alarm clock rings to wake us up, we are able to contact powerful consequences through language. We may think, "I can't wait to meet my friends in town for breakfast" and already begin to smell the coffee, taste the delicious French toast, or picture your friends' faces. Our "imagination" (the transformation of functions due to relational framing) sparks our motivation to get out of bed.

This is an example of another major symbolic process identified by RFT: *augmenting*. Augmenting establishes new consequences (so-called formative augmenting) or alters our interest in existing ones (so-called motivative augmenting). One way augmenting works is by bringing distant consequences to the present via language.

A short detour through the RFT lab will help us understand what this means more concretely. In 2008, Ju and Hayes came up with an experiment that demonstrated how motivation can be established through relational learning. First, the participants learned that if they pressed the space bar while there was a green light on the screen, a pleasant picture would be displayed. In other words, they learned that a specific cue indicated the availability of a specific reinforcer. This is similar to what happens when you go to a restaurant and look at the menu. If your favorite dish is on the menu, then you know that you can order it. If it's not on the menu, you likely can't.

Next, a relational network ($A = B = C$) was built to establish a relation of equivalence between a pleasant picture and two new stimuli that had no particular meaning prior to the experiment. For example, a relation of equivalence was established between a picture of a beautiful landscape, the figure ◊, and the letters *VUG*. This is equivalent to when a child who loves chips learns that his favorite food is called by the sounds "chips" and written by the letters *c-h-i-p-s*. The actual food becomes symbolically equivalent to the two other stimuli, even though their appearance is not particularly similar. In the final phase of the experiment, the researchers presented the green light either alone or in the presence of the symbolic stimuli related to a pleasant picture. The results showed that the participants chose to display the picture more often when there was a symbolic stimulus on the screen in comparison to the green light alone. This means that the availability of the reinforcer alone was not as motivating as with the presence of symbolic stimuli related to the reinforcer. Imagine that you are at the restaurant with a friend, and as you are wondering what to order your friend says, "Oh, salmon burger, I bet that is delicious!" The statement would increase the probability that you order the salmon burger—that effect would likely be based on augmenting.

Augmenting increases the probability that we act to produce a given consequence. What is crucial about this process is that it allows us to be influenced by distant consequences, even if they come long after our actions. Jean-Louis Etienne, a great French scientist and explorer, once said that he took a cold shower every morning for months in preparation for an expedition to the North Pole. As you can imagine, this was not a very pleasant experience at the time. However, the thought of being prepared for the cold several months later provided enough motivation for him to face the aversive sensations of a cold shower. Augmenting helps bring distant consequences to the present, which turns language into a powerful ally. It helps to direct our behaviors toward advantageous consequences that we wouldn't come into contact with otherwise. It can even allow us to contact consequences that we will never directly experience. When parents save money that will be inherited by their children after they pass away, they know that they will never see the consequences of their actions. The thought, "With this money, our children will have a secure life," has the power to motivate them to do so. Thoughts such as "I have to get rid of my anxiety to be happy," or "I should never trust people so that they can't betray me" can motivate action in much the same way. Most suicide notes suggest that death will remove pain (e.g., "I won't suffer any more if I kill myself"), which may be literally true but at the cost of life itself. No one alive knows what it is like to experience dying. However, the symbolic relations included in this kind of statement change the function of dying so that it now has desirable consequences. The pain associated with hurting oneself is therefore overshadowed by the hope of being relieved from suffering. Hence, even when it seems that we can use language to our advantage, its inherent traps are never far away. For this reason, the only way to avoid these traps is to pay attention to direct experiences and to use language in ways that promote lasting sources of satisfaction.

Motivation Based on Language Can Lead to "Adaptive Peaks"

The capacity for augmenting is key to the human ability to identify and build values, to solve problems, to care about the future, or to protect others, but it can create harmful insensitivity as well. There is a concept in evolution science that explains how this can happen. Adaptive peaks are the advantageous results of an adaptation that fails to provide a platform for advantageous future development. Behavioral adaptive peaks can form, for example, when we strive for short-term gains at the expense of long-term benefits. This strategy may be successful in chaotic environments where consequences are hard to predict, even though resulting behaviors may appear impulsive or illogical to others. The behavior of children in abusive homes might be an example (e.g., avoidance of vulnerability). The problem comes when the environment changes (e.g., the child is now an adult and is in principle able to control the environment) and the formerly adaptive behavioral patterns continue. In order to progress, she needs to learn new strategies, many of which will pay off only in the longer term, not in the short term. This kind of learning is difficult: it means walking down the adaptive peak in the interests of finding another peak to climb that will take her much higher.

Augmenting can establish this situation symbolically. A person who is determined never to be hurt by others, or never to feel insecure, or never to be wrong, or never to be alone (and so on) can develop patterns of action motivated by these verbal goals that trap them on adaptive peaks. Suppose drug use removes feelings of insecurity for a person symbolically committed to avoiding those feelings. The behavior "works" in that using makes this person feel less insecure; but it creates an adaptive peak that is limited and isolating. Symbolically established means–end relationships that are empirically incorrect (i.e., not adapted to relevant consequences) are especially prone to this problem. An adolescent might purge to be ultrathin because that state supposedly will lead to being loved by others; a workaholic may spend all hours working because financial success will supposedly lead to happiness. Failure to achieve these ends may result in even more emphasis on the same means. Thus, sensitivity to consequences can change symbolically by the ways language establishes consequences as meaningful, or diminish or augment the effectiveness of existing consequences.

The process of augmenting leading to adaptive peaks shows that psychological problems are not always a matter of avoidance. Many ineffective behaviors seem to be instances of approach toward a positively reinforcing consequence which leaves us stuck, away from more meaningful goals. Being right, using performance-enhancing drugs, seeking intense sensations, or feeling in control are some examples of situations where positive reinforcement may be limited or costly.

LANGUAGE IMPLICATIONS FOR PSYCHOTHERAPISTS

Symbolic Relations Are at the Core of All Human Mental Concepts

Psychology and psychotherapy contain many ideas about human mental life, including consciousness, meaning, purpose, intention, feelings, understanding, empathy, self-compassion, and so on. From an RFT perspective, these concepts are ways of speaking about psychological processes that involve symbolic relations. By seeing this connection, the reader can take RFT principles and use them directly to understand how the history and context of symbolic behavior might impact the particular focus of their psychotherapy work, from any clinical tradition.

We are not writing this book with the purpose of changing readers' basic theoretical approaches. We are writing the book from a contextual behavioral standpoint, but most orientations to psychology and psychotherapy contain many ideas about human mental life, and those that lead to evidence-based and effective practices should comport with RFT—or there is something wrong with RFT.

Therapists Cannot Avoid Language

As described above, symbolic relations are everywhere, and they are central to human functioning. Clinicians cannot avoid language and cognition, even if it is not a central focus of their therapeutic approach. There are approaches to psychotherapy that aim to get beyond words, reaching deeply into emotion and experience. RFT actually explains why that might be a good idea, but it is not a good idea *because* it avoids language and cognition. Symbolic relations are not merely "words"—they are deeply intertwined with anything that is meaningful to normal human beings: images, memories, bodily awareness, and consciousness itself involve symbolic relations. Symbolic relations build upon a vast number of bodily and behavioral functions, and there is more to human beings than symbolic actions or higher cognition. Still, no approach to psychotherapy or human behavior change can prosper without a good theory of symbolic relations.

Furthermore, although symbolic behavior is based originally on contingency learning, *it alters the impact of all forms of learning.* Symbolic relations can change what is a consequence, what is an antecedent, or what is an eliciting stimulus. Let's look again at one of our examples. Suppose a person learns that $P > Q > R$. Now suppose we shock that person every time Q appears. What will happen when P appears? We know the answer because the study has been done: the person will be *more* aroused when P appears than when Q appears, even though P has never led to shock (Dougher et al., 2007). Such findings mean that no amount of knowledge about behavioral principles can be enough to understand human psychology if it doesn't include symbolic relations. What has happened to humans matters—we cannot fully interpret human functioning by only using processes that are 520 million years old (operant or classical conditioning) or that are even older (habituation). Clinical problems typically involve an interaction between symbolic behavior and other learned and unlearned processes. Psychological assessment and psychotherapy need to attend to and manage these interactions.

The Outcomes Are Complex, but the Processes Are Much Simpler

From an RFT perspective, symbolic skills consist of deriving relations among events and changing their functions under contextual control. That's it. A wide variety of relations can be learned, after which any event can be "placed into them," much as pictures can be placed into frames—thus the name relational frame theory. In the broadest terms, the goal of empirical approaches to psychotherapy is to empower the clinician to know how to predict and influence what their clients do so that the goals of therapy can be met. Our challenge in this book is to show that RFT is a tool that can help clinicians predict and influence what their clients do, regardless of the clinical approach being used. To the extent that we are successful, we are demonstrating that human complexity emerges from a small and manageable set of relational processes.

The framework and the tools we derived from these processes will be presented in detail in the next chapter. Many techniques we present in this book may already be in your repertoire if you are an experienced therapist familiar with a variety of clinical traditions, but our goal is not to teach a new psychotherapy model. RFT is a universal language that should help you integrate techniques coming from different approaches into a coherent framework and do what works for your clients with greater awareness and precision. Our goal is to help you use language as a therapeutic tool by applying what we have learned from research on relational framing.

Language Alters Context Sensitivity

Symbolic relations transform the function of psychological events and influence our responses; they can increase or decrease our sensitivity to elements of the context. For example, a simple instruction such as "watch out" orients our attention toward a potential danger and, at the same time, decreases our sensitivity to other experiences that are less crucial at this moment. In therapy, a client might be asked to observe his physical sensations or to think of what he cares about in his life. These symbolic interventions are chosen to alter the client's sensitivity to key elements of his psychological life, depending on what is most useful in a given context (e.g., increase motivation, reduce avoidance).

When therapists use language to help their clients change, they need to remember that language is particularly powerful at creating insensitivity (a phenomenon that has generally already played a role in the development and maintenance of clients' psychological problems). Using rules and instructions can be helpful because it allows clients to learn new responses faster, but it can lead to overgeneralization and persistence despite a lack of effectiveness. In contrast, using language to orient clients to the contingencies influencing their behaviors (e.g., with questions, reflective listening, or metaphors) helps them draw their own conclusions and foster experiential skills that are more flexible and autonomous (see Chapters 5 and 8). It is actually possible for therapists to use rules in order to promote experiential skills, if these rules contain their own antidote against maladaptive insensitivity. For example, a rule such as "pay attention to the consequence of your behavior in order to make better decisions" describes an overarching principle that is experiential in essence and thus is likely to support the observation of contingencies relevant to effective decision making (see Chapter 9).

There Is No Delete Button

"Unlearning" is not a psychological process. There are many learning processes known to weaken actions (e.g., forgetting or extinction), but symbolic networks are the results of an individual's learning history, and history works by addition, not by subtraction. Even something that has been forgotten can be relearned more readily than truly new material; extinction is a matter of inhibition of learning, new learning, or response flexibility, not unlearning. This principle is particularly important when dealing with thoughts (i.e., symbolic relations) because derivation processes make inhibition of thinking more difficult than inhibition of other behaviors. It is possible to inhibit the behavior of walking or eating for hours, but it is impossible to do the same with thinking. This doesn't mean we don't have any control on thinking, though. It is possible to intentionally contact a particular thought, for example. But focusing only on this thought for a long period is impossible because it would require durably inhibiting other thoughts.

Thus, when a symbolic relation contributes to psychological problems, clinical interventions can't be a matter of erasing it. What we need is to decrease its relative chance of occurring or limit its impact, often by strengthening alternative, more useful symbolic relations. In the symbolic area, clinical interventions aim to alter the context of thinking with cues establishing new relations, or cues transforming the functions of existing relations, or both. It is important to keep track of both processes so that functions are not inadvertently altered in a negative way in the attempt to alter the form of symbolic networks. The expected outcome of these interventions is not the absence or presence of any particular thought in an absolute way, but a capacity of redirecting one's own thinking toward useful symbolic relations through a cumulative and inclusive process. In understanding psychopathology, we need to remember that clients themselves try to apply the common-sense solution of finding and applying a delete button (e.g., trying to forget a trauma or to suppress a judgmental thought). This leads us to our last general implication.

It's Not Logical, It's Psycho-logical

Human symbolic behavior is the basis of human logic, but symbolic actions are not merely logical. They are psychological.

To better understand this idea, suppose you believe initially that *A* produces *B*, but later on come to the conclusion that A actually *does not* produce B. Logically, that is the end of it. *A does not produce B. Psychologically*, it is not so simple, *even if you truly now believe that* A *does not produce* B. In part, it is because the relationship between *A* and *B* is learned behavior, and learning persists. For example, a child might believe his father died because the child thought, "I wish he would just die" shortly before that happened in fact. Even when the child is told this is not true, he may still have the thought that he is responsible. There is no delete button—that action (the thought "I did it") will be forever in his repertoire at some strength. He may feel guilty about it. He may avoid reminders of his dad. Many of the things that seem logical or coherent in dealing with this bothersome thought (argue with it; distract yourself from it; get reassurance from others about it; avoid triggers that make you think it) have a chance to *increase* the impact of the thought and even its frequency. In order to restore coherence without deleting the thought, we need to include the child's history in the analysis: it makes sense that he thinks he is responsible for his father's death, given that he once had this thought and that thoughts can't be erased.

There is another reason why therapists need to be cautious with coherence: coherence per se doesn't guarantee well-being. We can find logical answers to existential questions and still be unhappy. Consider a mother whose child was injured in a car accident while she was driving. As she reflects on this event, she thinks, "I am responsible for his injury." Regardless of the specific circumstances of the accident, it will always be possible to find a coherent justification of this thought. If she was driving too fast, it is easy to logically conclude she was indeed responsible. But even if she was driving safely, it would still be possible to conclude that she was responsible because she could have taken another road that day, or she could have avoided the other car by paying more attention, and so on. Coherence can be found anywhere, but it can be useless or harmful if it doesn't lead to effective actions. Psychological interventions thus can't be guided by any kind of coherence. They need to include a sense of purpose and a sense of effectiveness toward this purpose, that is, a form of *functional* coherence.

Human symbolic behavior is a double-edged sword—it influences human action for best and for worst. It can increase or decrease our sensitivity to the relationship between our actions and their consequences. It can encourage change or lead us to persist in ineffective strategies. It can help us solve problems, or it can structure our life as something that will begin only when our problems are solved. It can help us know and commit to our values or help us ruminate uselessly about the unfortunate past or feared future.

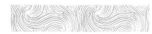 **CHAPTER SUMMARY**

In this chapter we have explored the implications of RFT for understanding psychopathology. Here are some of the key elements to remember:

- Fluency and flexibility in relational framing are linked to many important areas of human functioning that are key to psychological health, including perspective taking, empathy, problem solving, and analogical reasoning.

- The capacity to build symbolic relationships makes it possible for anything to become a source of pain. Even positive experiences can cause suffering due to the bidirectional nature of relationships. Once you know what you want, you also know what you don't have. If you find something that makes you happy, you must live with the threat of loss.

- All creatures tend to avoid sources of pain and danger and humans do the same with symbolic threats. Although avoidance is generally useful in the case of intrinsic danger (e.g., keeping your hand away from a hot stove), it is almost impossible to completely and durably avoid symbolic sources of pain because it can always re-emerge through derived relationships (e.g., watching a funny movie to avoid being sad can quickly trigger the thought "When the movie is over, I will be sad again.").

- Experiential avoidance is both a logical response to unpleasant symbolic relationships *and* a primary source of psychological suffering. Symbolic relationships are the result of an individual's learning history and history works by addition, not by subtraction. Thus, attempts to avoid or rid ourselves of symbolic relationships that cause suffering (e.g., memories of trauma, worries, low self-esteem) often have paradoxical effects, because they activate and expand the exact symbolic network we are trying to avoid.

- Since experiential avoidance is unlikely to work in the long term and takes great effort to maintain, avoidance of symbolic events can take us away from areas of our lives that matter to us (e.g., avoiding intimate relationships to stay away from memories of trauma).

- Humans can learn by experiencing contingencies or by contacting *descriptions* of contingencies (rules or instructions). Learning via rules and instructions is often more efficient, but tends to make us insensitive to changes in the contingences (e.g., picking a restaurant using reviews and not noticing that the quality of the food goes down over time).

- Insensitivity to changing contingencies can lead to persistence in ineffective behaviors (e.g., waiting for depression to improve by staying in bed all day, even though depression actually gets worse).

- Language, as a network of symbolic relationships, is inherently coherent and requires from us that we maintain that coherence through logic and sense making. Most of our interactions with the world are filtered by language, which can lead to three kinds of clinically relevant problems:
  - Bending our experiences in order to maintain the coherence of our ideas and beliefs (e.g., avoiding situations that make us feel insecure or ignoring criticisms to protect self-confidence).
  - Learning and solving problems only through language when contact with direct experience would be more effective (e.g., ruminating over past mistakes instead of repairing the actual damage done).
  - Letting coherence (i.e., sense making) per se become our primary guide and neglecting to assess the effectiveness of our actions (e.g., fighting over who is right even when it damages intimacy in a romantic relationship).

- Our ability to build symbolic relationships allows us to find motivation in distant and abstract consequences. This can be a major source of satisfaction, as when doing hard work that will pay often years later or connecting with one's values when immediate and concrete consequences of actions are painful (e.g., when satisfaction is accompanied by significant costs or when it limits access to greater sources of well-being). It can also lead to adaptive peaks, where the advantageous consequences following a behavior are associated with significant costs or limit access to greater sources of well-being (e.g., following a very restrictive diet can provide a satisfying sense of control but also damage health and prevent one from enjoying a meal shared with others).

- The RFT approach to language leads to key implications in psychotherapy:

  ○ Symbolic relationships are at the heart of all complex human cognition and mental concepts, including memory, mood, belief, self-regulation, sense of self, consciousness, intention, and purpose. Thus, all forms of human psychological suffering can be analyzed with RFT principles.

  ○ All forms of psychotherapy use language, even when they limit the use of words, rules, and instructions. Thus, regardless of your clinical tradition, RFT principles should be relevant to your practice.

  ○ The basic principles of RFT are relatively simple but the combination of these principles allows therapists to understand and intervene at a high level of complexity.

  ○ Language is a powerful tool for orienting and focusing attention, which can cause insensitivity to other parts of the context that may contain useful information. When responses are not sufficiently sensitive to relevant aspects of the context, they become overgeneralized, rigid over time and across situations, and difficult to modify. In order to avoid rigidity and across overgeneralization, therapists should use rules with caution and use language in a way that promotes experiential skills (e.g., through questions, reflective listening, metaphors, or rules encouraging the observation of contingencies).

  ○ Therapists can't help their clients deal with psychological problems by removing or replacing symbolic relations (i.e., thoughts can't be erased). Instead, clinicians can use language that establishes new symbolic relationships or transforms the function of existing relationships. This allows additional sources of influence to compete with the dominant symbolic relationship(s) and new or different responses to emerge.

  ○ Therapists can't rely on logic alone to help their clients deal with problems rooted in symbolic relations. They need to take into account the context that leads to problematic symbolic responses, and they need to foster forms of language and cognition that promote well-being.

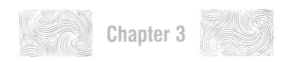

Chapter 3

Symbolic Tools of Change

How does human behavior change happen? With verbal adults at least, the answer largely lies in language, or the symbolic tools of change. In our previous chapter, we emphasized the deleterious effects of language, but it is worth noting that counteracting these effects most often requires the *use* of language.

Although language, the "new kid on the block" evolutionarily speaking, seems dominant in regulating human behaviors, evolutionarily older processes are not unimportant to change. An enormous amount of good can be done in psychotherapy by working with much more ancient processes— social learning, habituation, contingency learning, and the like. But even with that kind of work, psychotherapy is dependent on language.

From an RFT perspective, the clinical conversation is not just about words. It is also about such things as meaning, emotion, and purpose. The effects of looks and smiles exchanged between two people will be impacted by what they mean to those people. The emotions we feel, and the sensations we sense, are deeply penetrated by what they stand for, what their ascribed features are, where they are thought to have come from, or where they are believed to be going. If we understand that the essence of language is deriving networks of relationships among events and thereby changing the functions of these events, there is nothing in human behavior change that remains untouched by symbolic abilities.

In this chapter we will examine the tools of the trade that we will use throughout the rest of the book to vitalize your work as a psychotherapist. Based on the implications of RFT, we will provide a framework and we will examine some of the individual language tools that can be used within this framework.

A FRAMEWORK FOR USING LANGUAGE IN THERAPY

Just as the implications of relational framing for understanding human psychopathology and failures to thrive, the symbolic tools of change cut in multiple directions. Language is a blessing *and* a curse. That is why we as therapists need to understand language in a deeper way so that we can wield those tools more as a surgeon and less as a butcher. It is possible to become expert in the clinical application of relational framing, without becoming a geek, because the details that matter are details that can be seen in psychotherapy itself. A great deal of this book focuses on how to use language tools, but we will begin with what they are and what they are good for.

The Overarching Goals: Flexible Sensitivity to the Context and Functional Coherence

Promoting Flexible Sensitivity to the Context

What Is Context Sensitivity? Context sensitivity designates the degree to which we notice and respond to the various elements of the context, or "sources of influence." Our actions can be sensitive to different kinds of sources of influence, some of which are intrinsic and based on direct experience, some of which are based on biological structures and their remote evolutionary history, some of which are symbolic and based on derived relations, and many of which are combinations of these. When we behave according to a given source of influence, we are, by definition, less sensitive to other sources of influence or else we would respond in a different way. We gave many examples of this principle in the first two chapters. The explorer Jean-Louis Etienne can take a cold shower every morning because he is more sensitive to the distant consequence of being well prepared for his trip to the North Pole than to the discomfort of feeling cold water on his body. Direct learning can lead to insensitivity, as is the case when a short-term consequence overrides a long-term consequence. However, language is even more prone to producing insensitivities, because it can construct or instruct contingencies arbitrarily. These can include sequences that may never have actually been experienced by anyone—but nevertheless work by diminishing more direct sources of influence.

The Relationship between Language and Context Sensitivity. The ability to construct or instruct contingencies with language is yet another blessing and curse. On the one hand, language can promote healthy insensitivity to certain contingencies. A person may ignore the pain that comes with getting up in the morning, working hard, trying, failing, and trying again in a chain of actions that is motivated by the symbolically produced hope of reaching a distant goal—perhaps one, such as justice for all or a world absent of abuse, that has never yet been achieved anywhere. Language can also *increase sensitivity* to certain useful contingencies. We can notice things that were not noticed before, as when hearing "watch out!" as a car is coming our way; we can learn and teach things that are too subtle, distant, or complex for direct processes to be effective, as when receiving a prescription from a physician, or learning about the universe from a physicist; we can generate and test alternatives, as when planning an expedition to the South Pole and reviewing different routes before leaving; we can think rationally, as when deciding to start a treatment for cancer, even though it is painful; we can connect to meaningful purposes such as alleviating human suffering even in the absence of immediate satisfaction; and so on.

The potential of language is immense in part because enormous behavioral variability can be regulated by contextual features of the world. This potential has been the very engine of human progress and ingenuity. Take the example of the creativity test that consists of presenting a simple object like a pen and asking the participants to come up with as many uses they can think of for this object. The pen could obviously be used to write, but with language, we can derive a number of other functions: it could be used as a tube to help someone breathe after a tracheotomy done in an emergency, or it could be used instead as a weapon to stab someone. The same object, completely different functions. To be able to see these alternative functions, your sensitivity to various contextual features must be flexible. When you need to write, you focus on the ink in the pen; when you need to help someone breathe, you focus on its shape and hollow interior; if you need to defend yourself, you focus on its rigidity and sharp point. These features need not be known by trial-and-error use: language itself will help abstract them.

Implications for Psychological Problems and Interventions. On the other hand, language can blind us to useful contingencies, which promotes persistence in actions that are *not* working. Most psychological difficulties probably involve this kind of ineffective persistence. A client may keep engaging in obsessive rituals thinking she needs to protect herself from contamination; another may avoid intimate relationships because he thinks he is ugly; another may stay in bed all day thinking that getting up would be too exhausting. In such cases, the imagined consequences of action can overshadow other sources of influence that could support more useful behaviors. It is like not being able to see beyond the writing function of a pen.

Fostering healthy flexibility using language thus requires fluency in the application of relational abilities (you have to be able to think quickly, clearly, and coherently), but it also requires *flexible sensitivity to the context.* That is, thinking needs to be sensitive to relevant aspects of the context in order to be effective, much like a GPS needs to receive the relevant information sent by satellites in order to guide us effectively. We need to allow our contact with the world to better guide what relations we derive and what functions we change. Said in another way, we want our minds to be guided by an improved ability to observe and describe the relationship between our actions and the context in which they occur. We need to notice what works and what doesn't; what is relevant and what isn't. We want to allow our thinking to be guided by experience, the current situation, and our purposes.

Given that psychotherapy is based on the use of language and that language is particularly quick and powerful at generating insensitivities, how can psychotherapists help clients be more in touch with useful sources of influence without creating more problematic insensitivity?

To begin to answer this question, imagine a well-meaning therapist who sees that a client is avoiding intimacy and who attempts to solve this problem by cautioning him about the costs of doing so. In other terms, she is using language to alter the client's perception of the consequences of his behavior. The hope is that the client will become more sensitive to the detrimental effect of attempting to avoid a sense of vulnerability that intimacy produces, or perhaps less sensitive to the short-term success of this strategy. Although providing the client with a new rule might teach him a strategy that is more effective in this context, it doesn't necessarily strengthen the skill of bringing thinking more in touch with experience. The client didn't learn to avoid the pitfalls of language and the deceptive contingencies of experiential avoidance; he only learned a specific response to a specific source of influence, which could generalize across contexts *regardless of its effectiveness.* And although being guided by a new rule from a therapist might lead to better outcomes, it could also strengthen unhealthy forms of pliance (e.g., the idea that authorities need to tell him what to do because his own ideas cannot be trusted). If a client learns effective rules from his therapist rather than to observe and trust his experience, there is also a greater risk that this will increase dependence on the therapist.

We are not saying, "Don't give clients rules," because even that rule needs to be context sensitive. Rather, we encourage you to consider when and how to provide rules that help the client contact the contingencies that will naturally support effective and flexible behavior. For example, a client suffering from depression may be encouraged by his therapist to engage in activities again that will eventually bring satisfaction. If he does so, the client may naturally contact new sources of influence on his behavior, and the risk of dependence or excessive rule-based rigidity will fade away. This transfer of influence doesn't always happen automatically, however; it is far more likely to happen if the therapist is using language while being knowledgeable of its possible downsides.

A skilled therapist senses these dangers and is cautious about crudely giving instructions such as, "You need to do more pleasurable activities." Instead, the therapeutic focus will emphasize open-ended questions about what might be enjoyable, reflecting back the client's experience of the unsatisfying effects of inactivity and isolation, drawing out the client's values, exploring opportunities to act, or focusing on how the success of behavioral changes might be assessed or tested. On that foundation, more general rules might be derived without the dangers of overextension, insensitivity, and pliance. Such an approach puts the therapist in the role of increasing the fluency and the flexible contextual sensitivity of the client's own language processes, even while seeking the benefits of new rules.

The overarching goal of increasing flexible sensitivity to the context thus consists of helping clients be more in touch with their experience in a broad sense—not a specific experience, but a variety of experiences—so that most effective behaviors can be chosen in response to a given context. Metaphorically, this work is like helping a child build a jigsaw. We encourage her to look at all the pieces, and to notice the colors and shapes, in order to select those that fit together. But flexible sensitivity to the context is not enough to support effective action in a world made of language. We don't just notice things and respond to these things according to their intrinsic characteristics. Each thing we notice has a limitless potential for symbolic functions. Thus, a piece of the jigsaw can be transformed and fit with any other pieces. Clients need to be fluent in how they think about events and how they think about thinking itself to put together the puzzle in a way that works and fosters lasting well-being.

Promoting Functional Coherence

What Is Coherence? Coherence is a core property of language and cognition defined by the relative consistency of relational responses. Symbolic relations must be sufficiently consistent with each other within the same network to allow for mutual and combinatorial entailment to occur. In simpler terms, we need to build symbolic relations in a consistent way in order to use language as a communication and influence tool. This process begins with the meaning of single words (if "apple" → round red object, then round red object → "apple") and extends to networks of relations that grow in complexity (e.g., if Bob is smaller than Joe who is smaller than Fred, then Fred is bigger than Bob). Language consistency is necessary, in part, because we use language to build mutual understanding and to influence each other. Such understanding and influence are possible only if the relations evoked by symbolic cues and the functions they imply work the same way for both speakers and listeners—we want what the speaker "means" to correspond with what the listener "understands." For example, when language training is adequate, the word "danger" shouted by someone is generally understood as the imminence of a threat. If danger unpredictably meant "be careful" at times, and "you are safe" at other times, without clear cues to indicate which meaning applies, it would be impossible to respond to this word appropriately.

For the social purposes of language to be accomplished, listeners need to derive relations both among symbols and between symbols and intrinsic features of the environment in a coherent way. A listener hearing "when the bell rings, get the cake out of the oven" has to derive consistent and expected conditional relations within the sentence (if bell, then get cake) so that the actual bell can have the behavioral functions that allow the speaker's purposes to be achieved.

Coherence Is Pervasive. Coherence is so central to the ability to derive relations that we go to extreme lengths to establish it, even among random events. As soon as we name these events, they enter our symbolic networks. Even if we don't understand these events, even if they don't make sense, simply saying "this doesn't make sense" or "I don't know the name or the meaning of this thing" is a form of coherence. These events now belong to the category of things that "don't make sense" or are "unknown" to us.

Earlier in this book, we compared symbolic relationships to constellations in a night sky. Once they are built, it becomes difficult not to see them, as if they were *really* there. But these constellations are not inherent to the way the stars are situated in the universe. They are symbolic arrangements we apply to the world, and alternative constellations can be drawn according to different shapes. A similar process can be observed in a game created by French surrealists in the early 20th century, called *cadavres exquis* ("exquisite corpses"). This game consisted of drawing pieces of sentences from a hat and creating meaning from what resulted. It was *always* possible to make some kind of sense of these random arrangements of sentence fragments. The sentence that originally gave this game its name was "The exquisite corpse shall drink the new wine." Reading this, you are probably able to create a meaningful picture based on the concrete things that these words evoke, even though they were combined into a sentence randomly.

This imposition of coherence on the world is actually happening all the time in normal thinking. Socially, we are generally expected to justify our thoughts, feelings, and actions in a coherent manner (e.g., "Why did you do that?"; "Are you sad because I'm leaving?"). The purpose of this process is pragmatic (i.e., mutual understanding and predictability), but it can become toxic if it leads to arbitrary justifications and rules seen as essential features of the world.

The extension of internal consistency to a kind of *essential coherence* appears when we try to show that our ideas are "true" or "correct" not only by making them fit with each other, but by showing their *intrinsic equivalence* to the properties of the world. This process actually begins as early as we learn language. Our ability to relate things symbolically is an arbitrarily applicable extension of our ability to build relations based on intrinsic characteristics. Thus, it shouldn't be surprising that we tend to justify the coherence of symbolic networks by comparing them to the intrinsic properties of the physical world. Suppose a child is told, "an apple is smaller than a watermelon" and derives the idea that "a watermelon is bigger than an apple." Such statements are internally coherent (if $A < B$ then $B > A$), but that alone is generally not enough to consider them true. They need to be accompanied by cues pointing to their intrinsic equivalence with features of these objects ("See, it *is* bigger!"). As it becomes a habit to build relations of equivalence between our symbolic networks and our direct experiences, we begin to defend our ideas like we would protect ourselves against a physical attack, as if the symbolic world had fused with the intrinsic world. Magritte's famous painting of a pipe above the words (in French) "This is not a pipe" was titled "The Treachery of Images," but from an RFT point of view it could just as well have been called "The Treachery of Symbols."

Implications for Psychological Problems and Interventions. Let's bring this discussion back to clinical practice. Clients often come into clinical work seeking coherence in what they experience. Clients want to know what is TRUE, expecting both internal symbolic consistency and intrinsic equivalence with the world (e.g., "Why am I like this?"; "Am I broken?"; "Is it true that people who have been abused will never completely recover?"). They are asking the clinician to provide them with an essential truth that will make sense of their experience, resolving the discomfort that comes with incoherence. *Essential coherence* is generally problematic because (1) maintaining internal consistency and intrinsic equivalence at the same time is possible only if potentially important elements are ignored and (2) it can override more useful ways of symbolically interacting with the world, such as with relations of *condition* (which point instead to the *utility* of our ideas). Let's explore these two problems.

Ignoring and transforming key elements of our experiences to protect or restore the consistency of our ideas is a well-known process in psychology (e.g., adaptation by assimilation, cognitive dissonance). Given the variety of our experiences, it is difficult to make all the pieces fit together *and* show that it is the only possible arrangement without leaving aside some elements. Many thoughts and ideas directly conflict. We have the thought that we are good and the thought that we are bad. We have a positive attitude toward the future and a negative attitude toward the future. We both love our work and hate it. But it is not uncommon for clients to feel that all of their thoughts and feelings need to agree with each other. The problem is that this approach can work only by their becoming more and more insensitive to aspects of their own cognitive and emotional lives. Consider the statement, "I am _____." Suppose you are asked to fill out that statement with three positive attributes about yourself that you believe. Let's say you put down "honest, caring, and a hard worker." The inconsistency inside such a statement can easily be rooted out by the simple questions "All the time? With everyone? In all situations?" The uncomfortable feeling you will experience when applying that question shows the overextension. No, of course not. Not all the time. Not with everyone. Not everywhere. How can someone be honest and still lie sometimes? How can someone be caring and still ignore the needs of others or abandon friends? *Any* attribute or trait is an overstatement. This exercise contains an important lesson: maintaining the intrinsic equivalence between consistent symbolic networks and features of the world requires insensitivity to some aspects of our experience. And if important aspects are ignored just to fit our ideas, these ideas become less useful to interact with the world.

Sometimes, maintaining the internal consistency of symbolic networks is achieved by *radically ignoring the intrinsic[1] world* rather than trying to maintain intrinsic equivalence. Instead of defending the essential truth of ideas, the relevance of direct experience to evaluate ideas is rejected. In our previous chapter, we mentioned a type of rule following called pliance, which consists of responding to symbolic networks regardless of the natural consequences specified in the rule, but based instead on social consequences for rule following per se (e.g., a child puts her coat on even if it is warm outside, just because Mom said so). In this case, the only thing that matters is to conform to the rule itself since reinforcement is delivered by the social community (or the rule follower himself) regardless of what happens when the rule is followed. Thus, what matters in this case is a kind of *social coherence*. Children who question social norms ("Why do we have to _____?") will often hear in return, "Because that's the way it is" or "Because I say so," meaning, in RFT terms, "The network is internally and socially consistent, and that is all that matters." If they agree, they will be praised, and if they don't they will be punished.

The problem with social coherence is similar to essential coherence: a loss of relational flexibility (you have to think and behave in a certain way) and a loss of sensitivity to direct experience (natural consequences of action are ignored). This leads us to the second problem linked to essential

---

[1]Remember that by "intrinsic" we just mean "nonsymbolic." We are not saying that because a feature is not symbolic, it is independent of our experience, or "objectively true." For example, the color of an object can be seen differently by different people. Thus, the color is not inside the object; it depends on our perception. Functional contextualism, the philosophy of science on which RFT is grounded, includes the principle of a-ontology. This principle consists of not making hypotheses about reality outside of one's experience (symbolic or nonsymbolic) (see Monestès & Villatte, 2015). Our use of the term intrinsic here must be read in this larger philosophical context.

and social coherence: the influence these kinds of coherence exert on our actions.

If essential or social coherence is the dominant goal, clients will seek it either by hanging on tightly to the intrinsic properties that supposedly match their ideas, or instead completely ignore them. Regardless of the impact that these ideas have on what they care about in their lives, clients will align their actions with these ideas to maintain these kinds of coherence. The world as clients conceptualize it, then, makes it impossible to move toward a meaningful life: "A romantic relationship is *impossible* because I *really am* unlovable"; "Anxiety *really is* unacceptable, and I won't do anything that makes me feel that way"; "My spouse *really is* wrong, so we cannot be together." If social reinforcement maintains these conceptualizations, it becomes even more difficult for clients to respond effectively to the natural consequences: "I *can't* share my feelings because *we don't* talk about feelings *in my family*"; "As a man, I am *expected* to provide for my family, so I *must* work even if I am sick"; "I *can't* tell my partner I want to spend more time together because *he thinks* it's silly." In each case, social coherence is more important than doing things that support one's own wellness.

How can we help clients reach coherence in the service of valued actions, while avoiding the traps of essential and social coherence? The answer is in linking coherence to flexibility and effectiveness. By doing so, coherence becomes *functional*: what is "true" is what works with regard to a given purpose. The different elements of a network still cohere with each other, but intrinsic equivalence or arbitrary social reinforcement is not what justifies coherence. The way elements fit together can change depending on the impact that these symbolic arrangements have on the world in a given context. A pen *can* be a tube if, in this moment, using it as a tube can help someone breathe. Thus, in functional coherence, the nature of the relationship between symbolic networks and the intrinsic world is primarily *conditional*. If symbolically turning a pen into a tube has an effective impact on the world, then coherence is achieved. There is no need to add that the pen was *actually* a tube or that its *real* nature is to be a tube. It can be used to write a thank you note a moment after, and still not be essentially a pen.

Guiding clients to step back from the language stream to a degree can help them undermine essential coherence. But that is not easy because once derived meanings are established, symbols carry them everywhere. We can't suppress symbolic equivalence with the intrinsic world, even though it is just a mental construction. Try to listen to a conversation in detail, without also hearing what it means. You will find it nearly impossible. As soon as you hear "milk," you picture a white liquid. A person listening to a foreign language for the first time will hear its sounds, but for a native speaker this is extremely difficult. Essential coherence is so deeply embedded in these symbols that it takes considerable effort to view the process of thinking in the way we view a flower or a double rainbow: just for its appearance rather than for what it means.

A wide variety of methods focus on helping human beings back away from language. Examples may include meditation, paradox, contemplation, chanting, silence, Yoga, koans, psychedelic drugs, spiritual rituals, dance, body work, defusion methods, and attentional training. Only a subset of these methods have been incorporated into evidence-based clinical practice, but at least some of them are now reasonably well supported by meta-analyses or mediational studies (see Hayes, Villatte, Levin, & Hildebrandt, 2011). These methods limit contact with symbolic functions and internal consistency temporarily, while increasing contact with functions based on nonsymbolic experience. When we do that, essential coherence is diminished, and alternative useful functions become more available. New ways of relating things become possible as symbolic flexibility increases.

Language itself can help decrease essential coherence and increase functional coherence—indeed, many of the methods listed above (e.g., paradox, koans, defusion methods, attentional training) are largely verbal. We can build relational networks in ways that both make sense of our experiences and increase the flexibility of our ideas, holding inconsistencies within any given network with more equanimity, while turning our eyes toward the effectiveness of our actions. In therapy, clients are encouraged to practice relational flexibility by exploring a variety of hypotheses and taking different perspectives, and by conceptualizing their various and often contradictory actions, thoughts, emotions, and sensations as psychological events that can be observed merely as parts of themselves; to practice functional coherence by tracking the functional relationships that link thoughts, actions, and consequences, and by connecting their goals to meaningful life directions. Methods such as contemplative practice can nest within these more obviously verbal interventions to help clients relate more effectively to their experience through language because the deep message of such methods that are focused on the transformation of functions of language is that all relational networks can be examined for their functional impact. That helps keep hypotheses as hypotheses; perspective taking as perspective taking; or self concepts as self concepts.

As we will see in the next chapters on clinical interventions, social and essential coherence are not always problematic, and they can even be useful when functional coherence is not well supported by observable contingencies. In some cases for example, a therapist might promote social coherence by encouraging a client to trust her rather than to observe his own experience because, in this moment, judgment might be impaired (e.g., when a client is hopeless or highly distressed) or because there is a lack of experience supporting effective actions. However, even in these cases, functional coherence needs to be eventually involved in order to foster autonomy (see

Chapter 5). Some degree of essential coherence[2] is involved in the notions of "self" and "meaning of life" because they require stability, even though these are symbolic concepts and thus malleable through relational framing. As we will see in Chapters 6 and 7, conceptualizing the self as a container of psychological experiences and identifying overarching goals and qualities of actions as broad life directions are good ways of maintaining flexibility even when symbolic constructions are seen as essential.

In summary, the overarching goal of promoting functional coherence consists of helping clients think and make choices based on wholeness and effectiveness, so that all psychological experiences are integrated into flexible networks and actions are taken in the service of meaningful living.

The Overarching Strategy: Altering the Context to Transform Symbolic Functions

Transformation of Symbolic Functions

Language influences the way we perceive and respond to our experiences. Several examples of transformation of function were given throughout the first chapters of this book, and we saw that this process has both advantages and downsides. Because anything can become anything with language, virtually any event in our lives either can provide us with the strength to move in valued directions or, in contrast, can create barriers that are difficult to overcome. Therapy work is effective if it allows for a change in function, that is, if it changes the meaning of the client's experiences and their impact on his behavior. The skillful use of language is to promote symbolic functions that support rather than block effective actions.

Language relates events, but it also selects the functions of events that are already related. Think of an apple. Now see if you can remember what it sounds like to bite into one that is fresh. Now focus on what it feels like in your mouth to chew a big bite of a crisp, cold apple—the texture of the flesh of the apple as it is chewed. See if you can remember what it tastes like.

None of these experiences are new. They were all available to you with the first sentence "think of an apple" but until additional words were added, the many functions of an apple were diffuse and flitted across your mind in a disorganized or an idiosyncratic way. We then augmented the functions of sound (the crunch of an apple), of texture, and of taste. We

---

[2]Note that we are not equating essential coherence with essentialism, even though essential coherence is the pathway to essentialism. Essentialism requires a step further than building intrinsic relations of equivalence between symbolic networks and intrinsic experiences: the justification of these relations of equivalence by an appeal to the structure of reality *outside* of experience (see Monestès & Villatte, 2015).

could have continued for a long time with weight, shape, texture of the skin, color, and so on. We could have reminded the reader of the metaphors that apples commonly participate in, such as "the big apple" or "the apple of my eye." In this context, we are doing this just to note how many functions are already implicit given the single word "apple," so the order and focus don't really matter. But an advertiser might be more selective, now using the crunch, now using the taste, or now using ascribed functions such as our cultural memory of Eve offering an apple to Adam— depending on whether the goal was to sell juice, computers, or trips to Las Vegas.

Clinicians face the same challenges. They need to use language tools to augment contact with the existing functions of a relational network that promote positive change, to diminish present contact with the existing functions that do not, to bring new functions in a timely fashion, and to link existing functions to new events so as to manage when functions are likely to be selected.

Take the example of intimacy. Fostering intimacy requires sharing of feelings, but the functions of such sharing are multiple. Sharing feelings with others can be appealing, for example, if it means developing a sense of deep connection, but it can trigger an aversive reaction and avoidance if it is linked to fear of rejection or to experiences of being judged. If sharing feelings is mostly perceived as a risk of being rejected, and not enough as an opportunity to improve connectedness, then feelings are not likely to be shared with others. Ironically, however, if we focused crudely on trying to remove the fear of rejection or somehow talk a client out of it so as to increase intimacy, we might be *augmenting* contact with the very functions that are preventing greater intimacy. The goal (increasing intimacy) would probably be better served by focusing on the yearning for genuine connection. In a paradoxical version of this approach, it might even be possible to use functions that would motivate avoidance as cues to notice functions that would *motivate approach* instead. An example of that can be found in this transcript of a session in which one of us (SCH) works with a woman who feels rejected and uncared for by her demanding father (Hayes, 2009; the transcript has been edited here for length and confidentiality[3]):

THERAPIST: So if you pick one of those conversations and if you slow it down, is there something hurtful in there?

CLIENT: A little bit. Okay. I'm on the phone, I'm talking to him and

---

[3]Here and in all the other vignettes that refer to actual clients, we are not reproducing the entire word-for-word exchange we had with them. Changes have been made in order to make our point and to protect their privacy. However, the spirit of the original exchange is preserved. Other vignettes are fictionalized.

I'm thinking it's gonna be all be about him. So I can feel a little bit of that. When he calls I know that it's not gonna be "Susan, what's really going on? How are you feeling?" I don't even think my father *knows* me, who I am. So maybe there's some hurt there.

THERAPIST: Okay. Now here's a thing that's kind of odd though in there. . . . Would it be fair to say that if you push that hurt part of you away then you're sort of doing to yourself the same thing? If it hurts not to be seen, not to really be looked at for the person that you are, when you get in there and these emotions that come up when you're interacting with your dad can't be seen, can't be made room for, aren't you sort of doing the same thing to yourself?

CLIENT: Say that again. I didn't quite get it.

THERAPIST: Okay. What I'm asking you is, is it okay to be you, with your feelings and with your thoughts as they are?

CLIENT: Aaah. (*pause*) Can I be okay with who I am and what I'm feeling? Is that what you're saying?

THERAPIST: Yeah.

CLIENT: That *is* hard for me. (*pause*) I'm realizing it as I'm saying it. . . . I'm always judging myself that I should be this or that . . . which is kinda the same thing I said *he* did. (*laughing*) I hate that about life!

THERAPIST: (*laughter*) But you know if you go into pain sometimes it teaches you things. And there's something in here that it has to teach you. What if this pain is a value to you in that it teaches you something about what you want? What you want from your father but also what you want . . .

CLIENT: For myself.

In this example, the therapist is guiding the patient to take the painful functions of rejection and judgment by a critical father, and using an existing link to wanting to be known and seen without judgment ("I don't even think my father knows me, who I am. So maybe there's some hurt there"), to roll those painful functions over into the possibility of greater self-acceptance, so that intimacy with her father is even possible. Using the metaphor of a "teacher," the therapist suggests that the pain of rejection and judgment teaches something about what the client wants—from others and (as the client herself adds) for herself. The intent is to focus on and augment the importance of openness, acceptance, curiosity, and connection, and using the fear of rejection itself as a cue for those functions.

One way to augment and focus on useful functions even more rapidly is to emphasize new functions using the same words that describe old ones. For example, a person who is avoiding feelings in the effort to "feel good" can be asked to slow down and attend to emotions in the effort to "*feel* good." A person who is overcontrolling in order to avoid feeling "out of control" might be encouraged to let go so as to feel what it feels like to be "*out* of control" (where the tone of voice says that you mean "out" in the sense of "out of all of that" or "outside of that issue"—in other words, what it feels like to have "control" off the table as a concern).

Selecting and changing functions of psychological experiences is thus key to effective therapy. The question that remains is how. If we could simply change functions as we change a light bulb, our work would be simple. But therapy generally uses less direct means.

Altering the Context

A behavior is regulated by its direct and symbolic context: its biological history, individual history, and the current circumstances. The therapist begins and forever remains just part of the context of the client's behaviors. Thus, it is an overreach to view changing what people think or feel or how they behave as a therapist's job. We need to be more precise. It is our job to *change the context* in which people think, feel, and do. A therapist is not inside another person's mind or body. In the area of thinking, when we model, instigate, and support useful change, we do so by altering cues that evoke new ways of relating things and that change the function (i.e., the meaning and impact) of these things on the client's behavior.

How do we alter the symbolic context of clients' behaviors? The basic mathematics of psychotherapy tell us that addition is far more useful than subtraction. We cannot remove pieces of clients' relational networks because learning does not work that way. But we can change the context in which the sources of influence occur, and we can expand networks to bring in alternative, useful sources of influence. This kind of expansion reduces the dominance of troublesome symbolic networks, much the way that adding fresh water to a glass of salty water will eventually make it drinkable.

The Internet is another good metaphor for understanding how the mind works through addition, not subtraction. Large servers save almost everything that has been put on the Internet. Even if it is later deleted from a particular page or website, a photo, note, or bit of data can still be accessed through saved past pages. When people are victims of rumors or falsehoods on the Internet, a good way to undermine the impact of this harmful information (regardless of whether it is true) is to drown it into other kinds of content. Immersed in a sea of alternative content, the annoying piece of information is still available, not deleted entirely, but its impact is weaker. Similarly, if a client is excessively controlled by a difficult thought (e.g., "I am so nervous in social interactions"), other thoughts can be generated in order to influence her behavior in a useful way, without attempting to eliminate anything (for example, by asking, "What would be the benefit of interacting with people?"). Cognitive reappraisal, when it means cognitive flexibility or cognitive generativity, and the goal is not so much to eliminate or challenge but to broaden and build, is an example of this approach. However, if reappraisal becomes a way of suppressing psychological experiences, its utility wears off (see Kashdan, Barrios, Forsyth, & Steger, 2006; Troy, Shallcross, & Mauss, 2013).

Expanding networks can also be used to accomplish the goals of interventions designed to promote functional coherence. Placing thoughts in a relation of hierarchy or inclusion with who is experiencing them is a good example. We might report our thoughts after saying "I am having the thought that _____" or our feelings after saying "I am having the feeling of _____," which will consist of labeling the category of experiences and noting the natural hierarchy between the observer of these experiences and the experiences themselves. Perspective-taking language is another example, which we cover extensively in the chapters on problems related to the self and on the therapeutic relationship. After the report of a difficult thought, questions such as "and who is noticing that?" can help create distance between the thought and the thinker.

Note that expansion of a relational network doesn't necessarily lead to a transformation of function. Talking doesn't always lead to effective change, and certain sessions can leave both therapist and client with a frustrating feeling that no progress has been made, even though a great deal of content was discussed. It is not rare that talking even leads to an expansion of the problem rather than to a change of the person's relationship to the problem. Thus, therapists must keep an eye on the effect of their interventions and assess moment by moment and over time whether the way clients respond to their experiences is changing as a consequence of an alteration of the symbolic context.

Conversely, transformation of function doesn't always require an expansion of relational networks. For example, silences, facial expressions, statements reformulated as questions, changes of posture, or moments of contemplation can alter the impact of clients' experiences without explicitly adding any new relations. Smiles, nods, laughs, or tears can be indications that the clients' experience is changing or that the client is looking at the world in a different way. Sometimes it is better not to add any word to this new experience.

Let's look again at the vignette we presented above and observe how the therapist altered the context to promote useful functions.

THERAPIST: So if you pick one of those conversations and if you slow it down, is there something hurtful in there?

The therapist alters the context by slowing down and adds to the context the hurt linked to the client's talking with her father.

CLIENT: A little bit. Okay. I'm on the phone, I'm talking to him and I'm thinking it's gonna be all be about him. So I can feel a little bit of that. When he calls I know that it's not gonna be "Susan, what's really going on? How are you feeling?" I don't even think my father *knows* me, who I am. So maybe there's some hurt there.

THERAPIST: Okay. Now here's a thing that's kind of odd though in there. Would it be fair to say that if you push that hurt part of you away, then you're sort of doing to yourself the same thing? If it hurts not to be seen, not to really be looked at for the person that you are, when you get in there and these emotions that come up when you're interacting with your dad can't be seen, can't be made room for, aren't you sort of doing the same thing to yourself?

The therapist adds to the context the hurt the client inflicts on herself when she pushes pain away.

CLIENT: Say that again. I didn't quite get it.

THERAPIST: Okay. What I'm asking you is, is it okay to be you, with your feelings and with your thoughts as they are?

The therapist adds to the context the possibility of the client's being in contact with her thoughts with openness.

CLIENT: Aaah. (*pause*) Can I be okay with who I am and what I'm feeling? Is that what you're saying?

THERAPIST: Yeah.

CLIENT: That *is* hard for me. (*pause*) I'm realizing it as I'm saying it. . . . I'm always judging myself that I should be this or that . . . which is kinda the same thing I said *he* did. (*laughing*) I hate that about life!

THERAPIST: (*laughter*) But you know if you go into pain sometimes it teaches you things. And there's something in here that it has to teach you. What if this pain is a value to you in that it teaches you something about what you want? What you want from your father but also what you want . . .

The therapist adds to the context the possibility that pain is linked to a value.

CLIENT: For myself.

As we see in this vignette, the techniques used by the therapist to alter the symbolic context can be verbal (e.g., questions, reformulations) or non-verbal[4] (e.g., change of pace and tone of voice); they can select already existing functions (hurt linked to talking with her father) or expand the client's network and build new functions (pain can teach something about values). Progress happens when a change in the context leads to a change in the current functions, toward more useful behaviors.

This section on overarching goals and strategy was designed to create a framework to guide the use of specific symbolic tools that RFT provides for psychotherapy. Therapists alter symbolic contexts, thereby transforming the function of sources of influence, in order to help clients be more sensitive to useful elements of their experience, make more effective choices, and engage in effective actions. This strategy relies on broadening and building behavioral repertoires (including in the area of language and cognition) rather than attempting to remove experiences.

A framework gives a direction, as well as some general indications on how to go in this direction. But we can provide more specific guidance by identifying how the different ways of relating things (i.e., relational framing) can alter the context and transform symbolic functions of psychological experiences. In the next section, we will explore several of these "symbolic tools" (i.e., the different types of framings) and give examples of their use. The examples in this chapter are not meant to be comprehensive since the rest of the volume will focus more in depth on their use. Here we will describe their potential just enough to be clear about what they are.

USING RELATIONAL FRAMINGS
AS THERAPEUTIC TOOLS

Relational framings are collections of language abilities that we are evolutionarily prepared to acquire with sufficient training. In therapy, they are the tools we use to alter the context of the client's psychological experiences, hoping for useful transformation of functions. We saw in the first two chapters that framing combines three functional features: mutuality, combination into networks, and transformation of function. We sometimes use the term "frame" (as in *relational frame theory*) to refer to the smallest unit of practical utility for speaking with meaning and listening with understanding. But relational frames are things we do, not things we have, and to remind us of that we will generally describe them with the gerund form: relational framings.

---

[4]Remember that by nonverbal, we mean "not made of words." However, cues that are not made of words can still be symbolic (e.g., a gesture or tone of voice can mean something).

Dozens of framings can be involved in one sentence, and we are not recommending that therapists pay attention to any single one of them as they interact with clients. In line with earlier propositions made by other RFT authors (e.g., Luciano, Rodríguez Valverde, & Gutiérrez Martínez, 2004), we suggest instead a focus on framings that are most important to the transformation of function leading to effective behavior change. Sometimes, in a whole turn of speech, a couple of framings will be central to develop useful functions as in the following example, "If you were your mom right now, hearing what you just told me . . . Take your time to really picture the scene in your mind as if you were her." Here the therapist targets mostly a change of perspective, or deictic framing, to help the client notice the impact of what she said. This perspective shift is possible because it is combined with other types of framing, of course, such as conditional framing ("*If* you were your mom"), but it is more practical to think of this whole sequence as a perspective-taking move.

As we go through the different types of framings, it is also worth remembering that the specific symbols we use to activate relations and transform functions can have various forms. For example, deictic framing as used in the previous example could be said, "Now listen to that from your mom's point of view," or "Say you are your mom right now and you hear this." It could even be achieved without words, for example, by switching chairs. What matters is the function of the cues we use to activate the different types of framings. Some cues might even acquire a new specific framing function after a therapeutic intervention. For example, while asking, "Is it consistent with what matters to you?" might originally lead the client to think about the impact of her behavior in terms of a specific goal (conditional framing), it might cue attention toward overarching goals (hierarchical framing) after some work on meaning and motivation (see Chapter 7). The examples of symbols cuing specific framings we show below are among the most typical in English, but therapists should always check whether the meaning they intend to convey corresponds to what is understood by clients. Often, using pictures, gestures, and metaphors can help make these different types of symbolic relations more concrete and easier to observe (e.g., "and what happened then?" accompanied by a movement of the hand from the left to the right). This way, both therapist and client can make sure they understand each other, and useful transformation of functions are allowed to happen.

Coordination and Distinction Framings

The two simplest kinds of relational framing skills are coordination (which includes equivalence, similarity, or coming together) and distinction (or difference). For example, one might say "I am anxious" (*I* and *anxious* are in relation of coordination), or "I am not ready" (*I* and *ready* are in relation of distinction), which give an indication of how this person is thinking and feeling about herself in this moment. In their most basic application, coordination and distinction framings establish equivalence or similarity between things on the one hand or difference and exclusion between things on the other. These skills emerge first in our developmental histories—both because they are simple and because they are central to naming things, which affords enormous cooperative benefits (it allows members of a same culture to communicate with symbols about objects that are not immediately present in the environment; see Chapter 1).

In therapy, these types of framings are often used to help clients communicate about and discriminate among their thoughts, feelings, and sensations. The language of emotion, for example, is a primary means of communicating our needs, desires, and probable future behaviors to others. If the skill of naming sustained by coordination and distinction framings is weak or idiosyncratic, it is hard to get what we want. Naming is also a key process in developing flexible sensitivity to the context. By observing and describing sources of influence on our actions, we are better able to notice and adapt to different contexts rather than persisting in actions that are no longer useful. Those who have weak naming skills often have difficulty predicting and understanding the causes and consequences of their behavior, interpreting and effectively responding to events in their world, or getting their needs met effectively.

Such problems can emerge in many ways. A person who comes from a family where emotions were not acknowledged or discussed may never develop an awareness or vocabulary for emotions. Nevertheless, children raised in these environments typically learn names for emotions over time, but the use of these names may be too inconsistent, unusual, or vague to ensure good interpersonal skills. A person who was abused as a child while being told that he was loved by his perpetrator will have a different understanding of what love and caring means compared to a person who was raised in an atmosphere of safety and nurturance. A person raised by explosive parents who became angry at a moment's notice may see anger everywhere, even in the faces of others who are bored, sad, or even happy (Penton-Voak et al., 2013). If expressions of emotions are strongly punished, children may suppress them. After all, it may be better to deny or ignore feelings than to express them and be punished. Any of these fairly common experiences could disrupt the development of a language repertoire that is broadly shared and understood within the individual's language community. Strong feelings of anger might be named "annoyance," sexual attraction might be experienced as "disgust," or boredom might be understood as "anger." Similar processes could lead to the suppression of emotional awareness and communication, since contacting the emotion symbolically through naming could cause confusing or painful consequences.

Problematic naming is both challenging and worth careful attention from clinicians because the terms used to name experiences quickly enter into vast relational networks, sustaining sets of actions and further challenging efforts to detect and root out problematic labels. The person who reads too many contextual cues as anger in others will likely respond with his own hostility, for example (Penton-Voak et al., 2013), which in turn may generate real anger from others and reinforce the problematic relational response. The person who labels sexual interactions with the term "disgust" even if she is sexually aroused in a biological sense may have a hard time functioning sexually (Cherner & Reissing, 2013), leading to difficulties in intimate relationships, less frequent sexual behavior, and even fewer opportunities to distinguish between arousal and disgust. Detecting and correcting weak description and discrimination skills is a fundamental therapeutic task, facilitated by understanding the implications of coordination and distinction framing skills and how they can be assessed and altered in psychotherapy.

Opposition Framing

This type of framing establishes a relation of opposition between two events. It is different from mere distinction because it is more specific. If you wanted to know the temperature, knowing that it was *other than* hot would tell you less than knowing that it was the *opposite of* hot.

Because opposition is fairly specific, it can be useful when exploring what is, from the client's point of view, incompatible among her experiences or what the presence of an experience entails for other experiences. For example, clients often put meaning and purpose on hold while they focus on fighting with psychological problems. Opposition can rapidly expand the current focus through statements such as, "What would you do if this was not a problem but an opportunity?" Clients who have chronically put meaning and purpose on hold will sometimes be unable to say what they want, much as clients who avoid emotional labels have a difficult time saying what they feel. In such a situation, going after what a person wants directly is likely to get "I don't know" as an answer, but using opposition allows the "hook" to be what is known rather than what is unknown. This can be especially useful if the clinician helps the client to use cues that tend to motivate problematic behaviors as cues for opportunities to do something more meaningful (e.g., "What if the urge to run away is a sign that you want something in this situation?"). Opposition can be used to help clients infer more about their motivation.

An example exists in the transcript of the same session we presented earlier with the woman who feels rejected and uncared for by her demanding father (Hayes, 2009; the transcript has been edited here for length and altered to protect confidentiality).

THERAPIST: Pain teaches you something about what you value—about how you want to be with yourself and with others. When people are interacting with you in a way that you're invisible, that hurts. You feel angry about it. What if we were to flip that over and say, okay, what does that tell you about what you would like to have in your life? You're hurt because you want something.

CLIENT: Okay. I get that.

THERAPIST: So what do you want? Let me state it this weird way. What would you have to not care about for you to not be hurt when you're invisible?. . . . You care about your father and the relationship, but you also want this relationship to be something, is that fair? You want it to be genuine; you want it to be real; you want to be known.

CLIENT: I do want that. Yeah. I do. True. That is very, very true. That's why it's hurting me.

Opposition framing (e.g., "What would you have to not care about for you to not be hurt") is far more applicable than it might appear. Effective clinicians help clients understand more about what is present by knowing what is not present; to know more about what they want to do, by flipping from what they have not been doing or cannot be doing. The indirect nature of opposition allows the clinician to reduce resistance and find ways into avoided or protected territory through a kind of back door.

Opposition framing is also at the core of paradox and irony, which can be useful to help a client be more willing to explore a painful experience if it is approached with well-timed humor or irreverence. For example, a therapist might use statements such as, "What a great experience, uh?" or "That was what you wanted, NOT" while talking about the difficult experience. Such statements can get around well-practiced avoidance because it reframes something difficult to do as something great or wanted, not just as something painful.

Conditional Framing

Conditional framing is useful to evaluate effectiveness, in particular to track the impact of behaviors or to identify which behavior could help reach a given goal. It's most obvious use is to extend into possible futures (e.g., "What will happen *if* you tell your partner that you love her?"; "What would you do *if* you wanted to get closer to your children?"; "What is the next step you can take *in order to* move toward this goal?"), but conditional framing is much more broadly applicable than this common problem-solving use. Conditionality can be used to normalize or validate clients' experiences, for example, by acknowledging the impact of contextual variables on their feelings, thoughts, or actions (e.g., "Given what you have been through, it makes sense to have these feelings"—i.e., *If* you go through this, *then* you have these feelings). It can be used to explore potential contingencies (e.g., "If you *did* do that, what do you think you'd feel?") or to understand the motivation of others (e.g., "What do you think your father hoped would happen when he did that?"—i.e., what *consequence* his behavior could have had?). Learning to notice conditional framing on the fly can be useful in helping clients detect implicit judgments or failures to be present as they unintentionally put their own self-worth or self-acceptance into a conditional relation (e.g., "But even as you try to get that approval, are you buying into an underlying rule? I will be okay when I'm _____.").

Cause-and-effect relationships generally unfold over time in psychology (i.e., an antecedent precedes an action, which precedes a consequence). For this reason, temporal framing (cued, for example, by "after" and "before") is often linked to conditional framing, the same way correlation is always present in causal relationships—but not vice versa. Thus, exploring a contingency with a client might begin with asking, "What happened after you did that?" followed by "and do you think that was caused by your behavior?" just like a scientist might explore correlation effects as a step toward clarifying causal relationships.

Comparative Framing

Along with conditionality, comparative framing is perhaps the most central feature of problem solving and reasoning—two general skills that are not only useful for meeting everyday simple goals and achieve great projects in life, but to guide therapeutic work. We can recognize comparative framing in phrases such as "What is most effective between getting up and staying in bed?" "What would be more meaningful between these two career paths?" "Do you feel more stressed or less stressed after you drink alcohol?" It is particularly useful in evaluating the effectiveness of alternative actions, but that is more likely to be true if the contextual cues regulating comparison can be tightly linked to experience. It is easy for comparison to be regulated entirely by arbitrary social cues, like when we say that a dime is more than a nickel, even though their intrinsic characteristics suggest the opposite. The direct consequences of an action regulated by arbitrary comparisons are not arbitrary, however, and clients can be misguided by what they expect, hope, or fear, while missing what their experience advises them to do. Suppose a client is considering a new job offer and seeks your help deciding whether to accept it. It might be useful to apply an experiential form of comparison, more directly linked to natural than to arbitrary features of the alternative options:

THERAPIST: Just as another form of input, it might be worth noticing how you respond when you think of the two alternative options. Take a moment to imagine walking into your existing job. Take the time to picture yourself walking down the hall, opening the door to your office area, saying "hi" to your secretary, and sitting behind your desk. Slow this down—sort of savor how it feels. Watch your body. Notice the thoughts that flit through your mind.

Now let's do the same thing with your new job. Picture yourself walking down that different hall, opening the door to your office area, saying "hi" to your secretary, and sitting behind your desk. And again, open yourself up to what you feel. Watch your body. Notice the thoughts that flit through your mind. Slow it down. . . . What do you notice?

CLIENT: My whole body feels heavy when I imagine walking into my current work setting. My thoughts are anxious in a defensive way. That actually happens—it's not just in my imagination. As I picture the new job, it is very different. I'm anxious there too, maybe even more so, but it is over my ability to step up to the opportunities. I feel challenged. I wonder if I'm up to it, but it is not heavy and old and predictable. It's new . . .

As with conditional framing, it can help to notice comparative framing on the fly in order to detect the presence of a misapplied problem-solving mode of mind. Comparisons, especially when they are not experientially grounded, can be the signs of judgmental thought, which often takes people out of the present into a feared past or evaluated future. That is fine when a problem-solving mode of mind is useful and desired, but not when it is merely automatic and doesn't lead to effective actions, as is the case when we ruminate about inaccessible events.

Deictic Framing

Deictic framing is based on the symbolic relations that imply points of view linked to person, time, or place (I–you; now–then; here–there), and is thus tightly connected to the ability of taking and shifting perspective. This type of framing is involved in many therapeutic techniques because it helps clients observe and describe their experiences with a sense of distance between themselves and the events. That sense of distance is a function-altering process—we put difficult sources of influence at a psychological distance so that they can have less automatic effects on our behavior and can be seen for what they are. The elaboration of deictic frames gives clinicians a range of methods to increase a sense of perspective by changing place, time, or person.

One common and generally applicable way to do this is through the therapeutic relationship. Questions like "How do you think I might feel, hearing that?" or "If you were me, what might you say to yourself?" use the "I–You" deictic relation to expand perspective taking.

Much the same thing can be done, however, using time. For example, a client might be asked to go into a distant, wiser future and then picture this very moment when things were so difficult, as if they were long ago. When using this method, we might take time to have the client picture herself in a sensory way (e.g., how her body was hunched over; what her hair looked like) before touching the emotions, memories, sensations, thoughts, and urges that are present. The therapist might then ask perspective-taking questions, such as, "What do you feel about this person? If there was one bit of advice you might pass back from a distant, wiser future, what would it be?" This can also be done with the client staying in the now looking back at herself struggling with much the same issue as a child.

The same basic device can be used to change spatial perspectives, such as in a guided meditation in which the client looks at herself from the other side of the consulting room, before being asked to look at how she is dealing with current difficulties from this different point of view. Empty chair techniques, psychodrama, and role playing make use of the same relational processes.

In addition to reducing automatic stimulus functions, when we change perspective, we often see things that we didn't see before. Perspective taking seems to help normalize and validate emotions, thoughts, and sensations; to bring about a greater sense of self-compassion, and to foster a flexible sense of self. We will deal with these issues extensively in Chapter 6.

Hierarchical Framing

Hierarchical framing consists of building relations of inclusion, ranking, or category. It can be recognized in phrases such as "What value would this action be part of?" (inclusion) or "So, what you were feeling was a kind of a sensation?" (category). This type of framing allows the creation of unity amid diversity and diversity amid unity. What is whole at one level is elemental at another; what is elemental at one level is holistic at another.

Any event can be seen as an example of a *class* of events—and thus all events can be included in a hierarchy. A person dealing with how stupid and inept she judges herself to be is also, at another hierarchical level, simply dealing with the thought "I am stupid and inept." Sometimes just noticing wholeness at another level can provide a way toward greater functional coherence— without necessarily challenging the issues (e.g., ineptness; stupidity) that exist at another level.

Any event has features; that is a hierarchy too. Sometimes an event is so overwhelming that its features dim and only the total gestalt is available.

A panic attack may be totally overwhelming, but it is possible that considered alone a rapid heartbeat is not; nor are urges to run; nor is shallow breathing; nor are scary thoughts; and so on through every attribute of a panic attack.

And as these features are noted, they are noted using terms that also place them into a hierarchy—a rapid heartbeat is a sensation (one of many), an urge to run is an urge (one of many), and so on.

All of these things are held in awareness of a conscious person—which is yet another hierarchy. In some sense of the term, "I" is more like a container than the elements in the container (i.e., "I *have* the thought that I am stupid" vs. "I *am* stupid").

These are all examples of the mutual nesting quality that we were pointing to by the phrase "unity amid diversity and diversity amid unity." This way of thinking gives clear clinical guidance. When the whole is overwhelming or blurring useful qualities, hierarchical description that breaks down that whole can create useful contact with the grit and grain of the moment. When an event is overwhelming and seemingly threatening to the whole, it can help to use hierarchy to see the whole at another level. We can move up or down levels at any moment, going up hierarchically to find the whole and down hierarchically to find the grit and grain of the present. We will say more about this process when we address building a flexible sense of self and creating meaning and motivation.

Combination of Framings

The vast majority of language strategies occur at the level of networks of relations that are based on combining different forms of framing. Even a single short sentence is generally composed of multiple forms of framing. In general, we don't need to label these different forms in RFT terms—focusing instead on the key framing activity—but there are some higher order forms of framing that deserve discussion as part of our description of basic relational tools.

Analogical Framing[5] (Analogies and Metaphors)

Analogical reasoning establishes a relation of coordination between two sets of relations. A metaphor is an incredibly efficient process because entire networks of relations can be transferred from one domain to another. In an apt metaphor, salient functions that tie together a vehicle and a target allow other dominant features in the vehicle that are currently missing or weaker in the target to be seen. For example, the statement "cats are dictators"

---

[5] Although analogy is not technically a type of framing but a combination of framings, we will use the term "analogical framing" for practical purposes throughout this book.

takes a shared feature of dictators (the vehicle) and cats (the target), the feature of demandingness, and uses it to establish a new idea that is obvious with dictators but not yet with cats. The metaphor evokes a rueful smile, especially among cat owners, because it adds the new idea of cats ruling others in the house for their own ends.

Metaphors can be used to describe subtle or relatively abstract experiences by modeling them on something more concrete (see Chapter 5). Almost all emotional terms were originally metaphorical, but once the verbal community learned to train members in how to label emotions, the metaphor was no longer needed. In order to understand it, we no longer need to think of a "want" as something that is missing, or an "inclination" as something that is leaning and about to fall. In therapy, it can be helpful to use metaphorical talk to create greater emotional knowledge. For example, a therapist can help a client describe an emotion by inviting him to talk about it as if it was a painting. Analogical framing can also be used to build and apply metaphors that establish new functions or to change the function of the client's experiences by relating existing functions in a vehicle domain to a target domain (see Chapter 8). For example, the statement "Anxiety is like quicksand" uses the salient similarity of the pull toward struggle in both situations to establish a new function of "laying flat on an emotion" the way one might lie out on quicksand to avoid sinking into it. This type of framing can also promote symbolic functional generalization, that is, the connection between what happens during a session and what happens in the client's life (see Chapter 4). For example, after noticing that a client suddenly changed the topic of the conversation, a therapist could ask him if he "just drank a six-pack"—linking avoidance in session to his habit of drinking a six-pack at home to avoid thinking about painful things.

Storytelling and Narratives

We make sense of most symbolic events inside narratives and stories. Once even a small set of framing abilities are established, symbols are used in conversations and chronicles. If we take words out of the context of other words, they can lose much of their meaning. The flip side of that same point is that the meaning and the impact of symbols change when they are placed in different narratives.

Awareness of that fact provides avenues of important classes of clinical interventions that are designed to place the facts of a person's life into narratives that have greater effectiveness. We often miss the flexibility of stories and narratives because of the necessary consistency of symbolic relations. As we saw earlier, symbols have meanings that must be consistent to be useful. As a result, once a symbol has been established to mean something, it becomes difficult to let go of that meaning even when it would be more useful to do so. Truth with a capital T is commonly the grounds to resist flexibilities in narratives. It is as if it is important not merely to acknowledge the facts as we know them, but to hold on to the narrative we have used to make sense of those facts.

The story is told of a Chinese farmer whose teenage son broke a leg. The villagers wailed about the sad tragedy, but the farmer would only say "we'll see." Soon soldiers came to gather the teenage boys in the village to force them into military service, and the farmer's son was passed over because of his broken leg. The villagers fawned over his enormous good luck, but again the farmer would wisely only say "we'll see." The story goes on with multiple rounds of good and bad fortune linked to the leg, but our point has been made: the meaning of an event depends on context. In the "story of life" one of the most important aspects of context is how we make sense of events. These narratives can explain why an extremely painful event such as sudden death of a loved one can lead to posttraumatic stress disorder or to unusual forms of psychological growth, especially if growth cognitions are linked to meaningful actions (Hobfoll et al. 2007). Stories and narratives can be powerfully transformative, when they shed light on useful functions that were missed before. For example, testimonies of people who were able to overcome psychological difficulties are often used to increase the chance that people will seek treatment or to model effective change in the course of therapy.

Rules and Instructions

We saw in Chapter 2 that many of our behaviors are learned through rules and instructions, and that rule following can have different functions. Tracking is rule following reinforced by the natural consequence of an action, as specified by the rule (the experienced sequence action–consequence is the same as stated in the rule). Pliance is rule following that is socially reinforced because the performed action is seen to correspond with the rule, regardless of its natural consequence.

Rules and instructions can at times be useful in therapy because they facilitate faster learning and may spare clients from unnecessary aversive consequences. Psycho-education and instructions included in exercises and skills training are good examples of their use in clinical work (see Chapter 9). However, therapists informed by RFT are careful not to take clients away from their own experience when using rules, so as to avoid insensitivity to useful contingencies and dependence on arbitrary social reinforcement (except when doing so is a useful step toward tracking). Thus, instructions are generally used as the means to reconnect clients to their experience (e.g., instructions in a mindfulness exercise or behavior experiment), and rules are accompanied by encouragement to observe the natural consequences of following them ("What did you notice when you applied this new strategy? Was that helpful?")

CLINICAL EXAMPLE

As an example of how we propose to examine the clinical conversation in the practical sections of this book, let's observe the interactions happening between a therapist and a client in the following vignette. You will see that the therapist uses language to alter the context of the client's experiences, thereby transforming their symbolic functions. As new functions are selected, created, and amplified through that process, the likelihood that the client will engage in effective actions increases.

This exchange happens during an initial session with a depressed female client who feels rejected by others due to her physical appearance. She sought therapy on her own but now refuses to talk with the therapist about the difficulties she is experiencing. This is a fairly complex situation. Our goal in describing this interchange isn't to demonstrate one single right or correct style of therapeutic work, although we think this style is likely to help engage the client and establish a good therapeutic relationship. Rather, our goal is to try to show how RFT principles can help guide the therapist. In particular, you will see how the therapist uses language processes to motivate the client to share her experience despite her strong reticence. Our comments will remain relatively limited at this point. We will present specific uses of RFT principles in more detail throughout the remaining chapters.

THERAPIST: Would you like to tell me a bit about what brought you here?

CLIENT: There is no point, you can't understand.

THERAPIST: What can't I understand?

CLIENT: People reject me because I am fat and ugly. Look at you, you're thin and pretty. You can't understand what it is like for me.

THERAPIST: If I were in your position, coming to see a therapist for a first session, and I thought that I couldn't be understood, that would be really hard for me. Is that hard for you right now?

CLIENT: What do you think? Of course it's hard. . . . I am ashamed to be here in front of you, talking about how much I hate the way I look (*now looking at the therapist*).

In this first exchange, there seems to be from the client's view an opposition between communicating about her needs and being understood and helped. The grounds for that relation of opposition are an appeal to weight differences, and given that form of apparent contextual control, challenging the relation directly is not likely to succeed. Instead, the therapist uses perspective taking to create a context more likely to foster commonality and mutual understanding ("If I were in your position . . . "). If the client becomes more sensitive to this sense of commonality, chances that she will share about her life with the therapist will increase.

THERAPIST: Thank you for telling me that. I know your experience is obvious to you, but because I am not in your position, I need to ask you. When you look at me and tell me how you feel, I feel like I see more of what it is like for you. Can I ask you more about what it is like for you right now. . . . What you are going through?

CLIENT: You can ask, but nobody can understand what I'm going through. Nobody is interested in me. . . . I can't find anybody interested in me. I don't even know what I'm doing here.

THERAPIST: On your way to come here, did you have that thought already? That you didn't see the point of coming here and that nobody can understand you, including me?

CLIENT: I don't even have to think it. It's just true.

THERAPIST: I don't know what it is like for you, but I imagine that if I were to go see a therapist for the first time and I was pretty sure that there was no point and nobody is interested anyway, it would be really hard to go at all. Can you tell me more about what led you to come anyway? I imagine that it must not have been easy.

CLIENT: I was hoping that maybe you could help me. . . . But I was pretty sure that it was not worth trying. And now that I see you, I know you won't understand.

This second exchange is much like the first but more elaborated. The client detailed the problematic issue from understanding in general to one more specific event of interest. The therapist doesn't get defensive but instead again uses perspective taking to further increase the client's sensitivity to commonality between them and to evoke functions of motivation. The frame of opposition between how hard it must have been and the fact that the client came anyway evokes functions about a desire to be helped. Framed that way, the very fact that the client is still talking is testimony to how strongly she wants help. Evoking such functions is meant to increase the client's sensitivity to the potential benefit of talking to the therapist.

THERAPIST: Yeah, it seems impossible to you right now. I appreciate that you still make the effort to explain. I feel like you are giving me a chance to try to understand. You said you were hoping that I could help you, and at the same time you had the thought that it was not worth trying. How did it feel as you were just about to come in anyway?

CLIENT: I was desperate.

THERAPIST: That's not something I could know if you didn't tell me. Feeling desperate can be a different experience for different people, but I know what it is like for me: I look away from others, I feel alone, and I feel like nothing is worth it; I want to cry. . . . And it is very hard to even talk about it. Is it the same for you or is it different?

CLIENT: Yeah, I look down. . . . I don't want to cross people's eyes. I know they find me ugly.

THERAPIST: I can see why you would feel that way, then. Can you tell me more about that feeling of desperation?

CLIENT: I don't want to talk when I'm like that. People laugh at me if I say that it's because I'm ugly and fat.

THERAPIST: It must be a hard thing to do, talking while you think people may laugh at you. Did you think this would happen if you told me how you feel?

CLIENT: Yeah . . .

In this exchange, the therapist keeps targeting motivation functions to help the client get unstuck in essential coherence ("I know you won't understand") and move toward functional coherence. She does so in particular by tracking the current benefit of sharing about her difficulties with distinction and conditional framing ("That's not something I could know if you didn't tell me"). This creates a context in which the client might be more sensitive to what motivated her to come to therapy.

Then, the therapist begins to evoke the client's observation and description of her sensations, thoughts, and feelings by questions and reflections based on coordination framing and perspective taking. Experiences are talked about in ways that are more observational than logical: "You had the thought that it was not worth trying." The therapist is interested in observing experiences during positive actions as well: "How did it feel as you were just about to come in anyway?" An open, observational approach allows for exploring contingencies potentially involved in the client's difficulties, and it creates a context where avoidance is undermined (describing an experience entails contact with this experience).

THERAPIST: There is something I really admire in what you are doing right now. You said you came while thinking that it was not worth it, and now you are also talking to me even while you think there is a risk that I may laugh at you. That has to be hard to do . . .

CLIENT: Yeah . . . I feel embarrassed.

THERAPIST: Embarrassed too. . . . That is another feeling that must make it hard for you to talk to me right now.

CLIENT: Yeah, it's hard to talk about my flaws.

THERAPIST: Sometimes when feelings are strong, even our bodies react. Can you tell me about the sensations in your body, when you feel embarrassed like right now?

CLIENT: It's almost like it beats in my head.

THERAPIST: Is that why you are squinting right now? Almost like it would hurt to come out and interact?

CLIENT: Yeah . . . I do that all the time.

THERAPIST: So talking to me brings on difficult sensations for you?

CLIENT: Yeah . . . That's very hard right now.

The therapist puts sharing, a sense of difficulty, and courage into a relation of coordination. This is meant to create a context where positive functions of sharing are more likely to be contacted by the client. She then continues to evoke observation and description of experiences through questions and reflections based on coordination and conditional framing ("Is that why you are squinting right now?"; "Talking to me brings difficult sensations for you?"). The goal is again to create a context where avoidance is undermined.

THERAPIST: When I do something that is hard, in general it is because there is something that is important to me. It is hard and I still do it. Like right now, it is hard to know that asking you these questions makes you feel embarrassed and I still do it because it helps me understand you and I think it can be useful. Is there something that motivates you to talk to me right now, even if you are not sure I can understand?

CLIENT: I don't know what else to do. . . . I want to feel better. . . . Right now there is nothing worthwhile in my life.

THERAPIST: This is why you came here?

CLIENT: Yeah . . .

THERAPIST: And talking to me even though it brings those hard thoughts and sensations, it is for finding a way to make your life better?

CLIENT: Yeah, I'd like to have an interesting life, like everybody.

In this last exchange, the therapist uses perspective taking again, both to continue fostering a context of commonality and to evoke functions of motivation to come to therapy and share about difficult experiences. In addition, the conditional framing (e.g., "This is why you came here?") was meant to give the act of sharing, even though it is hard, the possible function of producing a better life. The concluding client's statement suggests that this change of function begins to happen and that coming to therapy and sharing start to make sense again (i.e., "I'd like to have an interesting life").

We meant this only as a brief example of how we might understand the clinical conversation. Doing therapy work based in RFT will require more than raw symbolic tools. A given case needs to be conceptualized and linked to strategies for intervention. It is to those issues that we now turn.

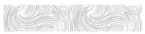 CHAPTER SUMMARY

In this chapter, you learned how to organize the principles of RFT and contextual behavioral science into a practical framework and a set of tools for use in psychotherapy. Here are the main points to remember:

- Our framework is organized around two overarching goals:
  - Promoting flexible sensitivity to the context, which consists of helping clients be more in touch with a variety of sources of influence so that the most effective behaviors can be chosen in response to a given context.
  - Promoting functional coherence, which consists of helping clients think and make choices based on wholeness and effectiveness, so that all psychological experiences are integrated into flexible networks and actions are taken in the service of meaningful living.
- The overarching strategy to achieve these goals:
  - Transformation of symbolic functions, which consists of selecting, amplifying, or creating new meanings of an experience in order to change the response to this experience.
  - Altering the context, which is the way transformation of symbolic functions occurs. It consists of using contextual cues to select or elaborate new relational networks or to undermine the impact of current relational networks.

- Relational framing is the basic unit of analysis of language. There are different kinds of framing, which allow us to alter the context and thereby transform symbolic functions in different ways. The main types of framings are:
  - Coordination and distinction framing (e.g., "It *is* normal to feel sad"; "What are the things you are *not* feeling right now?").
  - Opposition framing (e.g., "What is it like for you when you stay in bed *instead of* getting up?").
  - Conditional framing (e.g., "What happened *as a result of* sharing your feelings?").
  - Deictic framing (e.g., "If *you were 10 years from now*, what would your life look like?").
  - Hierarchical framing (e.g., "What are the things you do *as part of* moving toward more independence in your life?")
  - Combination of framings:
    - Analogical framing (e.g., analogies and metaphors).
    - Storytelling and narratives (e.g., tales, movies, and anecdotes).
    - Rules and instructions (e.g., "If you pay attention to the consequences of you actions, you will be more able to make effective decisions"; "Take a moment to notice the sensations in your body").

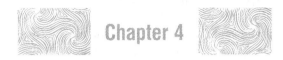

Chapter 4

Psychological Assessment

In this chapter, you will be introduced to a contextual behavioral method of clinical assessment that is rooted in an experiential approach to therapeutic change. You will learn how to use experiential language to conduct a functional assessment that facilitates therapeutic collaboration, nonjudgmental self-awareness, acquisition and generalization of adaptive behaviors, and maintenance of therapeutic gains. You will also learn to assess specific language markers indicative of psychological struggle and improvement, including the flexibility/inflexibility of context sensitivity and the ways coherence is established. Our aim is to help you use experiential language and functional assessment to inform dynamic case formulations and treatment plans, including those based on nonbehavioral treatment models. Therefore, we will not recommend specific domains or targets of assessment. We assume readers will draw on their own clinical training and expertise to guide their identification of clinically relevant behaviors, hypotheses about treatment mechanisms, and monitoring of treatment process and outcome goals.

CREATING AN EXPERIENTIAL CONTEXT FOR ASSESSMENT

The Client's Experience Is Central

Participating in a psychological assessment is nothing less than an act of courage. By sharing their private experiences and admitting they need help understanding and managing them, clients willingly open themselves up to judgment, misunderstanding, and rejection. When therapists remain acutely aware of this vulnerability, assessment is transformed from a precursor to treatment into an ideal opportunity to communicate respect, engender trust, and set the stage for collaboration.

An experiential approach to clinical assessment immediately establishes therapy as a collaborative process, something that is done *with* the client, not *to* the client. Together, the therapist and client explore the variety of experiences related to the client's reasons for seeking treatment and identify behaviors and contexts that seem clinically relevant. The client's participation in this process is essential: he is the only one who can decide what is meaningful to him, and only an analysis grounded in the client's experience can reveal whether a given behavior takes him toward or away from what matters most.

Experiential language is that which orients clients to their behavior and its context, encouraging open awareness and description rather than judgment. It allows clients to see their thoughts, feelings, sensations, and actions as products of contexts, while progressively developing a sense of self that transcends these psychological experiences (see more in Chapter 6). This approach creates a safe place from which clients can witness psychological storms, thereby undermining the natural tendency to avoid thinking and talking about painful events—important elements of both assessment and intervention. Experiential language, through the bidirectional transfer of psychological functions, brings "outside" events into the therapy room, allowing them to be jointly observed and their influence on current behavior to be mutually explored, even if they occurred long ago and far away. In this way, experiential language transforms each clinical conversation into in vivo assessment and practice, which facilitates learning and mastery, allows the therapist to provide performance-based feedback, and facilitates generalization of treatment gains beyond the therapy room.

An experiential approach to behavior change means that clients are encouraged to contact contingencies rather than just follow descriptions of contingencies (rules). Doing so promotes autonomy and self-efficacy because clients are involved in the process. It promotes flexibility because the skill that is learned (observing one's own experience) is generalizable to any context without the risk of becoming rigid. And it ensures that every observation fits the client's individuality because universal rules are limited to overarching principles such as "observe what works and do what works" (see also Chapters 9 and 10 on this topic). In practice, encouraging clients to observe contingencies means asking questions that orients them to different aspects of the context. We will explore this approach in great detail in Chapter 5, but some techniques will be reviewed in this chapter for the purpose of assessment.

The assessment process needs to have a quality of openness about it; otherwise social worries and concerns can dominate all other sources of speech. Clients have to have a sense that you are not judging them. As clients talk about their difficulties, they naturally often experience painful feelings in the room or report how badly they felt in a given situation. Noticing and explicitly acknowledging these difficulties are key to building mutual understanding and trust, to demonstrating credibility as a person who can help, and to removing the needless push to present only a sanitized view of the current situation. For an example, recall the final vignette of the previous chapter, where the therapist used *deictic framing* (i.e., perspective taking) to acknowledge the client's difficulty (e.g., "If I were in your position, coming to see a therapist for a first session, and I thought that I can't be understood, that would be really hard for me. Is that hard for you right now?"). To aid in perspective taking and empathy, a clinician needs to explore how the client is feeling while staying open to the possibility that clinician guesses may not be accurate (e.g., "That must be hard for you right now. *Is it?*").

Clients often want to talk about something other than specific questions you may draw from an intake form—which means that assessment cannot proceed effectively if it follows a too rigid structure. If a client is asked to expand on what she cares about in order to explore sources of motivation, she may avoid the area because it is too anxiety provoking. Pushing further is one option, but by seeing the avoidance, you might usefully explore it by asking the client more about how she is feeling right now, whether she often experiences this feeling, what she usually does to manage it, and whether that works in the short and the long term. Being sensitive to such issues is one way to help clients keep their own experience at the forefront of their therapy work, without being overwhelmed by the idea.

Connecting the Therapeutic Process to the Client's Life

The gap between what happens in psychotherapy and the rest of our clients' lives can feel enormous. Both therapists and clients can list a host of reasons that contribute to this impression, including the short amount of time in therapy relative to other activities, the somewhat artificial setting of a therapy room, or the fact that the therapeutic relationship is not intended to be reciprocal. Yet there are also compelling reasons to believe that the clients' behaviors you observe in therapy are directly relevant to their functioning in other areas of their lives, and that the therapeutic relationship has features that mirror other important interactions. Think of the socially anxious client who has difficulty making eye contact with you, doesn't show up for sessions when he feels ashamed, and constantly seeks reassurance that he is not disappointing you. Imagine a client who is suffering from posttraumatic stress and refuses to talk about her past, has difficulty trusting you, and subtly shifts the conversation when it feels too emotional, yet seeks therapy because she wants to develop more intimate relationships.

The obvious differences between therapy and "real" life may hide the wealth of situations that are functionally similar to treatment targets in areas of clients' lives that matter most—every one of them is an opportunity for therapeutic change. Specific behaviors can differ dramatically in form and still be part of the same functional class; that is, they share many of the same causes and consequences. Tracking such behaviors and recognizing them as clinically relevant often requires careful attention. This approach has been extensively developed in functional analytic psychotherapy (FAP; Kohlenberg & Tsai, 1991), but it is true of many other psychotherapy models (e.g., Gestalt therapy, relational psychodynamic therapy) and it is consistent with the functional contextual point of view presented in this volume.

For example, suppose a client expresses her satisfaction after doing exercises recommended by the therapist. The client may indicate that this is a kind of compliance by her word choice (e.g., "I did the exercises like you told me"), by an unexpected lack of information about her experience (as if the point is less about communicating an experience and more about producing an effect in meeting the expectations of the therapists), by paralinguistic cues (e.g., speed of response when asked about the homework, as if ready for the question; or disfluencies about the actual experience, as if it had not been thought about), or other subtle cues that indicate she is following the therapist's rule regardless of the natural consequences. This pattern would be particularly problematic if the client's excessive dependence on others or attempt to obtain approval from others were an issue in her life. In such cases the therapist's superficial, content-based impression may be that the client is progressing because she took advantage of suggestions for homework and had success doing so, while at a deeper functional level, this report of success may itself be a reflection of problematic processes.

Unfortunately, there is no simple recipe for recognizing the functional similarities shared by what happens in the therapy room and what happens in the client's natural environment. The function of a behavior is dependent on the context and the learning history of each client. It is only by observing the effect of a behavior in relevant situations that you can clearly unveil its function. What RFT adds is a focus on relevant relational frames, a consideration of some of the contextual events that need to be tracked, and techniques of language that help make connections between the therapy room and the client's life.

Improving your ability to recognize a behavioral and symbolic issue *in the room* takes practice, but you can be helped by the client himself. Elaborating hypotheses in a collaborative manner will contribute to the client's involvement in the therapeutic process, even if the client is not able to step back and describe where patterns of action come from. Techniques supporting this collaborative exploration are not new to most experienced therapists, but it is useful to consider their specific function within a functional contextual framework. For example, imagine a client suffering from depression who reports a number of thoughts that are preventing him from doing meaningful activities (e.g., "I am too tired," "It is going to be boring," "It's not worth it," "I'm not good at it anyway"). As you ask him to explain the situation further, he may express little motivation to do so and have a hard time expressing to you in more detail how he is feeling. Remembering to consider verbal reports not just in terms of their content, but also as statements about the relationship, samples of similar social situations or verbal habits, functionally defined actions, and so on, allows a kind of second-order focus to come into the conversation naturally. The clinician may realize that this response may be an example of behavior that is functionally similar to the problems that the client encounters outside the room—for example, excessive control by thoughts preventing him from contacting meaningful experiences.

In a sense, the current clinical situation is an analogy or metaphor for the client. Analogy relies on frames of coordination between entire sets of relations, and the clinician can draw attention to it in the hopes of increasing generalization: "It seems *like* it is difficult for you to talk right now. Do you feel the *same way* when you try to engage in activities and then start having the thought that it is not worth it?" If this situation is encountered with some regularity, the clinician can suggest a more sensory metaphor or, better yet, listen carefully for metaphors in the client's spontaneous speech that capture this symbolic set. For example, if the client mentioned feeling like being in a cage, the clinician might double down on that idea, suggesting that maybe her thoughts were like bars on a cage. If that suggestion resonated, now a single visual image could be used to link these sets of relations and to bring them into the situation when the client was showing avoidance in the session itself (e.g., "And right now . . . are the bars on the cage back up?" or "Instead of waiting for these bars to go down before we can work, would it be okay if I joined you in there and we can talk about what it feels like to be behind these bars?").

Perspective taking activated by deictic framing is another powerful tool to bring events happening in the client's life to the therapy room. Things that happened in the past, will or could happen in the future; things that happen in different situations, and even things that happen or could happen to others, are all immediately available if the appropriate symbolic context is created with relational framing. For example, a therapist might say, "Could you tell me what happened as if you were showing me the videotape of that moment? Just as if what happened there and then was happening here and now." In this example, the combination of perspective taking with a metaphor enhances the experiential contact with the event. Using the present tense, gestures, and postures that bring the characteristics of the distant event to the here and now will also contribute to connecting more closely with the client's life outside therapy (see also Chapter 8).

Thinking about assessment as a process of noting sources of influence over action (including symbolic actions) expands the assessment tools to include evoking potentially relevant behaviors by creating the appropriate context. Careful use of this process can allow greater precision about the sources of influence involved because they are being explored in direct experience and both the clinician and the client can see the result directly.

For example, imagine a client who comes to therapy complaining about her inability to keep a long-term relationship due to repeated and intense fights with her partners. Suppose it is your hypothesis that these fights emerge when the client feels out of control or seemingly vulnerable to hurt or rejection, leading to entanglement with thoughts that focus on issues of control such as "This is all just what he wants" or "I have no say over my own life in this relationship" and finally to withdrawing from the relation. If this same pattern were to extend into the therapeutic relationship, you might expect that ambiguous steps taken by the therapist involving conflict or interpreted as controlling might evoke thoughts of leaving, getting another therapist, or actions that undermine therapy such as extended silence, missing appointments, or superficial chatting. Conversely, you might hypothesize that minor disagreements might be constructive if the client is given full control over when and how these disagreements are discussed. Given that set, you may observe what happens if you express a disagreement with something that the client says but with a lot of control provided over the conversation (e.g., "Is it okay if I suggest a different opinion here? I can put it off until later unless you feel open to it") versus even minor attempts to control the situation such as suddenly changing the topic of conversation and a few minutes later asking, "Can I just ask something here? Do you have a sense of distance between you and me? Are you having thoughts like 'he just wants to talk about what he is interested in' or 'I'm not being listened to'?

ASSESSING CONTEXT SENSITIVITY

General Approach

Assessing context sensitivity consists of exploring the client's awareness of and responses to the sources of influence (intrinsic or symbolic antecedents and consequences) on clinically relevant behavior, based on reports about what is happening in the client's life, on your direct observation in the therapy room, and, ultimately, on response to intervention.

Such investigation involves asking a number of questions to determine the chain of events organizing the client's psychological life, essentially building a set of coordination (to name events) and of *conditional* (to identify functional relationships among events) framings. Antecedents are identified by exploring what happens before a behavior (temporal framing): "Where are you when you have those urges?"; "What do you notice right before you do that?" Consequences are explored by inquiring about what happens after a behavior occurs (temporal framing): "What happens next?"; "Does it stay like this for a while?"; "For how long?" Comparative (which allows to quantify) and distinction framings are particularly useful in assessing the strength and pervasiveness of a source of influence and the variability of responses: "How often do you feel disgusted after you eat?"; "Would you say that you procrastinate every time you have a deadline?"; "Is the result the same or is it different each time?" These questions may seem basic, but it's worth noting how new (and difficult) it can be for clients to think about their thoughts, feelings, and actions in this functional contextual way.

As you assess the client's awareness of and response to the antecedents and consequences, you will need to pay attention to their nature (symbolic or intrinsic) and identify which features of the context are most influential. In some cases, the client's behavior is influenced by elements of the context that the client is aware of (e.g., a client suffering from addiction uses drug when she has urges, and is aware of this pattern of response); in other cases, the client is not aware of the influence that elements of the context exert on a behavior (e.g., a client uses a drug when she feels anxious but is not aware of that feeling and its impact on her drug use). If we rely only on self report, the sources of influence that the client is not aware of are difficult to identify, but conducting an experiential exploration (see more in Chapter 5) and carefully observing instances of clinically relevant behaviors in session will help to progressively discover these sources of influence. Let's review the specific ways antecedents and consequences can influence behavior and its function.

Sensitivity to Antecedents

An antecedent is any event that sets the occasion for a particular behavior to occur. In many clinical disorders, certain antecedents become dominant and repeatedly trigger similar behaviors in similar situations, regardless of other features of the context that could trigger different responses. These triggers can be bodily sensations (e.g., cravings experienced by those struggling with substance use disorder), emotions (e.g., the anxiety felt by a person with agoraphobia), thoughts (e.g., predictions of humiliation by a person with social anxiety), memories (e.g., flashbacks of a trauma survivor), or external situations (e.g., the end of a meal for a person trying to quit smoking). When certain antecedents become dominant, behaviors are less responsive to other potential sources of influence within the context, including those that would lead to more adaptive responses.

In people with typical language capabilities, most antecedents stimulate behavior at least in part due to symbolic influences. This changes our consideration of antecedents in several ways. First, an antecedent that acquired its stimulus functions through symbolic relations can cue behavior that has never before occurred in its presence. A person may have a panic attack on an elevator and avoid all future elevators by association, but may also avoid taking phone calls, going on dates, or committing to a new job "because you can be trapped there too." These situations share no formal properties with the elevator. This is not a case of typical stimulus generalization; it is a case of symbolic generalization.

Second, the rapid expansion of relational networks and our tendency to establish and maintain coherence inside these networks can cause us to bend external situations to fit our preconceptions. These mental experiences often override our direct experience of the world. A client who grew up with a selfish father may feel hurt when his girlfriend doesn't consider his needs and preferences, while interpreting her kind and caring actions as manipulative and self-serving. The couple is locked in an unwinnable argument, where both generous and self-centered behaviors "prove" the client's belief that people are selfish.

Third, symbolic antecedents can control actions by producing consequences that have never been experienced before. Consider a former client who suffered from obsessive–compulsive disorder. Because she feared she would poison loved ones, she was constantly demanding that her children avoid new things. For example, her bedroom was suddenly off limits. Why? Because a cleaner had placed a cardboard box in the bedroom for a few minutes; but the box contained a bottle of Windex; but the bottle had been in the garage; but the garage had a caterpillar in it; but a caterpillar had been seen in a tree in the front yard; but the tree was near a flower bed; but the flowers had been fed with fertilizer that contained poison to kill bugs. The consequence of her children getting sick and dying due to her actions was entirely constructed, but that horrible imaginary consequence carried through several distinct "if . . . then" relations (conditional framing) such that walking in the room where a box had been was seemingly potentially lethal.

Relational learning thus undermines the clean dividing line between antecedents and consequences. When dealing with symbolic functions, motivation can be entirely controlled by antecedents but can function as if it were established by consequences.

Just as clients can be excessively influenced by some antecedents, they can be insufficiently influenced by other antecedents. This happens in a dramatic way when a medical condition or the use of drugs impairs the ability to perceive cues, but it happens in a more common way when we fail to notice changes in our health patterns, fail to detect the reactions of a partner, or miss a child's lack of educational progress. Symbolic events can be central to this kind of inattention either because we are "living in our head" or because we do not have the information necessary to detect important changes or milestones.

Sensitivity to Consequences

There are times when clients are too influenced by consequences, especially when short-term consequences conflict with long-term life satisfaction.

People suffering from addiction to drugs, alcohol, sex, or gambling are generally in situations in which pleasant short-term consequences overpower the long-term aversive consequences, for example. Often, however, situations like these also involve avoidance—for example, avoiding withdrawal symptoms, feelings of insecurity, or states of boredom. A similar kind of behavioral trap occurs when actions that have immediate pleasant consequences nest with alternative actions that are initially followed by unpleasant consequences. For example, procrastinating instead of studying, or watching TV instead of exercising has a combination both of approach toward pleasant distractors and avoidance of effort and work, at the cost of long-term benefits.

Symbolic consequences are especially likely to become excessive because of the arbitrary potential of language and cognition. For example, a person suffering from depression may be highly motivated to avoid painful thoughts or feelings even if doing so by withdrawal and inaction leads to depression in the longer term. Similar examples might be lying to self-aggrandize at the cost of genuine self-esteem; undermining intimacy to avoid painful rejection at the cost of committed relationships; or constantly fighting to gain social status at the cost of social cooperation and friendships.

A client might be insufficiently influenced by consequences when they are delayed, probabilistic, or contacted infrequently. These are often the flipside of the kinds of self-control situations we have just discussed, such as procrastination and drug use. The lack of influence by consequences also occurs when clients are learning new and more effective behaviors—if they do not see positive results quickly, they may be tempted to give up. For example, a person who is more frequently asking his partner about her interests in order to feel more connected to her might be discouraged if she is not very responsive at the beginning.

Monitoring Improvements in Context Sensitivity

Improvement in context sensitivity is measured by a change in awareness of and response to contextual variables, generally from observations and responses that are overly broad or too limited to observations and responses that are linked to relevant contextual features in a more flexible way. It is the sign that the client becomes less influenced by certain variables and more influenced by others. For example, a client might express a lot of negative judgments about his marital relationship during the first few therapy sessions but do so in a broad or overly general way. At the beginning, when asked whether he also sees positive things in his marriage, he responds, "No, there's nothing good in our relationship." A few sessions later, as the therapist asks, "How do you feel about your relationship now?" the client responds, "It's better. In fact, I can see how I was focused on all the negative things earlier because I was really upset. There are a lot of good things too, of course, such as how he supports my work career." This example is simple, but it illustrates what we are looking for, moment by moment and over time, in any kind of clinical work: a change of response to contextual variables.

In session, the therapist needs to observe in particular responses to aspects of the context that were previously ignored and richer responses to aspects of the context that were already noticed. As seen in an example from the previous chapter, it is like noticing that a person begins to be able to look at a pen and to use it as a tube or a weapon instead of noticing it for its more traditional writing function (i.e., the person is sensitive to new functions). Anything new that the client is showing in session is generally a sign of change (whether it is new in comparison to what she has been doing in the past sessions or in just the past minutes). A different tone of voice, a shift of posture, or a new facial expression are examples of nonverbal cues of change (e.g., a client who begins to smile when talking about his partner might be more in touch with the positive aspects of his relationship). Reports on what the client is doing outside the therapy room are more explicit cues; even though they are not the same as direct observations, they constitute the majority of the "data" that therapists analyze to assess improvement in context sensitivity. For example, the client might say, "I had a good conversation with my wife yesterday. It was one of these typical discussions that usually lead to fights. But this time, I just listened to her and realized I had never really understood what she was trying to say about the children before." Clients' reports also often pertain to what is happening *in* session. For example, as a therapist asks, "What do you notice in your body right now?" a client might say, "nothing" at first. But as observation and descriptions skills improve (see Chapter 5), the client begins to report sensations of tension in her muscles when they talk about certain topics. In other words, the client begins to be more sensitive to certain aspects of the context.

Obviously, evaluating whether or not the change of response is effective is a matter of clinical goals, which depends on each client's situation. In the next chapters on clinical interventions, we will present criteria to assess progress that are more specific to different psychological issues (e.g., awareness, decision making, self-identity, life meaning, and motivation).

ASSESSING COHERENCE

General Approach

Assessing coherence consists of exploring how clients integrate their experiences into networks of symbolic relations. You can use a number of questions cueing different types of framing to evaluate relational flexibility and fluency (e.g., conditional and deictic framing: "What would you think if you heard what you just said from one of your friends?"; conditional and opposition framing: "If you didn't use drugs, what would your life look like?"). Some questions will help assess the extent to which the client's conceptualizations are directed by functional, essential, or social coherence. In particular, exploration of conditional relations linking rules to effectiveness of action will give you information about the client's focus on functional coherence versus more essential coherence (e.g., "When you act upon this belief, does that help you reach your goal?"). Exploration of hierarchical and deictic relations linking the self and psychological experiences (see Chapter 6), and exploration of hierarchical relations linking actions to values (see Chapter 7) will reveal the client's ability to find wholeness and distance in self-concepts and to focus on overarching processes when engaging in actions (i.e., other dimensions of functional coherence). Exploration of relations of coordination between concepts and experiences will give you a sense of the client's attachment to his ideas as being essentially true (e.g., "How much do you believe this?" "Is it possible that your partner's view has some truth too?"). Exploration of social reinforcers for acting upon rules will help you assess social coherence (e.g., "If everybody approved what you do, regardless of what you choose to do, would you still choose to live according to this belief?").

As you assess relational fluency and flexibility, and the various forces driving coherence, you will get a sense of how clients' relational framing transforms their perception of the context and what interventions you can choose in order to help them build more useful ideas and concepts. Let's review in more detail the different aspects of assessing coherence.

Relational Fluency and Flexibility

Most clinical assessment is focused on the content and context of what is said—what clients think and how they respond to their thoughts. However, the clinical assessment can also target the flexibility and fluency of language processes themselves. RFT allows for such an assessment by targeting relational framing: the derivation and combination of symbolic relations into networks under contextual control, and the transformation of functions of related events also under contextual control. Framing skills can occur at different levels of speed and accuracy; they can be applied as a small or large set of relations; and the contextual control that regulates these skills can be strong or weak, flexible or rigid.

Experimental measures of fluency and flexibility in the relational framing process are beginning to emerge (O'Toole & Barnes-Holmes, 2009; O'Toole, Barnes-Holmes, Murphy, O'Connor, & Barnes-Holmes, 2009). They have been used primarily in the educational context, where training in relational framing fluency and flexibility increases IQ scores, even among developmentally delayed students (Cassidy et al., 2011). In the clinical domain, psychologists have developed laboratory methods that measure the degree to which deictic relations (I–you, here–there, now–then) are appropriately regulated by contextual cues (e.g., McHugh et al., 2004). Studies show that lack of flexibility and fluidity in deictic framing is common in those with underdeveloped social understanding, such as children with autistic spectrum disorder (Rehfeldt et al., 2007), and those with social anhedonia—an inability to experience pleasure from social interactions (Vilardaga et al., 2012; Villatte et al., 2008, 2010a, 2010b). With training, deictic framing skills can become more fluid and flexibly applied (Rehfeldt & Barnes-Holmes, 2009; McHugh & Stewart, 2012). When they are applied, disabled children begin to show somewhat better theory of mind skills—that is, they show better understanding of others' perspectives (Weil et al., 2011).

The flexibility and fluency of relational framing can be assessed in psychotherapy within a typical clinical interview. By posing questions that alter the context of reasoning, we can assess whether a client can use such things as temporal, conditional, hierarchical, or deictic relations; whether functions change strongly as a result; and whether these very processes can be augmented or diminished at will. Here is an example with a client who had an argument with his wife:

THERAPIST: What were you trying to accomplish by saying that?

The therapist tests conditional framing by exploring goals.

CLIENT: To get her to back off. It just wasn't fair.

The client's way of conceptualizing his experience seems driven by essential coherence (i.e., a pull to being right over being effective).

THERAPIST: Let's slow this down and try to notice some things. How did you feel once you said it?

The therapist explores changes in functions—potential change in the client's feelings—and the ability to shift attention under the control of temporal framing by slowing down and cueing comparison before/after.

CLIENT: I was waiting for the counterattack. I felt like I was going to have to defend myself.

The client points to functions apparently linked to the current argument but potentially controlled by other symbolic contexts.

THERAPIST: Can I ask an odd question? How old did you feel yourself to be when you said it?

The therapist uses a metaphor based on the "now–then" deictic frame to explore history.

CLIENT: Maybe 9. (*laughs*)

The client is able to apply this deictic frame.

THERAPIST: Well, when you were 9 you had very little control over your life. Maybe you needed to push back a bit. But now you are 39 and it is worth thinking about who is being defended now and for what reason. If you put yourself in your wife's shoes, what you do think she heard?

The therapist points to possible historical functions of the client's action in a conditional way. He then uses an "I–You" deictic frame to explore current social consequences of the client's action.

CLIENT: That I was mad and she needed to back off.

The client is able to apply this deictic frame.

THERAPIST: What do you think that pulled from her?

The therapist explores changed functions from 'I–You" framing.

CLIENT: Probably wanting to run away. Or attack back I guess, but knowing her she'd want to run away.

The client is able to describe new functions.

THERAPIST: Is that scary?

The therapist probes possible changes in functions.

CLIENT: That's why I get mad I think. I'm afraid she will. I was feeling afraid.

The client applies a conditional frame that results in changes of emotional function.

THERAPIST: So if she understands the rightness of your position, she will want to stay and what you fear won't happen.

The therapist underlines the conditional relationship ("if . . . then") included in the rule and implicitly attracts the client's attention to the incoherence between the purpose of action and the likely experienced consequence of this action.

CLIENT: I guess so.

THERAPIST: How do you feel when you are around someone who has a purpose of getting you to see the rightness of their position?

The therapist uses deictic frames of time, place, and person to further explore the incoherence between purpose of action/experienced consequence of action.

CLIENT: Usually I want to find an excuse to leave. I want to get the hell out of there.

The client is able to apply deictic frames and track a desired consequence.

THERAPIST: And when you see someone who is afraid?

The therapist evokes a new shift of perspective taking with deictic framing in a new context.

CLIENT: Usually I want to reach out to them.

The client shows fluency in changing context and capacity to track a desired consequence.

THERAPIST: So what if you took this down another level—all the way down to the deeper motives that were underneath "fairness" and "back off." What would have happened if you could have gone there . . . maybe even sharing your fear?

The therapist uses conditional framing to explore alternative actions that may actually lead to the desired consequences.

CLIENT: I don't know, but I don't think the fight would have ever happened. But that is hard for me. It feels out of control. Maybe I *am* out of control.

The client is able to see an effective and coherent resolution, but the coordination between "I" and "out of control" suggests a self-concept that acts as a barrier in this context.

THERAPIST: Yeah. The 9-year-old shows up. And some of that is hard to feel.

The therapist validates why it is hard based on history, using the client's deictic skills.

None of this is unusual clinically, but a practitioner guided by RFT would now know that the client has relatively good skills in understanding and generating rules that are based on the flexible applications of deictic frames (perspective taking) and temporal/conditional frames (before–after; if . . . then). He can sense the changed functions that occur when different frames are applied. That fluency gives him a lot of symbolic tools that the clinician can use going forward. His problem is that goals are driven by essential coherence (e.g., doing what is "fair") and their function is avoidant (avoiding feeling out of control, like he did when he was a child) and thus lacks vitality. Functional coherence (following rules that work) needs to become more central, but that requires slowing down and noticing the consequences of action, and being more flexible in exploring alternative perspectives and courses symbolically.

The words clients use to describe events can also provide significant cues about the way they conceptualize their experiences through relational framing. In many languages, there are several ways to express any given thought; that is especially true of English due to its mongrel history involving the influence of several languages. Word choices can be more or less common, however. For example, it can be worth noting when uncommon words or metaphors are used, especially if there are particular connotations or related words that seem meaningful. If this happens repeatedly in multiple areas, probes can assess more directly the possibility that certain types of relational responses are at high strength. For example, if a person describes his addiction using words that have violent connotations (e.g., getting hammered; getting slammed), issues of anger might be explored.

In formal textual analysis, actual word frequency and "collocates" (the frequency of words appearing nearby) can be used to assess unusual word choices (e.g., see the Corpus of Contemporary American English, *www. wordfrequency.info* for an example of such a resource). In clinical sessions, these discriminations need to be made by the therapist in flight, but the general issues occur frequently enough across clients that it is possible to become much better in actually noting unusual word choices.

Over the past decade, RFT has also developed tools to assess so-called implicit cognition, or the kind of thoughts we are not well aware of because they are produced very rapidly and hidden by more elaborated ones. For example, people might not be aware that they have negative attitudes toward members of an outgroup if the community punishes prejudice: their first negative cognition is hidden by a more acceptable one, produced over a slightly longer time frame (e.g., a man who implicitly has a long history of thinking that "women are not good leaders" might further think that "women have proved to be good leaders" and only notice this second more elaborated thought). Assessing implicit cognition can be useful because it can sometimes predict future action better than overt self-report ("explicit cognition") (Hughes, Barnes-Holmes, & Vahey, 2012).

In order to conduct such assessment, RFT conceptualizes implicit cognition as brief and immediate relational responses (BIRRs) and explicit cognitions as extended and elaborated relational responses (EERRs). BIRRs tend to be low in complexity and in derivation (Hughes et al., 2012)—they are simple and well-practiced. EERRs are more complex and extended and thus have more time to reflect competition between different viewpoints, or responses to such things as current audience effects (as when we filter out rude statements so as to not offend our in-laws). There is nothing magical about BIRRs over EERRs—both are relational responses—but because they happen under different contextual conditions, in some conditions BIRRs are more predictive and useful than EERRs and vice versa.

Those kinds of relational differences are why extended and elaborated measures of illegal or taboo behaviors such as drug use or sexual attraction toward socially sanctioned targets sometimes have less utility (Ames et al., 2007). In other words, self-reports sometimes fail because their assessment of EERRs allows many other functional dimensions to come into play. These same areas can often be usefully explored using measures that target brief, immediate relational responding, including those from RFT, leading to gains in the ability to predict clinical outcomes (Carpenter, Martinez, Vadhan, Barnes-Holmes, & Nunes, 2012; Dawson, Barnes-Holmes, Gresswell, Hart, & Gore, 2009).

RFT has developed a powerful computerized methodology for the assessment of such responses—the Implicit Relational Assessment Procedure (IRAP; see Barnes-Holmes, Barnes-Holmes, Stewart, & Boles, 2010)—which is arguably more flexible, reliable, and applicable than any existing alternative (Barnes-Holmes, Waldron, Barnes-Holmes, & Stewart, 2009). One key feature of the IRAP is that it allows for testing a variety of relationships (not just "association"—i.e., frames of coordination, as in the Implicit Association Test [IAT]; see Greenwald, McGhee, & Schwartz, 1998), and it tests those relations directly rather than by inference. In brief, the principle consists of presenting contradicting statements (e.g., "Women are good leaders" and "Women are not bad leaders" vs. "Women are not good leaders" and "Women are bad leaders") to a participant who must respond alternately true and false as fast as possible regardless of his or her actual attitude toward these statements. For example, during a first trial, participants would be required to respond according to a positive attitude toward women as leaders. In this case, they will need to respond "true" to "women are good leaders" and "women are not bad leaders" and "false" to "women are bad leaders" and "women are not good leaders." Then, they would respond according to the reverse attitude (i.e., negative attitude toward women as leaders). The speed and accuracy of response are then compared across trials; if faster and more accurate results appear for one of the trials, it is interpreted as BIRR (or implicit cognition) toward this attitude (e.g., faster and more accurate response for "women are good leaders—true" would indicate an implicit positive attitude toward women as leaders).

We already know that the IRAP is a significant step forward as compared to the associative approaches to implicit assessment such as the IAT because of the increased range of beliefs that can be assessed (e.g., see Gawronski & de Houwer, 2014). Recent research suggests that even more progress may be possible. For example, new versions of the IRAP (Levin, Hayes, & Waltz, 2010) allow item-by-item assessments that appear to increase the predictive utility of the IRAP (e.g., see Smith, 2013) and that hold out the possibility of implicit versions of a wide number of existing self-report devices.

Although RFT researchers are only beginning to explore applications of this work to clinical assessment, they have already published a series of studies relevant to mental health practitioners. For example, Carpenter et al. (2012) found that IRAP measures of the relationship between cocaine and being popular (at the time of admission to treatment) predicted treatment dropout in a cocaine treatment program and did so better than explicit measures. The IRAP detected a decrease in experiential avoidance resulting from a mindfulness intervention that was not detected with a questionnaire (Hooper, Villatte, Neofotistou, & McHugh, 2010); BIRRs measured by an IRAP related to fear of spiders predicted overt avoidance behavior with a live spider (Nicholson & Barnes-Holmes, 2012); BIRRs can be used to create measures of clinical depression (Hussey & Barnes-Holmes, 2012); and a recent study (Jackson et al., in press) found that statements that had been vetted by an IRAP to detect individual motives for exercise in fact produced harder exercise when presented during a cycling class. Thus, we are coming close to the time when sensitivity to antecedents, sensitivity to consequences, and well-practiced rules can all be detected to a degree using RFT-based methods that focus on brief, immediate relational responses.

Rules and Rule Following

As we saw in previous chapters, relational frames combine to form complex networks. Among these networks are rules, or descriptions of contingencies (antecedent–behavior–consequence) that can become powerful sources of influence on actions. The way these rules are elaborated and whether or not they are followed are crucial sources of information about the way clients develop coherence.

Sometimes a relatively complete behavioral sequence is described: "When I am alone at night, I need to drink or I'll get depressed." Other times the therapist needs to bring out the client's formulation. For example, if the same client had said, "At night, I need a drink," the therapist might have had to draw out with conditional framing—for example, "So as to . . . ?"— to which the client would respond, "Keep from being depressed." It is also possible that the client is not able to identify the whole behavioral sequence. In this case, using oppositional or distinction framing may be useful. Imagine the client answers to the previous question ("So as to . . . ?"), "I don't know, I just need a drink." You may simply ask in return, "What would happen if you didn't get a drink?" (distinction framing). The client could answer something like, "I don't know, I would feel horrible." The therapist could ask, "What kind of 'horrible' do you fear most?" to which the client might respond: "Feeling depressed, I guess."

Noticing how clients qualify behaviors commonly indicates the presence of rules underneath. For example, saying, "Drinking at night is necessary" likely indicates that the client's drinking is influenced by a rule even if it is not explicitly stated because the concept of "need" or "necessary" includes the idea that something is essential, required, or requisite (e.g., "If I want to be okay at night, I need to drink").

Many rules like these can influence client behavior, even if the client is not aware of them and thus not able to state them. Often, as you explore antecedents and consequences together, rules are formulated for the first time (the client may even say, "I had never realized I was drinking to feel better; I was just doing it as a habit").

When rules are not spontaneously expressed, it is still possible to explore them by asking clients about their thoughts as they prepare, perform, or justify an action. Take the example of a client who has difficulty developing close relationships. As you review an example of situations where problems occur, the client explains that when she meets a new person, she tends to avoid saying anything about herself, and as a result, nobody seems to find her interesting. To explore whether the client might be following rules, you may ask her: "What do you think about as you are talking to this stranger and don't say much about yourself?" To which the client may answer, for example, "I think that if I talk too much about myself, they are going to find me boring." Although asking about thoughts may not immediately reveal explicit rules, you will often find cues indicating the presence of implicit rules (e.g., "I feel like I don't want to talk about me"), which can be further explored with other questions based on conditional framing (e.g., "What would happen if you talked about yourself?").

Four main kinds of rule following typically contribute to psychological problems: pliance, inapplicable tracking, inaccurate tracking, and tracking leading to "adaptive peaks."

Pliance

Pliance is driven primarily by social coherence and consists of following a rule because social consequences are added for doing so, regardless of the correspondence between the consequence stated by the rule and the experienced consequence. The verbal community has to know we were exposed to a rule and has to see if our behavior corresponds to it. The consequences do not reinforce the action outside the context of rule following; instead they reinforce our compliance or noncompliance with the rule per se. Thus, the key dimensions of pliance are knowledge of the rule, knowledge of the action, knowledge of the correspondence rule-action, and social management of the consequences.

Certain cues in clients' language typically suggest that pliance is involved. When a client expresses a rule but doesn't state the consequence (e.g., "I have to stay with my husband." or "I should spend more time with my friends.") it is logically not possible to check the correspondence between the natural consequence and the consequence included in the rule.

However, it could be that the client is just not explicitly stating this conse-quence and is simply not expressing it aloud. In order to check if the client is engaging in pliance or in fact tracking a natural consequence, the therapist can ask "For what purpose?" or "What for?" If the client then states a con-sequence, it becomes possible to explore whether this consequence is what reinforces rule following. If the client struggles to find an answer, it is more likely a case of pliance. Sometimes, a client might answer by stating a cause that is more an antecedent than a consequence (e.g., "Because that's what I am supposed to do," or "Because she asked me to"). That is also a sign of pliance, given that there is still no consequence stated in the rule.

Pliance can also be assessed by symbolically altering the supports for pliance and seeing if the behavior changes, at least in imagination. Let's consider the example of a young college student working hard to have good grades in biology so that she can go to medical school later. If her motiva-tion is based on not disappointing her parents who have expressed their desire for her to be a medical doctor, she may keep working for years until she realizes that she is not doing what she really cares about.

Some of the kinds of questions that can help assess pliance in this case might include:

> "And if your parents loved you no matter what you do, do you think you'd feel the same way about your major?"
> "What if no one could know you were at school, getting an educa-tion?"
> "Suppose you could become a medical doctor but you could not tell your parents you made it? How would that impact you?"
> "If you were magically someone else—with a different name and appearance—what would you most want to be doing?"

Inapplicable Tracking

Inapplicable tracking is driven primarily by essential coherence or func-tional coherence relying on poor context sensitivity. It consists of attempt-ing to follow a rule that accurately specifies the natural consequence of an action (i.e., the consequence follows the action regardless of social approval for following the rule per se) but unfortunately, this action can't be done. Since the rule is accurate, following it is considered the right thing to do, even though it is not effective. For example, a person suffering from post-traumatic stress disorder might ruminate about events of the past and try to change what she did in order to prevent what happened. She might think, "If I had not decided to go out that night, I would not have been attacked"; "If I could go back in time and make different choices, my life would be normal now." These rules describe a behavior and its consequences, and they may even be essentially correct, but they are impossible to apply. It is not possible to go back in time—the world in which the rule applies exists only in imagination. Rumination, or excessive planning to prevent uncontrollable events from happening, is an example of inapplicable tracking. So are rules that promise positive outcomes based on the behaviors of *other* people. Imagine a client who thinks that she would be much happier if only other people had more consideration for her. The problem is that this rule doesn't say anything about what *she* can do to be happier. It all depends on others' behavior, and as a result, the only thing the client does is to complain that people don't have more consideration for her.

Some of the kinds of questions that can help assess inapplicable tracking might include:

> "If we just go with that thought, exactly what does it suggest you do right now?"
> "Is this a rule for you to follow, or is it one for others to follow?"
> "What is the next step, then?"

Inaccurate[1] Tracking

Inaccurate tracking is driven primarily by essential coherence or functional coherence relying on poor context sensitivity. It consists of following a rule pointing to a functional relationship antecedent–action–consequence that doesn't match actual experience.[2] This mismatch can be difficult to check because as soon as the rule is stated, our perception of the environment may become filtered by the rule itself. In other words, we tend to see what we expect to see. This disguised effect is more likely to happen

---

[1] Talking about accuracy might seem contradictory with the functional contextual approach we are using in this book. Indeed, we are never looking for external, objective truth when exploring experience and describing it with language (principle of a-ontology; see Monestès & Villatte, 2015). We are simply interested in the utility of our descriptions. By accuracy, we mean that the way a person labels an experience needs to be relatively consistent with her usual way of labeling similar experiences (and as much as possible with the way her verbal community labels similar experiences, so as to facilitate communication and social adjustment). Suppose a person's concept of anxiety is comprised of a set of sensations such as fast heartbeat, tremors, and tension in muscles. We would expect her to label how she is feeling as anxiety when she has these sensations. If she labeled her experience as fatigue instead, this would be somewhat inconsistent with her own way of conceptualizing her experiences. In that sense, her description would be inaccurate and could lead to inaccurate tracking. That could be due to a failure to notice certain sensations (poor context sensitivity) or to a failure to integrate certain sensations into consistent symbolic networks (poor coherence).

[2] Inaccurate tracking is different from pliance because what reinforces the action is not social approval of the correspondence between the action stated by the rule and the performed action, but other natural consequences not stated or imprecisely stated by the rule.

if the rule is vague or doesn't take into account short-term *and* long-term consequences. For example, a person who thinks that he must distract himself from obsessive thoughts to feel better can easily miss the inaccuracy of the rule, both because "feeling better" is not precise enough and because it specifies only the short-term consequences of thought distraction. Conversely, an inaccurate rule can weaken an effective behavior by predicting an aversive consequence or an absence of pleasant consequences even though advantageous consequences could actually be experienced. For example, a person suffering from chronic pain may be reluctant to engage in certain activities because she anticipates future fatigue or painful sensations that she will contact after a few hours of exercising ("It is going to make things worse!"). This makes the activity much less appealing, even though on a longer time scale it could actually increase her quality of life. Overgeneralization is another frequent kind of inaccurate tracking. The rule states the connection between a behavior and its consequence in a way that matches some but not all contexts. For example, a client might say, "I always end up betrayed when I trust people," while her experience is actually much more various than that. A rule expressed this way hides the positive instances where the client trusted another person. In other cases, the rule used to be accurate, or is accurate in certain domains, but it is now applied in a context where it is not effective to do so. This often happens when people were victims of abuse and learned to protect themselves from others. Even when the threat is no longer present, they might still withdraw from intimate situations.

Some of the kinds of questions that can help assess inaccurate tracking might include:

> "What does your experience tell you about thoughts like that—do they help you actually live more effectively?"
> "So, you seem to say that it is a good approach in the short term. What about in the long term?"
> "If you were to rate this strategy like a movie or a restaurant on a website, how many stars would you give it? Is it up to your expectations?"

Tracking Leading to Adaptive Peaks

Tracking leading to adaptive peaks is a subcategory of inaccurate tracking and refers to motivation toward consequences that provide some gains, but at the cost of a longer term path forward. A typical situation leading to adaptive peaks is when our actions are positively reinforced, which makes us believe that our actions are optimal. As a result, we ignore the cost of these actions and the potential gain from other sources of reinforcement associated with other actions. For example, a person might use drugs to enhance performance at the cost of her health, and another might abuse his partner to satisfy his needs at the cost of her own needs and of the relationship's quality.

Some of the kinds of questions that can help assess tracking leading to adaptive peaks might include:

> "As you've focused more on that goal, do you have a sense you've put your life on hold? Like life itself can start after this goal is achieved?"
>
> "It seems that it has had some payoff—some benefit. The question is, is that payoff worth all this energy invested in it?"
>
> "If you back up and look broadly, is this the kind of life you wanted to live? Are there any things you deeply care about that you have pushed to the side or put on the shelf?"

We described above the general approach to assessing relational flexibility/fluency, and rule/rule following. In the next chapters focused on interventions, we will present ways clients conceptualize their experiences that are more specific to different areas of psychological problems.

Monitoring Improvement in Coherence

Improvement in coherence is measured by a change in the way the client symbolically relates his experiences. Positive changes in fluency and flexibility are reflected by faster and more accurate relational responses (e.g., a client becomes more able to take the perspective of others when invited to put himself in their shoes). An overall ability to build alternative networks is also the sign that the client is less attached to one conceptualization of his experience and is thus more able to adapt his thoughts to the context. For example, a client might begin therapy thinking that "trusting always leads to betrayal." In further sessions, if she acknowledges that "trusting can also lead to intimacy," this would indicate that she is able to build a greater variety of symbolic networks about trusting, which may now become a possibility in certain contexts.

An increased tendency to hierarchically frame the self as a container of psychological experiences (see Chapter 6) and actions as part of higher order goals (see Chapter 7) indicates greater wholeness and sense of meaningful purpose. For example, a client might begin therapy describing herself as shattered and might be distressed by contradicting emotions and thoughts. Statements emphasizing the inclusion of a variety of psychological experiences into a stable and flexible self (e.g., "I have positive and negative thoughts"; "I am greater than my thoughts"; "I am still here") would reflect improvement in coherence. Some of this should be evident in actual speech in therapy; in fact, existing studies already show that changes in the tendency to see thoughts as literal expressions of the truth versus possibly useful guide (i.e., the shift from essential coherence to functional coherence) in therapy transcripts predict long-term outcomes (e.g., Hesser, Westin, Hayes, & Andersson, 2009).

Improvements in elaborating rules can be measured through an increase of conditional framing linking actions to meaningful goals, and a decrease of intrinsic coordination framing between thoughts and characteristics of the world or the self (see Chapters 5 and 6). For example, a client might begin therapy saying, "I can't apply for a job. I don't have enough self-confidence" (a sign of essential coherence) and later say, "If I don't look for a job, I won't be able to provide for my family" (functional coherence).

Improvement in rule following is measured by an increase in accurate tracking and a decrease in inapplicable tracking, inaccurate tracking, tracking leading to adaptive peaks, and pliance (except in some circumstances—see Chapter 5). Responses to rules can be reported by the client or observed in session. In both cases, rule following tends to be more effective when the client's action is reinforced by the consequence described in the rule. For example, a client might begin therapy saying, "I spent all night drinking because there was no other way to bear my anxiety" (inaccurate tracking) and later report, "I was feeling anxious all night long, but I decided not to drink to stay healthy" (effective tracking). Improvement in rule following is also measured by increased flexibility toward ineffective rules or more flexible sensitivity to the context of following rules. In the previous example, the client is not only following a new rule ("don't drink to stay healthy"), he is also *not* following the rule "Drink to bear the anxiety." Thus, whenever a client reports an ineffective rule but does not follow it in order to pursue meaningful purposes, an increase of functional coherence can be noted.

As for context sensitivity, more specific targets of assessment for coherence will be detailed in the next chapters on interventions.

FITTING RFT INTO SPECIFIC PSYCHOTHERAPY MODELS

This chapter provides an overview of language processes that bear on clinical assessment in general, but we have purposely eschewed any attempt to link them to specific assessment targets or techniques in particular treatment models. It is certainly possible to do so, however, and we have found such efforts clinically rewarding. In motivational interviewing, for example, it can be helpful to observe which symbolic relations emerge in response to reflections or open-ended questions, or whether particular types of framing tend to inhibit or evoke change talk.

We have also limited our discussion to assessment within clinical interviews or dialogues, though numerous standardized measures and neuropsychological tests are compatible with RFT and can inform a case formulation approach that incorporates symbolic behavior targets. For example, if cognitive therapists wish to assess potential cognitive mediators of treatment, implicit assessment may overcome challenges inherent in clients' self-report, such as social desirability concerns or lack of self-awareness motivated by experiential avoidance. The myriad implications of RFT for specific treatment approaches cannot be explored in the current volume, but one of our goals is to empower readers who are interested in specific models to explore these connections in both the therapy clinic and the lab.

CLINICAL EXAMPLE

The following conversation takes place during a first session with a 32-year-old man. The comments will help you identify where the client's struggles are matters of context sensitivity and coherence.

> CLIENT: I had to see a therapist because I can't live like this anymore. I am exhausted.
>
> THERAPIST: What's going on?
>
> CLIENT: I am scared that I might do something terrible. I think about it all the time. I can't stop thinking of all the ways I'll do something really bad.

In this first sequence, the client's desire to escape and avoid thoughts indicates that excessive influence exerted by some antecedents might be a central issue.

> THERAPIST: Are you bothered by your thoughts? Would you like to tell me more about what kind of thoughts?
>
> CLIENT: I think that I am going to hurt somebody. It's almost all the time. At first, I was just nervous when I was around knives and sharp objects. I was scared that I could hurt somebody by accident when I drive. Now it's almost everything. I can't be around people, or I am afraid I will hurt them.

In this second sequence, the therapist explores antecedents of escape/avoidance: the client is scared of knives, sharp objects, driving, and being around people. This reaction is triggered by symbolic cues: knives, sharp objects, and driving are in a relation of coordination with danger; he also seems to be following a rule that encourages avoidance through inaccurate tracking ("I can't be around people or drive or I will hurt somebody").

THERAPIST: Is it difficult for you to be here? Are you having these kinds of thoughts right now?

CLIENT: Yes. It's hard.

THERAPIST: I can imagine that it must be difficult to share that with me.

The therapist acknowledges the client's difficult experience (coordination framing to name experiences).

THERAPIST: Can I ask you to tell me more about these thoughts that are present in the room?

CLIENT: Right now? I am afraid that I might hit you. . . . Or take a book on this shelf and throw it to your face.

In this sequence, the therapist explores connections between the room and the life outside, looking in particular at antecedents of escape/avoidance. This connection is confirmed by the client who identifies more symbolic antecedents (which is a sign of awareness but inflexible response to these contextual variables).

THERAPIST: When you have these kinds of thoughts, what do you usually do?

CLIENT: I leave, or I try to stay as far away as possible from people.

The therapist explores responses to the antecedents using conditional/temporal framing (the client escapes and avoids people). The client shows awareness of his response to antecedents triggering fear but this response lacks flexibility.

THERAPIST: Are you having urges to leave right now?

CLIENT: Yes.

THERAPIST: If I had similar thoughts right now, I would not feel comfortable either. I really appreciate your efforts to stay with me, even though it is very difficult for you, because it helps me understand your situation better

The therapist improves collaboration by acknowledging the client's difficult experience through perspective taking (deictic framing) and by stating the benefit of staying engaged.

THERAPIST: Is it because you are afraid of hurting me that you pushed the chair away from me before sitting?

CLIENT: Yes, it worries me to be close to people.

The therapist explores further connections between the room and the client's life outside: antecedents (urges) and responses (pushing the chair away) are present here and now.

THERAPIST: Can you give me some examples of situations where you have thoughts that you might hurt somebody?

The therapist explores other antecedents in the life outside using spatial cues in order to assess the breadth of the client's difficulties.

CLIENT: Public transportation is the worst. I used to drive my car, but driving is very dangerous. It's easy to get into an accident. I never had one, but I know it can happen anytime. So I stopped using my car and started using the bus, but it's too difficult to be surrounded by people I may hurt. I always go by foot now.

Worries in public transportation and while driving a car are other symbolic antecedents influencing avoidance. Rules are also spontaneously expressed and suggest inaccurate tracking ("driving is very dangerous"; "it's easy to get into an accident"; "it's too difficult to be surrounded by people" are all evaluations of behaviors and thus suggest implicit rules that overgeneralize the consequence of driving and being around people).

THERAPIST: How does that impact your life?

CLIENT: It takes me hours to go somewhere, and I can't go everywhere I would like to.

THERAPIST: What are the places where you can't go anymore?

CLIENT: I can't see my brother as often as I would like. He lives 50 miles away from here. I used to visit him pretty often. Now it's only when he has the time to come, but that's not very often.

THERAPIST: That must be hard for you (*improved collaboration by acknowledging the client's difficult experience with coordination framing*). Are you close to your brother?

CLIENT: Yes, very close. It makes me very sad that I can't see him more often because of my stupid thoughts.

In this sequence, the therapist evaluates the impact of avoiding thoughts on the client's life using conditional framing ("How does that impact your life?"). The client is able to identify aspects of the context that are important to him (seeing his brother) but missed because of higher influence from fear of hurting people.

THERAPIST: Do you try to take your car to visit him sometimes, even if you have the fear that you might hurt somebody?

CLIENT: Yes, I tried a couple of times, but after a few miles, I didn't feel like it anymore.

THERAPIST: You didn't feel like it, or it was too hard to have these thoughts?

CLIENT: I am so stressed out in a car that I have terrible stomach pain and headaches. Driving is so dangerous for me that I don't see the point of putting myself in such a stressful situation anyway.

In this section, the therapist explores the lack of effective behaviors: the client doesn't drive to go see his brother, even though it would likely bring him satisfaction. This seems to reflect insufficient influence from distant sources of reinforcement (seeing his brother), excessive influence from intrinsic antecedents (stomach pain and headaches), and inaccurate tracking (i.e., following the rule "driving is dangerous" by not driving at all, as if driving inexorably led to bad consequences).

THERAPIST: It seems like you are suffering a lot from this situation

The therapist improves collaboration by acknowledging the client's difficult experience (coordination framing to name experiences).

You said earlier that you can't stop thinking. Is it something that you have actually tried to do?

CLIENT: Yes. If I could stop thinking of hurting people, I wouldn't be scared all the time.

The therapist asks further about problematic avoidance to begin to explore sensitivity to consequences. Notice the client expressing an inapplicable rule ("if I could stop thinking").

THERAPIST: What have you tried to do?

CLIENT: When I started to have these thoughts, I just tried to think of something else. If I saw a knife, I looked away.

THERAPIST: Did it work?

CLIENT: At first yes, but now I have to leave the room anyway because I keep thinking that the knife is there and that I could do something dangerous.

THERAPIST: Does leaving the room work?

CLIENT: Generally, it calms me down.

In this sequence, the therapist uses conditional framing to explore the consequence of attempting to avoid thoughts. Because of the symbolic nature of the antecedent, looking away worked only in

the short term. Leaving the room is followed by a decrease of the worries ("It calms me down"), but this strategy has a cost, since the client has to leave the room. The client's awareness of these different consequences is a sign of relatively flexible sensitivity to the context, but he is still more influenced by the short-term relief of avoidance strategies.

THERAPIST: Is it for the same reason that you were thinking of leaving this room earlier? To make the thoughts of hurting me go away?

CLIENT: Yes. It's the only thing I can do to feel better.

The therapist explores connections between the room and the life outside with analogical framing, focusing this time on the consequence of avoiding thoughts. Notice the rule expressed by the client, a rule fairly vague (feeling better) and narrowed at the same time ("the only thing"), which makes inaccurate tracking and pliance more likely.

THERAPIST: Do you always feel better when you move away from situations where you could hurt somebody?

CLIENT: It's hard to say. . . . There are moments when I can think of something else for a while. It gives me some rest. But often, I just don't know what to do anymore to clear my mind.

The therapist explores if the reinforcement of escape and avoidance is variable, which seems to be the case. The client shows awareness of this variability.

THERAPIST: Did you have the same experience when you took your car to visit your brother but then decided to go back home?

CLIENT: I felt relieved when I got home.

The therapist explores the consequence of avoidance in the context of driving using comparative framing. Again, the client mentions a decrease of his worries, thus showing some awareness of this consequence.

THERAPIST: Would you say that you felt better in the end?

CLIENT: Yes. I mean . . . Not really. I felt less scared, but I was sad that I didn't get to see my brother.

The therapist explores the consequence in terms of satisfaction on a larger scale of time with comparative framing. Although the client feels relieved in the short term, he also doesn't reach an important source of reinforcement (seeing his brother). The client shows some awareness of these different consequences, but the short-term consequence has more influence on the client's behavior at the moment.

THERAPIST: And what about the thoughts of hurting someone on the road? Did they go away when you got home?

CLIENT: I was relieved at first when I left the car, but then I got scared that maybe I had hit someone and didn't notice it.

The therapist explores the consequence in terms of worries with conditional/temporal framing. The worries decrease in the short term but come back later. Again, the client seems more influenced by the short-term consequence than the long-term consequence but shows awareness of these different consequences.

THERAPIST: That must have been really hard for you not to see your brother and be scared that you may have hurt someone at the same time.

The therapist improves collaboration by acknowledging the client's difficult experience and underlines the problematic consequence of avoiding (coordination framing to name experiences).

CLIENT: I was feeling horrible.

THERAPIST: How was that in comparison to when you were in the car?

CLIENT: Probably worse, but I just couldn't stay in the car anyway.

The therapist explores the possible counterproductive effect of avoidance using comparative framing (not only doesn't it work, but it makes things worse). The fact that the client holds on to the rule "I can't stay in the car," despite the awareness that it makes things worse, suggests possible pliance (i.e., the rule is followed regardless of the consequence) or inaccurate tracking (i.e., rule following is reinforced by natural consequences not stated by the rule).

THERAPIST: In these conditions, I imagine that it is difficult for you to find satisfaction in your life. What do you do when you are at home?

CLIENT: I spend my days playing video games. It helps me not getting totally depressed, and it is the only thing I can do without risking hurting somebody. I have started to play more and more since things have gotten worse.

THERAPIST: You seem sad as you say that.

CLIENT: Yes. I really like video games, but I know it is taking me away from people even more. It is a lonely activity.

In this last sequence, the therapist asks about sources of satisfaction in the client's life as a way of revealing a possible problematic approach toward short-term reinforcers. The client finds some satisfaction in playing video games, but this behavior has harmful consequences in the long term (it takes him away from people even more). Short-term consequences thus seem to exert excessive influence, whereas long-term consequences don't influence enough. In addition, the formulation of certain rules suggests tracking leading to adaptive peaks: "It helps me not getting totally depressed" (a rule lacking precision and masking long-term effects), and "It is the only thing I can do without risking hurting somebody" (inaccurate rule).

In most psychotherapy approaches, the assessment is never really over as long as a case is in process. At the beginning, assessment allows us to orient toward intervention, but later it helps us to evaluate the effectiveness of the techniques we chose to implement and to readjust our choices throughout the therapy. From the perspective of the framework we are using in this book, the assessment phase already activates clients' change because it contributes to shaping their ability to observe their behaviors and the sources of influence surrounding them. Improving this crucial skill further will be at the core of the next chapter, in which we lay out the first set of intervention principles based on RFT.

 **CHAPTER SUMMARY**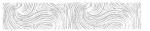

In this chapter, you learned to use RFT principles in the assessment of psychological problems and psychological change from a contextual behavioral perspective. Here are the main principles to remember:

- Since a central goal of therapy is to help clients develop their capacity to observe their own behaviors, and the sources of influence that maintain it, assessment needs to be conducted from the client's perspective as much as possible. This approach is supported by promoting functional contextual observation through:
  - Experiential techniques.
  - Questions asked with openness and genuine curiosity.
  - Involving the client in the assessment phase.
- Assessment can be informed by what is happening outside the therapy room (generally reported by the client) and what is happening in the here and now of the therapeutic relationship. In order to connect these two clinically relevant arenas, you can:
  - Use analogies that explore parallels between the client's life outside and inside the therapy room.
  - Use metaphors to explore symbolic generalizations across various contexts.

○ Use perspective taking to bring events happening there and then to the here and now of the conversation.

○ Evoke potentially relevant behaviors by creating the appropriate context in the therapy room.

• Assessing context sensitivity consists of evaluating the client's awareness and response to the sources of influence on behaviors. The main areas you can assess are:

○ Sensitivity to antecedents, which come before the response and act as a cue or trigger.

○ Sensitivity to consequences, which follow the behavior and determine whether or not it is likely to occur again in that context.

• Monitoring improvements in context sensitivity consists of tracking awareness of and new responses to contextual variables. You need to pay attention to:

○ Increased awareness of various contextual variables.

○ New responses to variables that are still present.

○ Changes moment by moment and over time.

○ Changes happening inside the therapy room and in clients' lives outside (generally reported by clients).

• Assessing coherence consists of exploring how clients conceptualize their experiences through different types of relational framings, and the degree of essential, social, and functional coherence involved in this conceptualization process. The main areas you can assess are:

○ Relational fluency and flexibility.

○ Rules and rule following.

• Monitoring improvements in coherence consists of tracking new ways of conceptualizing experiences, new rules, and new responses to rules. You need to pay attention to:

○ Increase in fluency and flexibility.

○ Increase in the formulation of rules that state complete contingencies and include meaningful purposes.

○ Increase in accurate tracking.

○ Changes in coherence moment by moment and over time.

○ Changes in coherence happening inside the therapy room and in clients' lives outside (generally reported by clients).

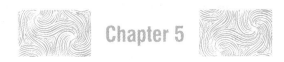

Chapter 5

Activating and Shaping
Behavior Change

The remaining chapters of this book will present various ways to use language, and the contextual cues that regulate it, to help our clients alleviate suffering and promote resiliency and psychological flourishing. In this chapter, we will explore how verbal interactions can be used to activate and shape behavior change. A primary task of intervention is to alter variables that regulate what our clients do. Often, we will focus on variables that directly belong to the area of language and cognition—such as what our clients think or believe. Other times we will focus on events that originate in the nonsymbolic world (e.g., sensations) but can usefully be touched by language and cognition. In either case, language of the client and language of the therapist are the main tools to promote positive change in psychotherapy. In particular, this chapter focuses on how to reconnect clients to their experience, help them develop a more effective way of making sense, and increase their response flexibility, with the goal of dropping problematic behaviors and engaging in more meaningful actions.

USING LANGUAGE TO ACTIVATE BEHAVIOR CHANGE

The behavioral problems that our clients face are influenced by elements of the context. Some elements carry too much influence, others not enough. In order to change our clients' psychological world, these sources of influence need to be altered in some way or another. Removing an element of the context or replacing it with another one is sometimes an option. For example, if a client can't get up in the morning because he feels too tired, removing his fatigue by going to bed earlier would probably make getting up much easier. As practitioners, we don't always have direct access to the elements of the context that regulate clients' behavior, however, and we often can't change them completely. Some symbolic and internal elements of the context are impossible to remove or replace. It may be impossible, for example, to remove the noise heard by people suffering from tinnitus, the pain experienced by people suffering from fibromyalgia, or the difficult memory of a trauma survivor. External or social elements of the context may be changeable but practically inaccessible. Although in the abstract we might assume we can improve the life of a depressed client who lost her job by helping her get her job back, in the concrete world this may not be possible. Even when the elements of the context can be directly changed, we often still need to activate the client's behavior so that he can make these changes himself. In our previous example, in order for the client to go to bed earlier to sleep more, the elements of the context motivating or preventing this behavior need to change first. Fortunately, when the elements of the context can't be removed or replaced, another approach is available. We can alter the impact of the context without attempting to change it directly. Language is probably the best tool we can use to that end because with language, anything can become anything. Although this limitless potential is often at the core of our clients' problems, it also leads to useful symbolic transformations of the context, such as when we turn a barrier into an opportunity to change.

Language operates as a filter between us and our internal or external experiences (i.e., our context). This filter can increase or decrease our awareness of these experiences, change their meaning and impact, and modify the way we interact with them. Although we have mostly discussed language as a variable influencing our behaviors, it is important to remember that language itself *is* a behavior. It is something we *do*. This means we can also *use* this filter to alter the perception of our experiences in order to change our actions. In a sense, language is *symbolic contexting*: a behavior that transforms the context symbolically, and thereby changes responses to the context.

Given that language is a behavior, it does not only transform the context and influence responses to the context, it is influenced by the context. In psychotherapy, we have to wonder what context can shape the client's language; for the most part it is the therapist's behavior, including her own language. A therapist's words, gestures, postures, and facial expressions are contextual cues that can evoke and strengthen new ways of symbolically relating to clinically relevant experiences. Through this process, the client progressively learns more effective ways to interact with these experiences, even when they cannot be intrinsically changed.

Imagine a client who engages in rituals to counteract obsessive thoughts and says, "I need to wash my hands." The therapist can change the context of the client's language by reflecting this statement back using a different formulation: "You're having the thought that you need to wash your hands." Framed this way, the client might begin to relate to this thought differently and the symbolic function of the thought might be transformed. Old responses might be reexamined and new responses might emerge: the client might begin to notice the process of thinking, instead of just responding to what the thought says.

In this section, we will cover three main processes based on RFT principles we can use to alter the impact of contextual variables on actions. These processes consist of using language to improve clients' functional contextual awareness through observation, description, and tracking of their experiences; using language to help clients make sense of their experiences in a way that is effective, not just coherent, by normalizing psychological experiences and assessing the effectiveness of actions; and using language to set a context that increases response flexibility.

Increasing Functional Contextual Awareness

The Goal

All actions occur in a context and are highly influenced by what is included in that context. Identifying contextual sources of influence is central to the assessment process, but altering the impact of those sources is necessary to activate behavior change. Clients need to learn to be good observers of their own inner and outer world and, based on what they see, to derive ideas about what would work.

Why This Is Important, from an RFT Point of View

Without healthy variation and selection by what works, behaviors do not evolve effectively. Any psychological event can be overextended once it is decontextualized. Without sensitivity to variations in the context, a single observation turns into a rule, a thought into a belief, a memory into a story, an emotion into a mood, and a behavior into a habit. This is particularly likely to be a problem with rules. The most flexible form of rules describes functional contingencies; that description is impossible if the person generating rules is out of touch with what he or she is doing, sensing, thinking, feeling, and remembering, and the internal and external contexts in which all of that occurs. Sometimes insensitivity to some aspects of the context is a clinical goal, but in the service of increasing sensitivity to more useful experiences, as when increasing motivation to overcome barriers (see Chapter 7). There are times when avoidance or even suppression can be useful, such as when facing the immediate demands of life-threatening disasters. But over time it is almost always useful to help clients get more in touch with their experience, whether it is intrinsic or symbolic, and to be more aware of the context of their actions in order to promote healthy psychological growth.

How This Method Touches on Various Clinical Traditions

Virtually every major clinical tradition tries to teach clients to be better observers of their internal and external world. Behavior therapists want to identify contextual variables influencing clients' actions in order to choose relevant targets in their interventions (e.g., chain analysis, or observation and description skills in dialectical behavior therapy). Cognitive therapists want to help their clients notice their own thoughts and the situations that give rise to them in order to reveal and ultimately change the cognitive errors these thoughts may contain. Humanistic therapists use a collaborative approach to help clients come more deeply into contact with their direct experience, and to resolve the conflict between their idealized and real self. Psychodynamic therapists want the person to have greater awareness of hidden urges, conflicts, mechanisms of defense, and desires and to learn to be more aware of them and honest about them. Existentialists seek to uncover the harm that comes from an inability to confront the anxiety that arises from confronting death, meaninglessness, and freedom. Thus, virtually all clinical traditions seek to improve the context sensitivity of observation and description.

How to Do It

In broad terms, the therapist uses language to encourage clients to observe and describe their actions and the various elements of the context that influence them. Obvious elements that are in the external context are relatively easy to observe (e.g., another person's facial expression, a change of temperature in the room), but a significant part of the clients' context is made of their internal experiences (sensations, thoughts, emotions). These elements are often missed because they are less tangible than external elements of the context and yet, they generally have a powerful impact on clients' actions. Thus, therapeutic work will often focus on increasing awareness of sensations, thoughts, and emotions. The process of observation and description then expands to the functional relationships connecting the various internal and external elements of the context to clients' actions. As functional descriptions are formulated, new rules of functioning are extracted. These new rules need to be followed with functional contextual awareness if we want to avoid the risk of applying them once more in an overgeneralized way. Clients should be encouraged to check the correspondence between the described or predicted and the experienced contingencies whenever they follow a rule. Thus, when psychotherapy is successful, it often provides a kind of learning laboratory for a more general skill: observing, describing, and tracking.

Metaphorically, clients can be encouraged to approach this process the same way that you would explore a place you have never visited before. Imagine you are taking a hike in a wild environment where there is no trail. You would have to attentively observe all the features of this place, such as concentrations of trees on your right, rocks on your left, or perhaps a river along your path. To remember what you noticed, you may draw a map and write your observations down as precisely as possible. You could also draw your itinerary on the map so as to remember the steps you followed to reach your destination. This would allow you to find your way again or show others where you have been. Using this map effectively would require that you check the correspondence between what is drawn on the map and what you see on the field. Blindly following the map would not likely get you where you want to go, especially if you are using a map drawn by somebody else.

Because the goal is the establishment of a more general skill, the role of the therapist in this process is preferentially to evoke rather than to provide observations and descriptions. This way, hopefully the client learns the overarching process of observing and drawing conclusions based on his or her own experience, rather than merely specific responses suggested by the therapist. Along this process, the therapist might use a variety of relational framings with different purposes, depending on what might be useful to observe and on the client's aptitude to become more aware of actions and the context of actions.

Observation. If the client is not in touch with his experience, and if we don't want to tell him what he is experiencing (so that an autonomous skill is more likely to be developed), we need to orient his attention toward potentially useful elements of the context. Orienting without giving answers can be achieved using *spatial* and *temporal* cues to direct attention to various features of the context. Nonverbal cues such as gestures, volume, and pace of voice can be used as subtle ways of evoking exploration. For example, the therapist might say "How do you feel there?" while placing her hand on her own chest. The therapist can speak slowly or quietly to help the client get more in touch with what is happening in the here and now. Verbal cues such as *where, here, there* (spatial) *when, now, then* (temporal), and more specific places and times (e.g., *in your chest, in your arms, at home, in the morning, tonight, a minute ago*) can be included in the natural interactions of a therapy session to increase contextually sensitive observation.

Sometimes the client is stuck, and basic spatial and temporal cues are not enough to help her notice some of her experiences. This could happen if she has never learned to pay attention to these experiences (e.g., due to family inattention, or invalidation, or to cultural factors) or has been avoiding her thoughts, emotions, and sensations for a long time (e.g., due to early trauma or avoidance within the family, such as sometimes happens in abusive situations). It also happens to most clients when more sensitive topics are explored. In these cases, analogical framing can be used to turn experiences into something more concrete and easier to observe. For example, the therapist could say, "Imagine that you are observing your feelings like you are looking at a picture" or "Imagine that your thoughts were recorded like the transcript of a conversation, and you read this transcript at the end of the day."

Deictic framing can also be useful by leading the client to adopt a different point of view on his experience and to notice things he couldn't see from his original point of view. For example, the therapist could say, "Imagine that you were seeing this panic attack with the eyes of your husband who was with you that day" (adopting the point of view of another on the client's own experience), or "Imagine your sister in the same situation, and observe what she is doing" (putting another in the client's point of view). This latter technique is particularly useful when self-awareness triggers painful experiences. It is often easier to talk about something or somebody else first, and then progressively notice the similarities with one's own experiences.

Description. Greater observation of psychological experiences naturally leads to broad increases in description, as cues orienting the client's attention begin to evoke verbal responses. Description is actually more specific than that, however, and describing is generally a skill that needs to be targeted specifically, especially when clients have difficulties putting words on their thoughts, emotions, or sensations. Clients need to learn to move away from judgments that hide useful features of their experiences. For example, a client who describes a sensation with a profusion of negative adjectives (e.g., horrible, unbearable, the worst thing ever) may have a harder time noticing other aspects, such as where he feels it, when it starts, what it actually feels like, or when it stops. Thus, in order to develop descriptive skill, the therapist often needs to help the client shift from judgments to more neutral descriptions. This can be done by using coordination and hierarchical framing to evoke the naming and labeling of experiences with limited judgment. For example, to a client saying "I feel horrible," the therapist could ask, "What does it feel like? What kind of sensations do you feel?" And imagine that this client answers, "I have horrible headaches, my mind is full of disgusting pictures." The therapist could again encourage him to describe his experience with more precision and less judgment, without having to directly address these evaluations (e.g., "Can you tell me more about these headaches? How would you describe these sensations?") or by leading the client to describe judgments themselves as experiences in more neutral terms (e.g., "What does horrible feel like?").

If the client has difficulties describing, it is possible to use analogical framing to build a parallel with something more concrete, and thus easier to define. For example, the therapist could tell a client who can't put words on a sensation, "If it was a color or a shape, what would that be?" or "If you were talking about a song, how would you describe this emotion?" He could also use physical analogies, like gesture mimicking potential characteristics of the experience as a first step before finding words (e.g., "If you were to put your body in a posture that reflects how you feel right now, what would it be? Would you be willing to show me?"). When clients struggle with describing, they often naturally begin to use a metaphorical language (e.g., "That's a heavy feeling"). The therapist should pay attention to these kinds of cues and help the client unfold the metaphor and refine the description of her experience with open questions that let her create her own metaphor, which is more likely to fit what she is observing (e.g., "Heavy like what? How heavy is that?"). If the client still struggles, the therapist can make suggestions while letting her decide if they fit the observed experience (e.g., "Heavy like a rock? Or more like a bag? How much space does this feeling take? Is it small but very heavy, or more diffuse?").

Deictic framing can also be used because the psychological distance it creates often opens the client to more ways of talking about his experience and reduces the immediate impact of symbolically involved experiences. For example, the therapist could ask, "Imagine that you were standing over there looking at the you who is sitting here, what would you see?" or "If you were watching a movie and the main character was going through the same events as you are going through, what kinds of emotions do you think he would be feeling? What kinds of indications would the director give to the actor so that he would be credible in this scene?" As mentioned earlier, this approach is particularly useful when self-awareness triggers painful experiences.

Since specific descriptions are generally more flexible than general ones, distinction and comparison framing, which helps the client to differentiate her current experience from experiences at other times and places, can often help behavior change. For example, the therapist could ask, "Is this feeling different from how you feel when you are alone at home?"; "Do you have this thought more often when you are surrounded by people?"; "Is this sensation stronger in the morning?" The point is not "gathering information" as if the client has to fulfill your curiosity or fill in a detailed form. The point is the client learning to look at experience and its context so as to promote context-sensitive behavioral, cognitive, and emotional agility. Questions and probes are designed to evoke curiosity in the client so as to help the client become a finer observer of her own experience.

It can actually be helpful to do this kind of exploration with obviously neutral events, such as eating a raisin, but in normal clinical work clients will be more open to the process if they see or sense a relationship between the experiences being examined and variables that might have an impact on clinically meaningful goals.

In the following vignette, we illustrate a variety of techniques aimed at improving the client's observation and description skills.

THERAPIST: You just stopped talking when I mentioned your relationship.

CLIENT: Yeah. I don't like thinking about it.

THERAPIST: What don't you like?

CLIENT: I don't know. I guess I just don't like thinking about it right now.

THERAPIST: Is it okay if I ask you how you felt when I mentioned your relationship?

CLIENT: It's okay, but I don't know what to tell you. It's kind of blank right now.

THERAPIST: Where is it "blank"?

CLIENT: (*moving his hand in front of his eyes*) Right there. Just blank.

THERAPIST: Do you notice anything in yourself as you say that?

CLIENT: Anger.

THERAPIST: Is it right there too or somewhere else?

CLIENT: Hmm . . . No, I think it's more in my jaw right now.

THERAPIST: How does it feel in your jaw?

CLIENT: I don't know how to describe it.

THERAPIST: If you were sitting over there, looking at yourself right here, right now, what do you think you would see?

CLIENT: I guess I would see a tense guy. I'm sorry. It's not about you. I hope you know that.

THERAPIST: Yeah, I know that. Thanks for saying that. So, tense, huh? In your jaw?

CLIENT: (*moving his jaw to release some tension, and breathing deeply*) Yeah . . . I had not really noticed that before you asked. I guess I'm a bit edgy now.

THERAPIST: Edgy? Like on the edge of something?

CLIENT: Yeah, exactly.

THERAPIST: The edge of what, do you think?

CLIENT: I don't know.

THERAPIST: If it was something concrete you can see, would this be more like the edge of a cliff, of a mountain, of a knife, of a diving board maybe?

CLIENT: No, not a diving board. Although . . . it does feel like I want to jump. Not at you. Just . . . I want to leave or something.

THERAPIST: Do you feel like leaving something or going somewhere?

CLIENT: Leaving something

THERAPIST: Any idea what?

CLIENT: This feeling.

THERAPIST: The blank (*moving her hand in front of her eyes*) or the anger?

CLIENT: The blank.

In this vignette, the therapist started with using coordination framing cues to evoke the client's observation of an experience that she suspected was getting in the way of the client talking about his relationship. When the client continued to struggle to identify what he felt, she used spatial cues, leading to the client initiating a metaphor (his hand in front of his eyes) that helped as a starting point for description ("just blank"). More coordination cues led to a feeling ("anger"). The therapist helped the client observe and describe with more precision by using distinction framing ("Is it right there too or somewhere else?") and deictic framing ("If you were sitting over there, looking at yourself right here, right now, what do you think you would see?"). Finally, she used another metaphor spontaneously brought up by the client ("edgy") to help him identify that he felt like escaping a feeling.

Tracking. Shaping tracking takes the client one step further by helping him consider the *functional relationships* that connect his experiences together. This is fundamental for the client to notice the conditions that evoke psychological reactions and the impact of his actions. As with the observation and description processes, the therapist needs to preferentially encourage clients to track on their own as much as possible. This has two advantages: on one hand, it limits the risks of pliance and counterpliance being disguised in the form of tracking; on the other hand, it limits the risk of dependence on the therapist and trains the client to observe and draw conclusions on his own outside therapy.

In the tracking process, the description of the client's experience is followed by questions based on conditional framing between antecedents, behaviors, and consequences (while including thoughts, feelings, and sensations in this contingency) as they are directly experienced. For example, the therapist might ask, "What happened right before you decided to leave the room? And what happened as a result?" Here also, analogical and deictic framings can help the client notice functional relationships that are more difficult to notice.

A number of metaphors can be used to improve the client's tracking by linking it to a concrete situation in which the contingencies are either already known or easy to observe. For example, a parallel can be drawn between a client's counterproductive attempts to escape his emotions and the effect of struggling in quicksand. Gestures that mimic a functional sequence can also draw the client's attention to the impact of the different elements included in a contingency analysis (e.g., a movement of the hand from left to right that represents the sequence antecedent–behavior–consequence). We will explore this process in more detail in Chapter 8.

Temporal perspective taking is often helpful given that functional relationships are laid out in time. For example, the therapist could ask a client who is struggling with noticing the impact of acting on urges to use drugs: "Imagine you keep the same approach to this situation. What do you think your life will be like a year from now? Just picture in your mind what your life might look like in a year. What do you see?" Interpersonal shifts in perspective taking can also help the client notice the impact of one's behavior on others ("If you look at this argument from her point of view, how do you think that made her feel when you said that?") or decrease defensiveness and self-judgments that get in the way of noticing the full contingency ("Let's look at this like it was happening to somebody else").

To gain more precision, the therapist can use comparative and distinction framing to explore short-term, long-term, and variable consequences. For example, he could ask "Do you feel better or worse after you decide to stay in bed? What about a few hours later? Is it still the same or different?"; "Do you always feel less anxious when you avoid discussions with other people?"; "Does it happen from time to time or always?" A variety of situations are also explored to assess to what extent the described contingency is representative of different contexts. This is particularly useful to avoid the overgeneralization that can accompany rule following—even tracking if it is not sufficiently contextually bound.

The following exchange illustrates the tracking process with a client suffering from posttraumatic stress disorder.

THERAPIST: Can you tell me more about these difficult thoughts? In what situations do they appear?

CLIENT: In particular when I am in confined places, with a lot of people. Like when I teach. It reminds me of when I was assaulted, even though I know I am not in danger in my classroom. It's oppressing to see everybody looking at me. I feel trapped.

THERAPIST: This must be a really difficult feeling. What do you do when you have these thoughts and feelings in your classroom?

CLIENT: Last time I went to work, which was weeks ago now, I left after 10 minutes, pretending that I was sick.

THERAPIST: How did you feel just after you left? Were you still thinking of your traumatic experience?

CLIENT: Yes. I couldn't think of anything else, actually.

THERAPIST: And how about feeling oppressed?

CLIENT: I felt better when I left the classroom. I was relieved not to see all of their eyes on me anymore.

In these first exchanges, the therapist encourages the client to describe her experience, emphasizing temporal and conditional framing to highlight the functional relationship between the antecedent (being in the classroom, feeling oppressed), the action (leaving the classroom), and the consequence (feeling less oppressed but still thinking of the traumatic episode).

THERAPIST: If it's okay, I would like to review step by step with you what you just said to make sure we are not missing something important.

The therapist prepares the client to reorganize the sequence of antecedent, action, and consequences that will lead to the formulation of precise functional descriptions.

CLIENT: Okay.

THERAPIST: So, first you went to your classroom . . .

CLIENT: Then I started to feel very anxious. I saw everybody looking at me. It reminded me of what happened to me. I felt oppressed. I couldn't stand this anymore so I left.

THERAPIST: And what happened next?

CLIENT: I felt relieved.

THERAPIST: Okay. And you said that you were still thinking of what happened to you, right?

CLIENT: Yes. That's the only thing I could think of.

THERAPIST: How did that make you feel?

CLIENT: Horrible. I couldn't get that out of my mind. I can't ever get that out of my mind.

THERAPIST: It's always in your mind. . . . That must really be hard for you. But were you still trying to get it out of your mind?

CLIENT: Yeah, I wanted to stop feeling oppressed.

THERAPIST: Is that what happened?

The therapist leads the client to assess the impact of avoiding by drawing her attention toward the consequence of escaping the classroom.

CLIENT: I didn't feel as oppressed.

THERAPIST: Have you felt oppressed again since then?

The therapist leads the client to assess with more precision the impact of avoiding by drawing her attention to long-term consequences.

CLIENT: (*sighs*) Pretty much all the time . . .

THERAPIST: Do you mean that you felt oppressed again even on that day?

CLIENT: I'm sure I did. I feel oppressed all the time.

THERAPIST: I see. Although, you said that you didn't feel as oppressed when you left the classroom, right?

The therapist uses comparative framing to gain precision.

CLIENT: Yeah. . . . But quickly after, I felt like everything was oppressing me again.

THERAPIST: I see . . . So it keeps coming back? When you leave the classroom, you want to feel less oppressed. Overall, would say that you feel less oppressed if you leave the classroom?

CLIENT: A little less oppressed . . . for a while.

THERAPIST: In the short term?

CLIENT: Yeah, in the short term.

THERAPIST: But not in the long term?

CLIENT: No. Obviously not.

In these last exchanges, the therapist helps the client observe the distinction between short-term and long-term consequence, and lets her assess this difference by herself.

THERAPIST: So you feel less oppressed only in the short term. And does it always make you feel less oppressed or only sometimes?

The therapist leads the client to assess variability in the consequence of avoiding.

CLIENT: I don't know. I'm not sure.

THERAPIST: I know, it's probably hard to remember. Have you for example ever left a place because you felt oppressed but didn't feel any better, even for a little while?

The therapist uses distinction framing to help the client gain precision.

CLIENT: I went to a concert once. I left before it even began.

THERAPIST: Okay. And what happened next?

CLIENT: I thought I would go out for a few minutes, just to calm down. But I was still feeling very anxious after half an hour, so I didn't go back inside and went home instead.

THERAPIST: So that time, leaving didn't remove the feeling of oppression . . .

CLIENT: No, not at all.

THERAPIST: Does that mean that leaving when you feel oppressed removes that feeling for a little while but even that is not always true?

CLIENT: Probably. But I don't always notice that because I just leave every time I feel oppressed. I am very upset in these moments. I don't really pay close attention to what happens next. I just feel like I can't stay there anymore.

THERAPIST: That seems understandable to me. It's hard to notice everything that is happening when we are very upset. In the end, would you say that leaving the places that make you feel oppressed removes that feeling?

CLIENT: I think it does a little, but not always. And not for long.

In this last exchange, the therapist accompanies the client in the formulation of functional relationship among her different experiences. The therapist lets the client draw her own conclusions as much as possible. If she doesn't take into account important aspects of the situation, the therapist can ask questions about her experience in this area while remaining open to any answer.

Sometimes clients are highly distressed or completely lost and require more guidance to track effectively. The need for direct guidance is greater in settings where the therapist can see his clients for only a short period of time. Early on in therapy it is common for more directive approaches to be used before they are faded out. Being precise and functional can undermine some of the risks of clinicians stating their own rules, but the goal is always to direct the client's attention toward her own experience. This is an area of concern because the practitioner needs to work to distinguish pliance and tracking in order to know what to support. For example, a therapist provides a homework exercise and asks the client to observe what happens. If the client comes back after doing the exercise and says, "I did like you said and it worked," we need to be careful about supporting this as if it is progress (e.g., "Excellent!"). This response could reinforce rule following regardless of what actually happened after doing the exercise because the natural and relevant consequence is not clearly stated and we do not know yet what controlled the action of rule following. Only the correspondence between the specified behavior (trying the exercise) and the behavior actually performed is underlined. Instead, the therapist has the possibility of redirecting the client to her experience in order to help her contact the consequences of her behavior and formulate her own observations (e.g., "When you say 'it worked' what do you mean? What did you do and what did you notice happened?"). Thus, to increase the chance of tracking, it is preferable to remain as precise and functional as possible, and to encourage the client to check the correspondence between the described or predicted contingencies and what was experienced. Let's observe this technique in the following exchange with a client suffering from depression:

THERAPIST: Last time, we looked at a series of activities that you could do during the week. Were you able to do some of these activities?

CLIENT: I did some.

THERAPIST: What did you do, for example?

CLIENT: I went to the movies last Monday.

THERAPIST: How was that?

CLIENT: I don't know. . . . I did it because you told me to.

Although the therapist might not have actually told the client to go to the movies, the client seems to have done this activity with the purpose of following a socially provided rule, regardless of what would actually happen. This is common with clients suffering from depression since they don't experience much satisfaction from doing activities in the beginning, and pliance tends to be higher at baseline. As a result, the client mostly focuses on the correspondence between the behavior that was planned in therapy at the previous session and what he actually did, without much attention to the full experienced contingencies.

THERAPIST: Can you tell me more about it? What movie did you see?

Instead of arguing with the client about the actual purpose of doing the activity, the therapist directs his attention to the experience of seeing a movie.

CLIENT: A science fiction movie. I forgot the title.

THERAPIST: Was that a good movie?

CLIENT: Not too bad.

THERAPIST: What did you like and what didn't you like about it?

CLIENT: I liked the story. I used to read a lot of science fiction novels. It made me think. I used to like that a lot. But the actors were not very good. It was hard to forget that they were acting. I like when you can totally forget that it's a movie, you know.

In this exchange, the therapist helps the client develop a more detailed observation of his experience with distinction framing (what did you like and what didn't you like) in order to increase contact with potential sources of satisfaction (a natural and relevant consequence of going to see a movie).

THERAPIST: Would you say that going to the movies was a positive or a negative experience, in the end?

CLIENT: Not negative, no. A little positive. Not too bad of an experience.

THERAPIST: Is it something you imagine doing again?

CLIENT: Maybe.

THERAPIST: What would motivate you to go again?

CLIENT: If I can find a good movie, maybe I could have a good time.

In this last exchange, the therapist helps the client formulate a contingency that matches his experience more closely and leaves aside the role of the therapist as a reinforcer (going to see a movie → having a good time). In this vignette, we see the importance of tracking also after the client does something new. Observing, describing, and tracking make up an ongoing process to apply throughout therapy. As the client becomes more sensitive to crucial aspects of the context, he begins to engage in new behaviors, which need to be observed with a functional eye in order to avoid pliance and following rules that are not effective.

Making Functional Sense

The Goal

Using language implies being coherent at least to some degree, and thus, using language to deal with psychological experiences implies that we are making sense of these experiences. In order to avoid the traps of coherence, however, psychotherapy needs to help clients make sense of their experiences in a way that is helpful, not just coherent. We may have disparate and uncomfortable thoughts, feelings, memories, and sensations, but we can relate them all to our history and the impact of the current context and be guided by what works best in dealing with this diverse internal world. Normalization and effectiveness thus become a primary criterion for making sense in clinical work.

Why This Is Important, from an RFT Point of View

Language itself pulls for making sense, simply because deriving relations and changing functions require some degree of coherence in our symbolic networks for these processes to occur. If a network is not coherent, it is not clear what to derive and thus what functions to change. If you say "a diet coke" when a waiter asks you what you want, both of you must derive that by "diet coke" you meant a particular sugar-free soda. If you actually meant a glass of wine, saying "a diet coke" would misdirect the waiter (that would not make sense to him). If he brought a glass of water, that wouldn't make sense to you.

The problem is that the internal consistency of networks requires some bracketing or restriction of the network if essential coherence is at the core of sense making. In that case, we can end up preferring being right about our conceptualization of the world rather than building useful ideas and making effective choices. Just like coherent scientific theories can be useless if they don't lead to practical and effective applications, rules and statements such as "This is not fair. I shouldn't have to carry that burden" can be true in a descriptive sense but useless or even harmful in a practical sense. We will see in Chapter 6 that coherence can always be found when all these experiences are hierarchically related to consciousness or a sense of stable perspective taking. In this section, we will focus on ways to approach coherence based on functional utility.

How This Method Touches on Various Clinical Traditions

An interest in making sense based on consciousness and effectiveness is reflected in many clinical traditions. For example, person-centered therapy uses genuineness to foster greater internal congruence of the ideal and real self in the service of human freedom. Jungian psychotherapy seeks "personality integration" through "individuation"—the process of integrating opposites by holding both of them in consciousness—for a higher spiritual purpose. There are many other examples; our point is that this goal is common in psychotherapy across a wide range of approaches.

How to Do It

Making functional sense of psychological experiences happens in two main ways: by normalizing and accepting thoughts, sensations, and emotions as responses to a history and a current context; and by focusing on the usefulness of ideas, concepts, and choices rather than their essential truth.

Giving up on sense making based on essential truth is a difficult thing to do because we are generally not used to thinking in terms of effectiveness *independently of being right*. It is liberating though, particularly inside a strong therapeutic relationship, because as therapists, we don't have to convince our clients that they are wrong. Focusing on what works puts the client's life at the center of our attention. This is something that clients and therapists are often grateful for once they have learned to focus on effectiveness.

When clients come to therapy, it is often because they suffer from experiencing a certain level of incoherence in their life. The discrepancy between what they want to do and what they are currently doing is generally very painful. The gaps between what they expected and what they experienced; or what they were told would happen and what did; or between what others seemed to get and what they got, all feed into this sense of incoherence, as if something is wrong and must be put right before life can proceed. Establishing effectiveness as the criterion for coherence can carry a sense of relief and welcome immediacy: they want to make their life *work* better now, and functional coherence is generally an entirely new idea.

The more automatic strategy for filling the gap between actions and aspirations is to try to eliminate or replace elements of the context, such as unwanted psychological experiences (e.g., by avoiding painful sensations, by suppressing urges). Clients often begin therapy believing that it is not possible to engage in a desirable activity if it brings aversive feelings too: the aversive experience needs to be eliminated or replaced first. For example, a sexual abuse survivor may want to be more intimate with her partner but feel painful emotions every time she tries to get closer to him. These emotions are experienced as barriers to getting more intimate. Therefore, she tries to eliminate what she experiences as incoherent, that is, a difficult emotion associated with a desirable activity. She attempts to suppress the emotion, and if it doesn't work, she avoids intimacy altogether. Looking for coherence in the correspondence between feelings and actions can also lead to difficulties when clients engage in a problematic approach *because they feel* drawn toward a harmful reinforcer (e.g., urges to drink) or give up on effective behaviors *because they don't feel* like engaging in these activities.

An alternative approach is to normalize difficult psychological experiences by linking them to the current context and the client's history. For example, coherence can be established between having a history of sexual trauma and feeling painful emotions in contexts of intimacy; having a history of addiction and feeling urges to drink in the presence of alcohol; and having a history of reinforcement deprivation and not feeling like doing anything. Once coherence is established in this part of the client's symbolic network (i.e., his way of understanding his experiences), fighting against elements of the context that can't be eliminated becomes unnecessary. Their meaning has changed. The problem is not a problem anymore, and the client can focus on finding coherence in effective actions.

Normalizing Psychological Experiences. Normalizing experiences is useful if the client currently sees his own experiences as incoherent and, as a result, tries to eliminate or change them (e.g., "I shouldn't feel so anxious. What's wrong with me? I need to do something to relax"). In this context, it is naturally better to avoid making him feel like we, as therapists, see his experiences as incoherent, which would often result in triggering shame or resistance.

Normalizing clients' psychological experiences consists of acknowledging their presence, being open to their nature and conditions of occurrence, and connecting them to the client's history and the current context of the targeted behavior using conditional framing. For example, as the client explains that she can't be close to her partner because she immediately feels anxious, the therapist tells her "You feel very nervous when you try to be more intimate with your partner (*acknowledges*). Given what happened to you (*links to history*), it makes sense that you feel this way when you try to be more intimate (*links to current context*)." Simple statements including coordination framing can also turn psychological experiences currently lived by the client as disturbing or confusing into normal experiences of human life (e.g., "That's normal"; "How hard!"; "That's totally understandable").

Deictic framing is very useful to normalize and accept psychological experiences. It helps create a sense of common humanity between the client and other people, including the therapist herself. For example, the therapist can say, "If I had been through the same life events, I would probably feel the same way." Such a response is often even more powerful than simply stating the normality of these feelings because the client can directly relate to another person's experience. Sometimes, the therapist can't tell if she would feel similar experiences in the same situation and with the same history because what is reported by the client is too foreign to her. Often though, that disconnection is at the level of facts (e.g., the therapist has never used a gun and is talking to a veteran who had to kill people). At the level of what it is like to be a human, there is no difference between the client and the therapist, regardless of their histories. In order to remain authentic and increase connection, the therapist can acknowledge that she does not know what it is like to be in the client's shoes, that she has never been through such events, but can connect to that same feeling, triggered by other events, even though that feeling is not as strong (e.g., a feeling of guilt triggered by something she wished she had not done). Or she can simply acknowledge that she doesn't know what it feels like to be in the client's shoes but would like to better understand through the client sharing more. The therapist can also acknowledge her own current psychological experiences as a way of modeling this new approach toward difficult feelings. For example, the therapist might say, "I feel like it is a difficult topic for you. It makes me feel sad that you had to go through such painful events in your life" (meanwhile, the therapist doesn't change the topic, which models acceptance of difficult feelings). When clients see that therapists are emotionally moved by their pain, a sense of validation can occur based on very few additional words.

Evoking Assessment of Response Effectiveness. To increase the client's sense of effectiveness, the therapist uses conditional/temporal framing focused on the relationship between his behavior and its consequence in terms of lasting life satisfaction. For example, if a client says, "I wake up in the morning and the first thing I think is that I won't make it through this day and I'd better stay in bed. So I stay in bed almost every day," the therapist might ask in return, "When you have this thought and you stay in bed, does that bring you closer or farther away from what matters to you?" Notice that the therapist doesn't try to convince the client that "I'd better stay in bed" is not true, nor does she try to replace this thought with another. Instead, asking about effectiveness sets a context to assess the utility of the client's *response* to the thought. Some clinical approaches explicitly use the assessment of responses effectiveness as a way of *normalizing* psychological experiences first. For example, in coherence therapy (Ecker, Ticic, & Hulley, 2012), the client is led to explore what she actually gains or hopes from engaging in the problematic response. In our view, this is a useful way of normalizing experiences while also contacting sources of reinforcement and extracting meaningful purposes. These meaningful purposes will then be served by alternative means if the client sees that her current response is not the best option (see Chapter 7).

The therapist also uses comparative and hierarchical framing to encourage the client to assess alternative options, and link effectiveness to sources of lasting satisfaction (see Chapter 7). For example, he may say, "On the one hand, when you drink, you say that it makes you feel better in the short term but ruins your family life. And on the other hand, when you don't drink, you feel very anxious and your family is safer around you. What option makes more sense to you in terms of what you care about in your life?"

The following vignette shows an exchange with a client suffering from fear of public speaking. Note how the therapist uses conditional framing focused on consequences to set a context in which making sense is linked to effectiveness. Notice also how the therapist uses conditional framing focused on historical and current context to normalize psychological experiences and thus bring more coherence in this part of the client's network.

CLIENT: I can't imagine giving that talk tomorrow. It is going to be the most horrible experience of my life. I am seriously considering not going.

THERAPIST: If you are frightened of speaking in public, I can understand that you are not looking forward to giving this talk. Is there any reason why you would do this presentation?

The therapist normalizes the client's experience (not wanting to give the talk) by linking it to his fear of public speaking through conditional framing. He then uses conditional framing again to explore sources of motivation for giving the talk.

CLIENT: I have to. . . . Everybody expects me to report the activities of my team.

THERAPIST: Is that an important moment for the company?

CLIENT: Oh yeah! It's a big deal.

THERAPIST: Why is that a big deal, exactly?

CLIENT: Well, you know, our team did a very important work this year on enhancing the performance of the company. We created a new website. We invested a lot of money in advertisements. So it's important that everybody in the company can see what we did. They need to know that we worked hard and that we are about to see great results from our efforts.

THERAPIST: Are you proud of this work?

CLIENT: Yes, absolutely.

THERAPIST: What do you think the company is going to think of your work?

CLIENT: I think they are going to love it.

THERAPIST: It sounds like this talk means a lot to you.

In this exchange, the therapist uses hierarchical framing to help the client connect his public speaking performance to a higher, more meaningful purpose (see more on this in Chapter 7). Notice that the therapist never tells the client what the best thing to do is, nor does he try to convince him that it won't be a horrible experience.

CLIENT: Yeah . . . But I am so scared of talking in front of hundreds of people. This is going to be horrible.

THERAPIST: Yeah, I know. It must be very scary for you. Is it possible that this talk may be a horrible experience and also a meaningful experience?

CLIENT: It is both, yeah. But right now, it feels mostly horrible, very stressful.

THERAPIST: Yeah, thinking about talking in front of everybody already makes you feel stressed; that's understandable and I'm pretty sure I would feel the same way in your position! What do you think would be the most useful for you? Not going so you avoid a horrible experience or going to have a meaningful experience?

CLIENT: Well I can't really imagine missing this moment. It's too important for my team.

In this last exchange, the therapist once again normalizes the client's difficult psychological experience, this time using deictic framing ("I would feel the same way in your position"). He then sets the context for assessing the effectiveness of alternative options to bring satisfaction with comparative and hierarchical framing. Once again, notice that the therapist never argues with the client about the credibility of his thoughts. He only encourages him to consider other functions of giving the talk, not with the purpose of changing this experience itself, but to better assess the effectiveness of his responses to these opposite sources of influence.

Clients are often open to looking at the bigger picture because they are currently not satisfied with what is going on in their lives. Even if they don't necessarily see things through the lens of effectiveness yet, they do want their difficulties to improve. However, it is not rare that clients are strongly attached to the idea that what they are doing is right and that they just need to put more effort in it, or that they blame others for the lack of success of these strategies. This is usually a sign of excessive influence from inapplicable or inaccurate rules. In such cases, the therapist can lead the client to evaluate the effectiveness of following these rules without questioning their credibility. This principle is similar to what we presented above, but the client's strong attachment to these rules requires the therapist to be particularly careful not to get pulled into their content. What matters is how the client responds to these rules, not what the rules say. Observe this technique in the following exchange with a client complaining that his wife doesn't show enough interest in him:

CLIENT: She never asks me anything about what I do at work. That's really frustrating. At the end of a day of work, I would love to talk about what I did, what's important to me.

THERAPIST: Do you bring the topic up yourself sometimes?

CLIENT: No, because if she was really interested, I wouldn't have to start the conversation. She would ask me first!

The client formulates a rule likely influencing his behavior. Since his wife has to ask first to prove her interest, he can't tell her about his work. Tracking is inapplicable here since it doesn't define the client's behavior, but rather defines that of someone else.

THERAPIST: So you wait until she asks you about your day?

CLIENT: Yeah.

THERAPIST: Does she ask you at some point?

CLIENT: Rarely.

In this exchange, the therapist leads the client to assess the effectiveness of following the rule "waiting until his wife asks about his day."

THERAPIST: I imagine that it must feel very disappointing. Did you tell her that you would like her to ask you more about your work?

The therapist expresses empathy to increase mutual understanding and prevent defensiveness, which is particularly useful when clients are following rules rigidly. Then, she explores alternative strategies that the client may have tried in order to assess the effectiveness of a range of possible actions in this context.

CLIENT: No. If I ask her, it's not going to be natural. It would sound fake. I want her to really care, not to ask me just to make me happy.

THERAPIST: What we are trying to do here is to find out what works and what doesn't work so you can choose what is the best for you, right? How about we look at this together in detail so that we better understand what happens in this difficult situation with your wife?

The therapist sets a context encouraging the client to approach his behavior through the lens of effectiveness. In the following exchange, she leads the client to track the sequence antecedent–rule–behavior–consequence.

CLIENT: Okay.

THERAPIST: So you said you come back from your day of work. . . .

The therapist evokes observation of antecedent by initiating the reformulation of the sequence but intentionally leaving her sentence incomplete (implicit temporal framing to explore what comes next).

CLIENT: I would like to talk about my day, to share what's important to me.

The client describes the Antecedent.

THERAPIST: And then, what happens?

The therapist evokes the next step of the contingency through temporal framing.

CLIENT: Nothing. I wait, hoping that she is going to ask me about my day but it never happens.

The client describes the sequence rule–behavior–consequence.

THERAPIST: How do you feel then?

The therapist evokes further consequence, in terms of psychological experience (temporal framing).

CLIENT: Very disappointed. Lonely.

The client describes the consequence of following the rule.

THERAPIST: Would you say that waiting contributes to having a conversation about your work with your wife?

The therapist evokes assessment of effectiveness with hierarchical framing.

CLIENT: No. But there is nothing else I can do.

The client notices the ineffectiveness of his response, but formulates a new rule limiting other options.

THERAPIST: What would happen if you started talking about your work without waiting for your wife to ask you?

The therapist evokes tracking of alternative response to the rule with opposition framing.

CLIENT: I don't know what would happen. But I don't want to do that because it would not feel like she is spontaneously interested.

The same rule is formulated again.

THERAPIST: And you said that it would be the same problem if you told her that you would like her to ask you about your work, right?

CLIENT: Yes. It has to come from her or else it won't mean anything.

The client formulates another rule preventing him from changing his behavior.

THERAPIST: So, let's try to figure out what works and what doesn't work, okay? You said that waiting doesn't work. You already know that because it is what you have been doing for a long time, right?

The therapist reorients the exchange toward assessing the effectiveness of the client's response to the rules.

CLIENT: Yes.

THERAPIST: Have you been able to observe what happens when you tell your wife about your work instead of waiting for her to ask?

The therapist orients the client to his experience. So far, he has refused to talk to his wife first because of the rule "She has to talk first or it won't feel like she is really interested." The therapist invites him to explore this different approach, simply as a way of observing what would happen.

CLIENT: No. I never do that, so I can't tell. But I know it wouldn't be the same as if she asked first.

THERAPIST: Would there be any risk in trying that, just to see what happens?

Notice how the therapist never contradicts the client's rule. She simply offers the possibility of trying, just to observe what happens.

CLIENT: No, there is no risk. It's just that it's not how I would like things to be.

THERAPIST: I know. This is frustrating when you really want something and nothing you do seems to help.

The therapist expresses empathy again (coordination framing to qualify the experience as frustrating), to create a context more favorable to the experimentation of other approaches with his wife.

CLIENT: Exactly. That's frustrating. I feel like I have tried to be patient, but it doesn't work.

THERAPIST: How about trying something different? This way, you can observe what happens.

CLIENT: I can try. I guess it can't be worse than what it is like right now, anyway.

Increasing Response Flexibility

The Goal

When an element of the context influencing the client's behavior in a problematic way can't be removed or replaced, it is still possible to increase the flexibility of the client's actions by transforming the symbolic function of that source of influence. Imagine, for example, a client suffering from chronic pain who fears that he can't stand his pain and that doing anything will make it worse and therefore doesn't engage in any exercise. Part of what is controlling his avoidance is the symbolic function of the pain (e.g., he thinks "it's unbearable"). The painful sensations are not *intrinsically* a barrier to exercising. RFT researchers have shown that remarkably short interventions can weaken the link between pain and avoidance of pain by altering its symbolic function (e.g., McMullen et al., 2008). Interventions of this kind can make it psychologically possible to experience exercise as something that is painful and yet both possible and beneficial. If we can help the client connect to different functions of what is currently perceived as a barrier, it will help him gain flexibility in the way he responds to his pain and thoughts about his pain. Instead of avoiding his pain, he may start exercising again.

Why This Is Important, from an RFT Point of View

Language attributes symbolic functions to our experiences, and problematic functions can dominate and narrow response flexibility. Removing these functions is a vain pursuit because derivation processes can always reinstall them in the networks. However, it is possible to alter the symbolic context of the sources of influence and develop alternative functions to evoke new responses.

How This Method Touches on Various Clinical Traditions

Many clinical traditions aim to alter the symbolic impact of contextual sources of influence to promote response flexibility. Humanistic therapies have long argued that encouraging clients to go into their felt sense of events increases a sense of openness and choice. Mindfulness-based traditions encourage similar awareness of bodily experience and learning to direct attention toward events voluntarily rather than automatically, in a more welcoming and less judgmental way. Cognitive therapy seeks to establish "distancing" so that the impact of thoughts will be less automatic (Hollon & Beck, 1979). Psychodynamic approaches encourage the exploration of difficult materials from an attitude of "dispassionate observation" so that choices can be more conscious. In all of these approaches there is an idea that stepping back changes automaticity and allow new forms of action. Other approaches consist of changing the meaning of psychological experiences in order to encourage different responses (e.g., reappraisal in cognitive traditions).

How to Do It

Increasing response flexibility can take different paths, but it always requires an alteration of the context. In this section, we will show two main approaches that both consist of altering the context even though in a sense they go in reversed directions. On the one hand, we can change the context around the source of influence currently controlling the client's response, which in turn can change the response. For example, a client who doesn't go to work as a response to the thought "I am too depressed" might be invited to look at this thought as a spam coming to his email box. On the other hand, we can change the context around the client's behavior in order to evoke a different response, which in turn will change the function of the original source of influence. For example, the client could be invited to experiment going to work while deliberately thinking "I am too depressed," which may weaken the impact of this thought.

Changing the Context around the Source of Influence. Increasing response flexibility by changing the relational context around the sources of influence aims to change their symbolic functions without trying to change their intrinsic characteristics. It is impossible to make an exhaustive list of the ways we can alter the context because the variety of framings and the combination of these framings lead to an infinite number of techniques. In this section, we will present some examples based on different relational framings.

At the most basic level, new functional cues can be presented that significantly change the way the client sees the source of influence and its effects. For example, shifting posture, or facial expressions, or using a specific pace and tone of voice can give a new meaning to things brought up by the client. The therapist can lean forward when the client talks about some important topic that she usually tends to avoid, or move his chair to the client's side to decrease resistance or pliance with what she is saying. The therapist could also gently smile and nod to convey a sense of curiosity about a difficult experience reported by the client—turning it into something interesting to observe rather than merely a barrier to action. Some therapists like to use music in therapy because it helps clients see things in a different way without having to say anything.

A person struggling with a difficult emotion or thought might be asked to distill that experience down to a single word and then to place it on the floor so that the therapist and client can talk about that feeling or thought. The metaphor of "seeing an object from a distance" may symbolically transform some of the functions of that feeling or thought. Mindfulness interventions rely on the same effect when they ask clients to view thoughts as clouds floating by, with consciousness per se being more like the sky. Many "defusion" methods used in acceptance and commitment therapy fit this overall pattern.

Simple relational framing such as coordination and distinction used to evoke describing can also lead the client to be more in touch with the intrinsic characteristics of his experience. As a result, the problematic influence exerted by symbolic functions may decrease. Imagine, for example, a client who avoids looking other people in the eyes because she immediately feels judged by them. Here, the eyes of other people have an aversive symbolic function. Since this avoidant behavior also appears during interactions in therapy, the therapist can encourage the client to describe what she sees while looking into his eyes, with words emphasizing intrinsic functions over symbolic functions such as in the following short vignette:

> THERAPIST: Try to describe what you see as concretely as possible.
>
> CLIENT: I see your eyes. They are blue.
>
> THERAPIST: What else do you see?
>
> CLIENT: There is also a white part. They are round. I also see your eyelashes.
>
> THERAPIST: What do they look like?
>
> CLIENT: They are brown and thin.
>
> THERAPIST: What about the movement of my eyes?
>
> CLIENT: They don't move much. Maybe laterally, a little.

In this approach, augmenting the intrinsic functions is done with the hope of balancing unhelpful symbolic functions, even without necessarily challenging or changing fears of social judgment directly.

Coordination framing can convey a sense of compatibility between things that are currently seen as opposite. Because of history, we can't replace one relation with another, but it is possible to establish a new relation and use it more frequently. For example, the therapist can take a client's habitual statement that opposes an emotion to an action ("I would like to invite her on a date but I am afraid") and use coordination framing instead. ("I see. You would like to invite her on a date and you are afraid"), which will immediately open up the possibility of new actions. This technique is not focused on subtracting or eliminating a current act of framing— language works through addition, not subtraction. Rather, adding alternative symbolic relations merely increases the variability of thinking, affording new and more effective responses to thoughts.

Opposition framing can be used to transform the function of problematic sources of influence in several ways. An example is humor and irreverence, which often help create distance from rigid thoughts. Imagine, for example, a client with social anxiety who went to a job interview and tells her therapist about the awful experience she had. The recruiter was very cold, asked her embarrassing questions, and even criticized the way she was dressed. As the client is stuck in the memory of this experience, and apparently unwilling to ever go to an interview again, the therapist says, "Wow . . . he was a really nice guy, huh? Not!" smiling with compassion. Of course, for this type of move to create distance rather than resistance or shame, it is important to make sure that the therapeutic relationship is solid and that the timing is appropriate. Another typical example consists of turning a cue that usually triggers a problematic behavior into an opportunity to try something more effective. For example, to a client saying, "I am frustrated right now. And when I am like that, I get angry, and I make things worse in my relationship. I become negative and judgmental, and I criticize everything about her," the therapist might say "Good catch. And now that you have noticed that, could this be an opportunity to actually improve your relationship? The very pull to do the usual thing can be a sign to try something truly different."

Using comparative framing to undermine the impact of problematic sources of influence can consist of bringing other potential sources of influence to the client's attention so that alternative responses become more available. In one example, the therapist can evoke the client's observation of a better outcome if another action was chosen (e.g., "Is this the best way for you to reach your goal?"; "Are there more effective approaches to resolve this problem?"). In contrast, poorer outcomes might be drawn to the client's attention as a way to help him persist in an effective action. For example, the therapist might say, "I see that it was hard for you to spend this whole night with urges to smoke. If you had actually smoked, how do you think you would be feeling right now?"

We will see in later chapters that hierarchical framing can transform the function of sources of influence by helping clients see the "bigger picture." On the one hand, hierarchical framing can help clients take some distance from experiences that influence them in problematic ways. On the other hand, they can be more in touch with experiences that serve higher purposes. A simple example of this strategy is to link an experience to a hierarchical category that has a different impact on the client's behavior. Observe in the following exchange how the therapist uses this approach to formulate the client's statements:

CLIENT: I'm so weak.

THERAPIST: It must be hard to have this thought. How are you feeling?

CLIENT: I'm crushed. I can't to do anything.

THERAPIST: And the feeling of being crushed shows up again, huh?

CLIENT: Yeah . . .

THERAPIST: And then the thought that you can't do anything. . . . It seems like these experiences happen in a sequence. Is that what you notice?

CLIENT: Yeah, it goes pretty fast, but I can see that.

In this simple exchange, the therapist is reformulating the client's statements as thoughts and feelings he *has* rather than things he *is*, which hopefully will override the relation of equivalence implicit in the initial thought

("I'm so weak"). Once thoughts and feelings are seen as events that can be observed at some distance, with openness and curiosity, other responses to these thoughts become more available than with the frame "I am."

Analogical framing can change the function of sources of influence in particular through the use of metaphors. Through this process, useful functions of objects, situations, or characters are applied to the source of influence in a way that changes the client's response. For example, to a client saying, "I am afraid all the time. I keep thinking that something bad is going to happen," a therapist might say, "I am afraid, something bad is going to happen. . . . You are hearing this song all day, huh?" This simple turn of a phrase helps her relate to her thoughts with more distance, as she would with the lyrics of a song. The use of physical props in the therapy room can have much the same effect. For example, if the client is talking about a painful self-judgment, the therapist might reach for a cup and bang it down on the table in front of her while saying, "So it's sort of like suddenly 'I'm an idiot' shows up [bang] and then you have to decide what to do with that thought." In this case, that parallel between a loud noise and a painful emotion increases the applicability of a physical metaphor. Once the metaphor is understood, the client's reaction to the presence of the cup and of a painful self-judgment creates a chance for new functions to emerge. The therapist might then say, "Maybe we can just let the cup sit there without drinking from it" as a way of saying, "Maybe we can just notice that 'I'm an idiot' thought without elaborating it."

Perspective taking (through deictic framing), can be used to help the client look at a source of influence from a different angle, along interpersonal, spatial, or temporal dimensions and, as a result, consider alternative ways of responding to this experience. For example, while preparing an exposure exercise, the therapist might say, "So, you are saying that right now your fear is more powerful than what you care about in your life. How do you think you will look at this once you go back home and you think of this exercise again?" [temporal perspective shift]. The therapist might also say, "Imagine that you were with your daughter, and as you are teaching her to swim, she says she is too afraid of going in the water. What would you tell her?" [interpersonal perspective shift].

When a transformation of function is effective, the client begins to respond in a new way to sources of influence. Sometimes, the change of response is sudden, similar to the emotional insights sought in many forms of therapy. More often, the client at first begins to show signs of greater flexibility through her way of speaking about the source of influence, or her posture and tone of voice, and over time, she actually changes her core response. These changes are signs that the intervention is working and therefore should be watched with attention. It can be useful at this point to help the client notice this change and the better outcomes that the new response produces.

Changing the Context around the Behavior. Another approach to increase response flexibility is simply to evoke a new response by using another source of influence while the original source is still present. Once the client has experienced that a new response is possible, the original problematic source of influence may start to lose its impact. Here also, it is impossible to provide an exhaustive list of the many language-based ways to evoke a new response, so we will present only some typical examples.

Often, evoking new responses takes the form of instructions in experiential exercises or, less formally, merely of invitations to try something different. For example, if a client is engaging in emotional avoidance, the therapist might say, "So, you have observed that when you do that, it works in the short term but not in the long term. How about trying something different right now? What if we took just a moment to observe together what happens if instead of thinking of something else, you allowed these thoughts to be there?" If the client is stuck in a single pattern of thinking, therapists often use questions to evoke cognitive reappraisal in much the same way: "And so that same familiar thought comes up again. If we were to step back and look at the whole picture, what other thoughts might be there about this situation?"

The way such invitations are formulated can make the new response more likely to appear. For example, setting a context for curiosity, exploration, or even playfulness can turn the response into something more attractive (e.g., "Let's look at this as an experiment"; "Imagine that we are exploring together a land that nobody has seen before"; "You practice yoga, right? Imagine giving space to this thought is like stretching your muscles a little farther than what you usually do. We just get at the edge, to gain some flexibility"). Showing empathy helps normalize the client's reticence to change his behavior, while maintaining the invitation to try something different (e.g., "You seem scared right now. That's quite understandable!").

Often, a new response can be presented rather casually and "by the way," even though it constitutes a genuine step toward more effective behavior. For example, as a client says, "I can't stand this feeling, I would rather not talk about it," the therapist may ask, "What do you feel when you notice that you don't want to talk about it?" The level of observation is shifted, but meanwhile the client stays in touch with this experience, which is already a sign of greater flexibility.

As the client engages in a new response, the therapist may want to help him notice this increase in flexibility so that the function of the original source of influence can change and sometimes even become a cue for an alternative response. For example, a client who used to stay in bed when she had the thought "I can't get up" now sees this thought as a cue for getting up and making coffee. The thought is still there, but the response has changed.

In the following vignette, you will see techniques that aim to transform the function of problematic sources of influence, and other techniques directly targeting the response instead.

CLIENT: I feel terribly stressed, and talking about my stress is even more painful. Can we talk about something else?

THERAPIST: I can see that it is really hard for you. We can change the topic of our conversation, of course. But is that what you want to do or what your stress wants you to do?

CLIENT: I don't really have a choice. . . . I feel very nervous, and that's really painful. I can't stay like that.

THERAPIST: Yeah, that's painful, I know. And it makes sense to want, to escape that. Would you like to have a choice though?

CLIENT: I would like to be less controlled by my stress, for sure . . .

THERAPIST: Because this way, you could do what you really want? You could decide to talk about something else or to keep talking, no matter how stressed you feel?

CLIENT: Yes. I'd rather not feel stressed at all though!

THERAPIST: I understand. And right now, the stress is there . . .

CLIENT: Yes.

In these first exchanges, the client's response seems controlled by painful sensations of stress and the thought, "I don't really have a choice." In response to the client's attempts to escape, the therapist sets a context encouraging the client to engage in a different response. She does so by increasing the client's interest in having a choice with conditional framing (i.e., if he was less controlled by stress, he could do what he really wants).

THERAPIST: How about we observe how much it is controlling what you can do or not do?

CLIENT: How?

THERAPIST: Well, perhaps we could start with this. It looks like since you said you wanted to change the topic of our conversation, you were actually able to keep talking about your stress. Did you notice that? I wonder if it is a sign that you can still decide to do what you want, even when you feel stressed.

The therapist encourages the client to notice the flexibility that has already begun to occur. In this context, stress and urges to escape may start to lose their function of antecedents controlling the client's behavior. They can progressively become sensations that the client can choose to react to or not.

CLIENT: So far, yes. But I still find this unbearable.

THERAPIST: You still have that thought . . . it is unbearable . . . Okay. What does this stress feel like? I know it is not easy to talk about it. At the same time, perhaps it could help us explore further how to be less controlled by stress.

The therapist labels the statement "it is unbearable" as a thought to help the client distinguish between intrinsic and symbolic functions of stress. She then encourages the client to describe the sensation as a way to transform its function (increased contact with intrinsic characteristics) and to engage in a different response than escaping.

CLIENT: I just feel tensed. Agitated. You can probably see that.

THERAPIST: The way you are moving your legs, for example?

CLIENT: Yes, when I feel stressed, I can't stop moving.

THERAPIST: What else?

CLIENT: I feel like out of breath. That's why I want to talk about something else.

THERAPIST: I see. It makes you want to escape. It is understandable. Can you still try to describe this sensation even if it is painful?

CLIENT: I'm breathing fast and my chest feels tight. . . . My belly is moving fast . . .

THERAPIST: What do you feel like doing?

CLIENT: I want this sensation to go away. It is unbearable.

THERAPIST: It feels unbearable. . . . How would you make this sensation go away?

CLIENT: I feel like leaving.

THERAPIST: How long have you had this urge?

CLIENT: Since I came in.

THERAPIST: So this sensation makes you want to leave, but you are still here. How do you think that is possible?

CLIENT: I guess I am not entirely controlled by it.

THERAPIST: But when you have that sensation, it feels like you have to do something about it, like leaving or changing the topic of our conversation?

CLIENT: Yes, it feels like I have no choice.

THERAPIST: So you can feel like you have no choice and still choose to stay and talk about your stress?

CLIENT: It is hard, but I am doing it right now I guess.

In these last exchanges, the therapist encourages the client to describe sensations of stress in order to contact their intrinsic functions. Pain in the throat, heart racing, and belly movements are not intrinsically controlling the client's behavior. It is the function that language attributes to these sensations that makes the client think that he must escape (i.e., "This sensation is unbearable"). Note that although these sensations are bearable, they still seem quite aversive. Thus, the therapist encourages the client to notice his increased tolerance to sensations of stress (greater flexibility).

Although psychotherapy work is essentially made of verbal interactions, before we leave this specific area we should note how simply new responses can be evoked without extensive verbal interactions. Shifts of posture (e.g., leaning forward or backward), facial expressions (e.g., smiling, frowning), or onomatopoeias (e.g., "ahah?" "ouch!") can lead the client to respond in a new way to events without saying much at all. Well-timed silence or reflective listening can evoke new action. For example, after a client says, "I can't talk about this topic because it's too painful," the therapist might take a moment of silence and then gently repeat with an interrogative tone "It's too painful?" thus showing interest and implicitly inviting the client to talk more about this experience.

Almost everything the clinician does when a client is engaging in previously problematic reactions is an opportunity to establish new reactions. Variability in the practitioner's responses is a major source of flexibility in the client's response, especially if the practitioner's response differs from conventional social exchanges. Clinicians need to watch out for their pull to do normal things because the power to establish new responses comes from out of that set. For example, suppose a client is confused. Suppose this happens with regularity and appears to be clinically relevant: expressions of confusion come with an implicit or explicit demand to do something, but focusing on that issue has a quality of predictability or entanglement in session. In normal social interactions, attempts will almost always be made to reduce the confusion. This can be easily tested by the reader: In almost any social interaction you have in the next day, randomly say "I'm confused" and watch how it leads to attempts to restate, clarify, reassure, understand, interpret, or dig out sources of confusion. Given this high base rate of responses designed to eliminate confusion when it is expressed, it is relatively unlikely that clinicians doing these same things will lead to new responses. But there are myriad appropriate clinical reactions outside of that normal social set. Let's list several to see how wide the range of possibilities might be to a client saying, "I'm confused":

"Great! I'm glad you are noticing!"
"Should we stop everything and chase that?"
"Is that okay?"

"Me too. Can we both just sit with that for a while?"

"Can we carry that reaction with us as we continue to look in this area?"

"What does that normally pull from you?"

"Etymologically, 'confusion' means 'poured together.' What is poured together right now?"

"Well, you say that as if you need to get clear—but it *is* clear. It is clear you are confused. So now that we are clear, what would be a good next step?"

We are not suggesting that you abandon the client in a state of confusion, or that confusion per se is useful. The suggestions listed above target the problematic function of asking for clarification in a specific clinical context. Applied inside a solid relationship in which the goals of therapy are clearly identified (see more in Chapter 10), this approach offers the client opportunities to respond in a new way to an old problem.

Our point is that to evoke a new response, something must change in the typical context. *Any* change in the context can potentially evoke a new response, so the ally of clinical work in this area is thinking outside the box. Doing what is normal and expected socially is unlikely to be helpful when problematic responses are well grooved because that *is* the typical context.

USING LANGUAGE
TO SHAPE BEHAVIOR CHANGE

In the first part of this chapter, we explored how to help clients better observe and assess their behaviors in order to alter the impact of problematic sources of influence. This is useful for encouraging clients to abandon ineffective strategies and envisage alternative actions that bring more satisfaction. We also reviewed a variety of ways to create a symbolic context that begins to increase the flexibility of clients' responses. Actual and sustainable change is often a longer process, especially if the client needs to learn new ways of acting in the world. Even when the actions naturally lead to more desirable consequences, therapists may need to use behavioral principles deliberately to support and shape more effective actions. Virtually all of these processes are conducted inside the clinical conversation, which is why they deserve discussion here.

The Goal

Shaping behavior change includes reinforcement of step-by-step progress, support of tracking over pliance when change occurs, and weakening of problematic actions. All of these involve language processes.

Why This Is Important, from an RFT Point of View

Not all human behavior is symbolic or rule-governed, but language touches virtually all behavior that is clinically significant. By using language tools deliberately, we can use other behavioral principles directly to shape behavior more by experience and less by rules, which should encourage greater response flexibility.

How This Method Touches on Various Clinical Traditions

The language of shaping and reinforcement is entirely behavioral, but the point of learning to do what works is embedded in virtually every clinical tradition.

How to Do It

Reinforcing Progress

Although the influence of the medical model on psychotherapy has led many clinicians to focus first on the reduction of behavior problems, in our functional contextual view the primary goal of therapy is to gain flexibility and broaden behavioral repertoires that sustain well-being. This approach suggests that our work should be mostly focused on reinforcing progress toward effective actions.

Reinforcing Step by Step. Shaping is one of the most effective principles we can use when supporting clients' progress. It consists of recognizing and reinforcing steps toward effective behaviors. Too often, we wait for a perfect action to occur before acknowledging an improvement. This is frequently the case in clients' real lives, where new consequences don't necessarily occur until a perfect behavior is executed. For this reason, the therapist ought to compensate for this lack of natural support during the early stages of learning. Consider the example of one of our clients who demonstrated problematic reactions to feelings of frustration. At the beginning of therapy, he would get angry very easily in conversations when people didn't understand what he meant. As a result, he would either quit the conversation or make mean comments to people he spoke with (both strategies that allowed him to escape from his uncomfortable feelings). Even though he was aware that his behavior was problematic, it was still difficult for him to let go of his feelings of frustration. After a while, he made some progress: he would stay engaged in conversations and wouldn't make any overt arch reproach, but he would still roll his eyes and sigh when others didn't immediately understand him. This expression of frustration would still bother people, so it was not easy for him to find satisfaction in the efforts he had accomplished so far. Our strategy therefore was to reinforce his progression toward more effective interactions, even though at this point, his skills still needed improvement. The following is a reproduction of a short exchange demonstrating how we can proceed:

THERAPIST: I am not sure I understand you. Are you saying that your friend was not listening to you or that he didn't understand you?

CLIENT: (*rolling his eyes*) He said that he didn't understand me, but what I'm saying is that I think he was not really listening.

THERAPIST: Ah, okay. Thank you for making it more clear for me. I know that repeating yourself is not an easy thing to do for you.

The therapist attempts to reinforce the effort by linking the client's behavior to a positive outcome (greater understanding) and acknowledges the difficulty it represents for the client.

CLIENT: I'm sorry. I know I rolled my eyes again.

THERAPIST: Yeah, it's not easy for me when I see you do that because it makes me feel like I bother you while I really want to understand you. But I do appreciate that you took the time to explain to me what happened again. It is really helpful and I feel like this way we can keep having a good conversation. What do you think?

The therapist distinguishes between effective behaviors and behaviors that are still problematic. Note that in both cases, the therapist points to the effects of the client's behavior, thus encouraging the client to track the actual consequences of his actions.

CLIENT: I wish I were less reactive. But I get frustrated so easily . . .

THERAPIST: I know. That's why I particularly appreciate your efforts.

The therapist reinforces the client's efforts again by mentioning actual consequences happening in the room.

In this last example, we saw that the therapist differentiated effective from problematic behaviors. On the one hand, the therapist acknowledged the progression and reinforced what is working, and on the other hand, he indicated to the client what can still be improved. This approach is often subtle and can lead the therapist to reinforce behaviors that are *apparently* totally inappropriate but that, in fact constitute genuine progress. In the first stages of therapy with this same client, it might be helpful even to reinforce his criticisms because he was at least engaging in conversation, which was a genuine improvement.

It is also important to note that the reinforcers used by the therapist were similar to the consequences occurring in the client's real life. As we noted in a previous chapter, it is helpful that there are often functional similarities between what happens in the therapy room and the client's life. This applies to shaping as well. To ensure that the behaviors learned in therapy will generalize outside the room, the consequences they provoke with the therapist need to be functionally similar to what will happen in natural settings. Thus, in the previous example, the therapist clearly stated that making the effort to explain again helped him understand and continue the conversation together. This is likely what will happen in the client's life if he keeps improving his skills.

Reinforcing Tracking over Pliance. Choosing appropriate reinforcers also entails taking into account the risk of encouraging pliance, since the natural consequences of a behavior can easily be substituted by the therapist's whim, even unintentionally. We saw in a previous example that a client suffering from depression went to the movies "because the therapist told him to do so." There is a good chance that going to the movies is an effective behavior for a person who is trying to engage in activities again. However, it won't bring much satisfaction, or not for long, if the only function is to comply with a therapist's rule. When delivering reinforcement, the therapist should therefore try to connect the client's behavior as closely as possible to its natural consequences. This can be done by encouraging the client to assess the correspondence between the predicted and the experienced contingencies, with particular attention to positive consequences. To this end, the therapist can use coordination, comparative, and distinction framing (e.g., "Did things go as you were expecting?"; "Was the consequence as you were hoping or different?"; "Was it better?"; "Not as good?"). Observe this approach in the following short example:

CLIENT: This week, I was very happy because I finally found the time to do the exercise at home, like you told me.

THERAPIST: I'm glad that you found the time to do this exercise since it was supposed to give you an opportunity to try a different, perhaps more useful approach to deal with your anxiety. What did you experience as you were doing this exercise?

CLIENT: It was interesting, very different from what I usually do, for sure.

THERAPIST: Did it seem like this approach was more, or less helpful than what you usually do?

CLIENT: I think it is still early for me to tell, but I think I felt less overwhelmed.

In this exchange, the way the client talks about her homework at first suggests that she may be mostly reinforced by the correspondence between her actual behavior and what was planned. In other words, she may have done what she was "supposed" to do regardless of the natural consequences (pliance). The therapist expresses genuine satisfaction too, but directly linked to the expected natural consequences. He then invites the client to describe her experience during the exercise in order to help her check the correspondence between the expected and the experienced contingencies (tracking).

When the behavior targeted by the therapeutic work is social by nature, it can be difficult to distinguish between tracking and pliance since the expected natural consequence often corresponds to a reinforcement socially delivered. For example, a client who wants to improve his relationship with his partner may choose to satisfy her request: "I would be happier if we spent more time together." This is a desirable natural consequence for him, but doing so could end up being reinforced just because he did what she wanted him to do (i.e., without tracking the correspondence between the consequence stated by the rule and the experienced consequence). This entanglement between tracking and pliance can happen in interactions between client and therapist too. This is not necessarily a problem as long as the client doesn't stop tracking altogether. To avoid this, it is useful to encourage clients to keep in mind the function of their behavior by formulating rules that make a clear connection between actions, antecedents, and consequences, and to limit arbitrary social reinforcement of rule following. The following example illustrates this approach with a client working on being more reliable in her relationships:

CLIENT: I was wondering if we could change the time of our next appointment because I am not 100% sure that I will make it at our regular time next week, and I don't want to bother you by canceling at the last minute.

THERAPIST: I appreciate that you are telling me that. It makes my work much easier when my clients ask to move an appointment in advance instead of canceling at the last minute.

Since the client only states that she didn't want to "bother" him, the therapist formulates the connection between the client's behavior and its natural consequence.

CLIENT: That's what I thought. And since I want to be more reliable . . .

THERAPIST: (*showing interest*) So you called me because you wanted to be more reliable?

CLIENT: Yes. I feel like you can trust me this way. I feel like I am acting more like an adult.

THERAPIST: (*showing interest*) And that is important to you?

CLIENT: Yes, very important. I want people to trust me. I want to be seen as a responsible person. And I know that for that to happen, I have to be more reliable.

In this exchange, the therapist helps the client connect her willingness to be more reliable with consequences that matter to her and not only to others. This is useful for maximizing her ability to track desirable consequences instead of arbitrarily following the rule "be reliable."

Watching for pliance doesn't necessarily mean eliminating it altogether. There are situations when clients are too lost or distressed to be able to observe natural contingencies on their own, and sometimes natural contingencies are not currently supporting effective change. For example, a client who self-harms in order to cope with intense emotions might not recognize that other methods are more effective because at first they are not. They often require practice to show better results. In these cases, the therapist might choose to increase her influence on the client's way of thinking and acting, as a first step before helping him observe, describe, and track contingencies on his own. For example, a therapist might ask a client to "trust her" or to "lean on her"—statements that could encourage pliance. We can think of this approach as an analogy to using anesthesia in order to conduct surgery. The goal is to temporarily remove a source of pain in order to perform the operation. In an analogous way in psychotherapy we may need to encourage pliance to temporarily insulate the client from the natural contingencies if they are too harmful and don't shape effective actions. Once the client is skilled enough to deal with the world more effectively, this artificially augmented form of social influence can be faded out.

We will see in Chapter 7 that pliance can also be explored to extract sources of meaningful reinforcement. When clients engage in actions "just to please others," it often reflects a strong interest in social connection. Once that motivation is better identified by the client, it can help her choose actions that are more effective to meet her needs, or engage in the same actions but with greater awareness of their purpose.

Weakening Problematic Behaviors

When clients make progress, they not only engage more frequently in effective strategies, but they also tend to abandon those that are not working. This often happens naturally since alternative strategies are generally incompatible. For example, not responding to urges to drink alcohol is incompatible with drinking alcohol. Hence, if the first is strengthened, the second is naturally weakened. However, problematic behaviors can remain present for a while in the behavioral repertoire of a client even when more effective behaviors are strengthened. This is particularly true in the early stages of learning a new behavior. In this case, weakening problematic behaviors directly at the same time as appropriate behaviors are being reinforced can help the client learn faster. Although our approach relies primarily on the reinforcement of useful behaviors, certain techniques can be used in verbal interactions to weaken inappropriate behaviors.

Delivering and Orienting Undesirable Consequences. When a behavior is followed by an aversive consequence, its frequency tends to decrease. Thus, if a problematic behavior occurs in the therapy room, the therapist can help the client track the consequences that follow. Imagine, for example, a client demonstrating difficulties with social interactions. During their first session, the therapist notices that she often interrupts her in the middle of a sentence, which prevents them from developing effective interactions. After another interruption, the therapist gently tells her, "When you interrupt me, it is difficult for me to understand your situation well. And I would like to ask you some important questions to have a better sense of the difficulties you are having." This would likely function as an undesirable consequence for the client since she probably wants to be understood by her therapist. In fact, this consequence was already present but didn't sufficiently influence the client's behavior. Therefore, pointing to what is happening can help the client track the consequence and adjust her behavior. Note that, as for the use of reinforcers, undesirable consequences need to match what is happening in the client's life. Even though the people she usually has conversations with may not tell her, they are probably also bothered by her frequent interruptions and have a hard time developing good relationships with her. Thus, the therapist doesn't use an arbitrary aversive consequence but helps her better adjust to the contingencies of her natural environment (although it would be useful to test this hypothesis by encouraging the client to observe the consequence of her interruptions during interactions with others).

Blocking. Another possibility is to simply make the problematic behavior impossible to perform (blocking). For example, a therapist can help a client suffering from posttraumatic stress disorder to be less reactive to the evocation of the traumatic episode by asking her to describe her emotions. By doing so, she blocks the usual forms of avoidance. Of course, the client actually remains free to engage in that action, but the context created by the therapist makes it less likely to happen. If the client stops her description and reengages in avoidance, the therapist can gently redirect her attention to these emotions as in the following example.

THERAPIST: Is it becoming difficult?

CLIENT: Yes.

THERAPIST: I noticed that because you stopped talking. Is that what you do when emotions become really painful?

CLIENT: Yes, it's like freezing. I can't speak.

THERAPIST: Freezing, okay. Do you feel that in a particular part of your body?

CLIENT: My neck and my shoulders.

Extinguishing. Another way of weakening the frequency of a behavior is to stop delivering the reinforcing consequence that has maintained it so far (extinction). This is often not easy to do during social interactions because an absence of response can be interpreted due to symbolic transformations of function. Imagine, for example, a client asking her therapist if she could die of a panic attack. At first, telling her that this is very unlikely seems legitimate. But the therapist may have to be cautious about not reinforcing reassurance seeking if she asks the same question again (it may then be an instance of problematic experiential avoidance). Simply not responding may not extinguish the response, however, because the client may interpret the therapist's absence of response as a sign that he doesn't care, or even as confirmation of her worst fears. In this situation, an alternative approach is to help the client notice the function of her question and let her choose to persist in avoidance or to extinguish her behavior herself. The following exchange illustrates this approach:

CLIENT: Do you think I could die of a panic attack?

THERAPIST: This question seems to bother you a lot. I think you also asked me last time, am I correct?

CLIENT: Yeah . . . I know. But that really scares me. I just want to be sure.

THERAPIST: I can answer your question. But I would like you to notice the effect that it might have on your anxiety. How did you feel when I answered last time?

CLIENT: I felt better, reassured.

THERAPIST: Okay. How long did you feel better?

CLIENT: I don't remember. . . . Not very long. I felt okay after our session, but when I went to bed, I started to worry again.

THERAPIST: Were you thinking that you may die of a panic attack?

CLIENT: I was scared about that, yes.

THERAPIST: What do you think would happen if I answered your question again today?

CLIENT: This would make me feel better. It is very hard for me to think that I could die.

THERAPIST: Do you think that it would last this time?

CLIENT: I don't know. . . . . I know what you are going to tell me anyway. I keep asking my doctor and my family too. Everybody tells
me that I am not going to die. But I can't stop thinking that it's
going to happen.

THERAPIST: I know it is hard, what you are experiencing right now.
That is completely understandable. What I can do is give you a
choice. I can either answer your question, which, as you say, will
probably make you feel better for a while or you can choose to
leave this question with no answer. This will be probably more
difficult at first, but it could give you an opportunity to observe
what happens when you are not immediately reassured. What do
you think?

If the client chooses to leave the question with no answer, this would
be a signpost that the client is making progress toward less reactivity to
her thoughts. However, it is possible that she will want to be reassured this
time again. In that case, the therapist can choose to tell her the answer but
also profit from this situation by helping the client to observe the consequence of this choice. In particular, the therapist can encourage the client to
describe the evolution of her anxiety as the session goes on and to take note
of what happens next. With time, a better awareness of the effectiveness
of this strategy may help the client make a different choice. Such methods
should eventually allow a lack of a response to extinguish seeking reassurance without the symbolic functions of the lack of a response overwhelming this direct contingency process.

CLINICAL EXAMPLE

In the following vignette, you will find a number of the principles we laid
out in this chapter. In this vignette as in most other vignettes of this book,
we don't intend to demonstrate a complete transformation in the client's
behavior. These kinds of changes rarely happen in a few turns of speech.
But significant improvements can be generated over time by these kinds of
interactions, as they set the adequate context for change.

Observe how they combine in a natural flow of interactions between
the therapist and the client. This exchange happened with a 41-year-old
man presenting with depression, anxiety, and addiction to marijuana.

THERAPIST: So, how did it go yesterday? You had planned to work on
the house, right?

CLIENT: Well, it didn't go as I wanted. I woke up feeling tired, and I
didn't think I could do a good job if I was tired.

THERAPIST: You felt some tiredness, and you had the thought you couldn't work well with that feeling, huh? So what did you do?

CLIENT: I thought it would be better to rest in the morning and work on the house in the afternoon.

THERAPIST: Is that what you did?

CLIENT: Yeah. I was nervous that I would mess up the work on the roof if I didn't rest first.

THERAPIST: I see. You were tired and nervous about being tired, is that what you mean?

CLIENT: Yeah.

THERAPIST: How did you feel after deciding to rest?

CLIENT: I felt okay. I thought I had a plan for the day. I was feeling pretty good actually, and I started to rest on the couch, listening to some music.

THERAPIST: Okay. You said things didn't go as you wanted. So, what happened next?

CLIENT: Well, I ended up smoking. . . . You know, when I am alone . . . and I listen to some music. . . . I can't resist. I just feel really good when I smoke. In the moment it's hard not to think of that feeling, you know.

In these exchanges, the therapist guides the client in observing and describing each step of his experience, reformulating the main points of the sequence antecedent/rule–behavior–consequence. The client's problematic behaviors were influenced by antecedents (feelings of tiredness, urges, inaccurate and imprecise rules: "I didn't think I could do a good job if I was tired"; "It would be better to rest in the morning and work on the house in the afternoon"; "I can't resist"; "I just feel really good when I smoke"). He was also influenced by a history of reinforcing consequences (anxiety about tiredness decreases and feeling good increases when he smokes). Conversely, the positive consequence of working on the house failed to influence his behavior.

THERAPIST: You have a long habit of smoking when you are alone and when you listen to music. It's understandable that you have those urges. And I know it is hard for you not to smoke when you have those urges. Does that mean that you didn't do what you wanted to do?

On the one hand, the therapist normalizes urges and acknowledges the difficulty of resisting, given the history of smoking. On the other hand, he helps the client assess the effectiveness of his response.

CLIENT: No. I'm disappointed. And my wife was probably too. She didn't say anything, but I'm sure she was. If only I could feel less tired in the morning and not have those urges, I could function like everybody, you know . . .

The client formulates an inapplicable rule.

THERAPIST: This must be frustrating. I remember you really wanted to do this work on the roof, so I understand you are disappointed [*normalizes feelings*]. If I summarize what happened yesterday, it seems like it all started with feeling tired and anxious about feeling tired, right [*evokes tracking*]?

CLIENT: Yeah. Then I thought I would rest, but that was a bad idea because urges to smoke always come if I stay like that on the couch, with the music and all . . .

THERAPIST: Are you saying that choosing to rest was not the most effective strategy if you actually wanted to work on the roof yesterday?

CLIENT: Yeah. That was not a good idea. When I do that, it just doesn't work I think.

In these exchanges, the therapist helps the client assess the effectiveness of his behavior.

THERAPIST: Okay, well this is useful to know, don't you think?

CLIENT: Well yeah, but when I feel tired, it's like I can't think right. I know it is not a good thing to go back to sleep or to smoke but in the moment, I can't resist the urge.

THERAPIST: Okay, I see. So you would like to change the way you respond to these urges, right?

CLIENT: Yeah. If they could go away, that would help . . . [*inapplicable rule*].

THERAPIST: Do you think they will go away?

CLIENT: I doubt it. I feel tired all the time. And smoking? If my wife was not around, I would be smoking all day!

In these exchanges, the therapist helps the client focus on the effectiveness of his response rather than the impossible removal of the source of influence (the urges and the tiredness will likely not go away, at least not until he starts to engage in other activities).

THERAPIST: Do you have urges right now?

CLIENT: I have been feeling tired since I woke up a couple of hours ago, yeah. And I would definitely smoke if I could.

THERAPIST: That's interesting. Do you mind if I ask you more about your urges right now?

CLIENT: Okay.

THERAPIST: I think it is interesting that you said, "I would smoke if I could." Why do you think you are not smoking right now?

CLIENT: Well, I'm not going to smoke in your office, in therapy . . .

THERAPIST: Okay. Does that mean you are more motivated to stay here than going home and smoking?

CLIENT: I . . . I don't know . . . I didn't think about it that way I guess.

THERAPIST: I find it really interesting that you are having urges right now but you are still here, talking to me, instead of being home on your couch, smoking.

The therapist underlines steps toward effective behavior to reinforce progress.

CLIENT: But when I am here, it is easier to resist because I am not alone, you know.

THERAPIST: I see, okay. Why do you think it is easier?

CLIENT: Talking distracts me from the urges.

THERAPIST: Okay. Interesting! It's like getting rid of the urges, in a way?

CLIENT: Yeah, pretty much.

THERAPIST: But right now, we are talking about these urges, so your attention is all on them. And you are still here . . .

CLIENT: I guess I can resist for a while.

In these exchanges, the therapist establishes a connection between what is happening in the moment and what usually happens in the client's life by asking if the client is feeling the urges. He then helps the client notice the increased flexibility of his behavior in the presence of the source of influence (despite the urges to smoke, he is not smoking) to help transform the function of the urges ("from impossible to resist" to "can be resisted").

THERAPIST: Is it hard to resist right now?

CLIENT: As we talk about it, yeah.

THERAPIST: Is that okay if I ask you more about it?

CLIENT: Okay.

THERAPIST: How does that feel exactly?

CLIENT: You mean, what the urges feel like?

THERAPIST: Yeah . . . What are those sensations like, exactly? Can you try to describe them as concretely as possible? Like you would describe a picture that I can't see.

The therapist uses analogical framing to help the client describe the urges.

[Here, the client describes the urges during several minutes, encouraged by the therapist to be as precise as possible and to focus on the intrinsic characteristics of the sensations.]

THERAPIST: It seemed you were able to stay in contact with your urges without smoking. What do you think?

The therapist helps the client notice the increased flexibility of his response to urges during the past minutes of describing his sensations.

CLIENT: Yeah. I usually don't go that far. I light a joint before . . .

THERAPIST: What do you think you are going to do when you leave this room?

CLIENT: Well, I guess I should start working on the roof. That's what I should do, right?

The client shows signs of pliance.

THERAPIST: I think that what is important is that you do what works best for you. What do you think will work best for you, when you leave this room?

CLIENT: Working on the house.

THERAPIST: Why?

CLIENT: Because I don't want to spend my days smoking on the couch. I need to finish that work on the house. I want to see my wife look at me in a different way tonight.

After having evoked the client's observation, description, and tracking, established effectiveness as a criterion for coherence, transformed the function of the sources of influence through describing urges and evoking a different response (staying in contact with the urges), and reinforced progress toward effective behaviors, the client is finally presented with an alternative choice. He chooses the effective behavior over the problematic behavior but expresses this choice in a way that indicates pliance rather than tracking ("That's what I should do, right?" asking for the therapist's approbation). Therefore, the therapist reframes the client's choice as a matter of effectiveness to reach his own goals, and encourages him to connect his behavior with a desired natural consequence (tracking over pliance).

Having presented the principles that guide the use of language to activate and shape behavior change, we now turn to an area of behavior problems that requires specific framing skills: issues with the self.

 **CHAPTER SUMMARY**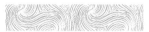

In this chapter, you learned to use language to activate and shape behavior change in the therapy room. Here are the main principles to remember:

- When the elements of the context influencing the client's behavior can't be removed or replaced, it is possible to use language to alter their impact. To this end, you can use language processes to help the client consider more effective behaviors. This consists of:
  - Increasing functional contextual awareness in order to adapt responses to relevant contingencies. You can:
    - Evoke observation of the client's experience.
    - Evoke description of the client's experience.
    - Evoke tracking of the client's experience.
  - Promote functional sense making through normalization and assessment of response effectiveness. You can:
    - Establish or acknowledge the coherence of psychological experiences.
    - Reframe the client's behavioral problem in terms of effectiveness.
  - Increase response flexibility by targeting current sources of influence or current responses. You can:
    - Change the context around the source of influence.
    - Change the context around the response to evoke a new response.
- To strengthen changes that begin to occur in the client's behavioral repertoire, it is possible to use principles of learning (shaping), while connecting what is happening in the therapy room to the client's life outside. This consists of:
  - Reinforcing progress. You can:
    - Reinforce step by step.
    - Reinforce tracking over pliance.
  - Weakening problematic behaviors. You can:
    - Deliver and orient to undesirable consequences.
    - Block behaviors.
    - Extinguish behaviors.

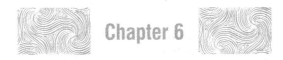

Chapter 6

Building a Flexible Sense of Self

The topic of "self" is key in many approaches to psychological intervention. In this chapter, you will learn how to use RFT principles to deal with issues related to the self. We will examine some of the typical problems faced by clients in this area, and we will explore how an RFT approach to the self can inform therapeutic techniques that foster variability, stability, functional coherence, and a healthy sense of responsibility.

THE CONCEPT OF SELF

A regular theme in this book is how our actions are highly influenced by the coherence of the relational networks that constitute our language. One area in which inadequate coherence can be particularly powerful and harmful is the way we conceptualize ourselves.

Even small children are encouraged to define themselves with labels that supposedly point toward relatively stable patterns of behaviors. Parents may deliberately encourage positive labels of this kind (e.g., "You are so smart!" or "You are so sweet"), but as these labels gain in importance, they may also be used almost as levers to coerce compliance with social expectations (e.g., "You are so sloppy! Look at this room of yours!" or "You know better than that! You are way too smart to do something that dumb!")

Symbolic behavior does more than describe overarching categories; it also encourages us to maintain behaviors that are coherent with the labels we use for ourselves. Personality traits are due to a variety of factors, including patterns of temperament that can already be observed at birth, but behavioral consistencies across time and situations are likely amplified and in some areas may even be due to the labels we apply to them. A child may be told that she is very shy based purely on her behavior around other people (e.g., she doesn't talk much, and she stays close to her parents when strangers are around). This definition constitutes a symbolic network that includes a relation of equivalence between the self and "shy" and a relation of hierarchy between shy and all behaviors that usually fall in this category. Although such a label might have started as a simple observation in a specific situation, it can become a new source of influence over future behaviors. When asked to play with other kids at school, the girl might think, "I'm too shy, I can't be around people I don't know." After several years, we forget that the label actually came *after* the observation of relevant behavior in particular situations. The girl herself may think she avoids strangers *because* she is shy, and she may offer this explanation to others—when it actually doesn't explain her behavior at all—it just labels it and in turn encourages it.

What we see in this example is that from a simple observation, a definition of the self can emerge and lead to rules about the self. If a person defines herself as friendly, this might be because she showed warmth toward others in the past, and they responded by complimenting her on her "friendliness" or calling her "friendly." Now that she *is* friendly in her mind, it is logical and coherent to conclude that she will show warmth in the present and in the future. And if she is friendly, she must show warmth toward most people. And if she doesn't, there must be something wrong with her because she is supposed to be friendly. Ultimately, the "friendly" label could prevent her from seeing the variety of her behaviors and experiences, which could have a cost (e.g., when feeling anger toward others could serve a useful role in reasonable limit setting). In a sense it is as if we try to *be* the label we live inside in order to maintain the coherence of self. Helping clients learn to "be themselves" with more flexibility will require backing out of this system.

PROBLEMS WITH SELF-CONCEPTS

The problem with maintaining coherence of the self by behaving according to self-labels is that it can dramatically narrow the variety of our actions and reduce our range of options in responding to people or situations. In particular, it often prevents clients we see in therapy from engaging in new and more effective behaviors, which could bring more satisfaction in the long term. For example, a person might say, "I have always been selfish. That's just the way I am and the way people see me." Because she really does want to help others and be seen differently, she starts to consider engaging in altruistic actions. However, as soon as she finds something she can do, she may think, "I'm only doing this because I want people to know I'm not selfish. But *that* is selfish. I will always be like that." In fact, it seems as though every time the coherence of a relational network is threatened, language restores it by transforming the function of events that seem to conflict with previously established concepts. Other labels such as "I am depressed," "I am a victim of abuse," "I am borderline," are all potential barriers to effective change because every action that contradicts these definitions can be transformed by language to fit the existing relational network. For example, as she imagines going back to work, a person suffering from depression may think, "I won't be able to work because I am depressed" (i.e. "A depressed person wouldn't go to work; hence going to work would invalidate my feelings"), and thus decide to stay home. A person who was a victim of abuse may think, "I can't have a normal relationship with my partner because I was abused" (i.e., "Having a normal relationship would mean minimizing the abuse and my suffering") and as a result avoid intimate physical contact. A person suffering from borderline personality disorder may think, "It's normal that I get angry at people since I am borderline" (i.e., "I wouldn't be borderline anymore if I was not getting angry at people, and my suffering wouldn't be recognized anymore") and as a result continue to start fights. In every case, relations built by language guide clients' behaviors so that coherence is maintained despite the problems that result from not going to work, avoiding relationships, or getting angry at people.

The problems caused by excessive attachment to definitions or concepts of the self are pervasive in psychological disorders. Some clients, whom we often categorize as rigid, identify so strongly with a label that they would seemingly do anything to avoid contradicting it. This is common when people have found "answers" in a diagnosis, even if the label might be perceived negatively (e.g., depression, psychosis, attention-deficit/ hyperactivity disorder). Other clients "label shop"; that is, they look for the right label that will finally help make sense of their history and responses and let them know who they really are. People suffering from problems in emotion regulation (e.g., borderline personality disorder, bipolar disorders) may end up identifying with more general labels, such as "unstable," or with the idea that "no one is as messed up as me." Clients also report a feeling of emptiness when they can't find the right categories. Some would adopt any definition, even negative ones, as long as it makes them feel whole—or coherent, in RFT terms.

When clients are unhappy with their lives, they naturally look for means to change it. Here again, the way they approach their self has an important impact on the solutions they try to apply. If they see themselves as "the problem," they might change the definition of the self and become attached to this new definition to bring coherence back into the self-network. For example, a woman who has learned to see herself and to behave as a perfect mother may attack herself through harsh self-criticisms if she fails even once in her role as a mother. She is now a "bad mother." This is painful, but in her eyes, it feels right and coherent to do so, and may paradoxically feel soothing (i.e., "I did something wrong, but at least it makes sense since I am a bad mother"). On the one hand, an excessive sense of responsibility can therefore lead people to ignore the numerous contextual variables that contribute to ineffective behaviors and to target instead the self even though it will make ineffective actions even more likely. On the other hand, losing a sense of responsibility, or self-efficacy, can lead to hopelessness, as is often the case for people suffering from addiction or depression. They feel like they have tried everything to make things work without success and thus come to the conclusion that they just can't do anything to improve their lives. Again, this is a coherent conclusion but may not be a useful way of approaching the self.

Coherence is necessary in the self, but if it is found at a narrow conceptual level (i.e., inside the closed categories), it leads to rigidity and instability because no such category can capture a human life. Narrow self-concepts can become an excessive source of influence over our behaviors, much like the other symbolic and intrinsic processes we saw in previous chapters. Since the concepts we apply to the self are *symbolic* sources of influence, problems linked to the self can often be approached with the same techniques we presented in Chapter 5. However, it is useful to devote a whole chapter to this topic rather than treating it as any other kind of symbolic source of influence because dealing with issues linked to the self involves a specific and extensive use of particular symbolic relations, namely, *deictic (perspective-taking)* and *hierarchical* framing.

AN RFT PERSPECTIVE ON THE SELF

In order to apply RFT principles to problems with the self, we first need to explore how RFT accounts for various senses of self. We will see in this section how stability originally builds up across multiple perspective-taking and hierarchical experiences and is then transferred to elaborate networks of self-definitions. Problems start to arise once we lose this sense of self as a point of view and superordinate term and begin to identify with labels of various supposed features of the self.

The Origin of the Sense of Self

It is useful to remind ourselves that human activities are interactions between an organism and a context. RFT applies the same approach to the self. The self is not considered to be an entity but a various set of relational activities controlled by contextual variables. It would actually be more technically correct, despite its awkward feel, to speak of "self-ing" rather than "the self." It sounds awkward because we often label activities with a noun rather than a verb (e.g., "language," "thought"). Indeed, we generally think of the self as a *thing*, almost like an object we could observe and touch. However, as soon as we point to something concrete that we think *is* the self (e.g., one's brain), we are disappointed because it doesn't seem to fully match our feeling of having or being a self. The self seems broader and more abstract. From an RFT perspective, this feeling is created by a relational activity applied to multiple experiences.

We generally think of the self as the agent of our behaviors, the conscious place where we make decisions based on what we perceive in the environment. Self is often viewed as a kind of control tower monitoring the relevant information and transmitting orders to behave in certain ways. RFT researchers believe this feeling of a self that centralizes information and gives orders likely begins as we learn to discriminate our perceptions from others' perceptions. A progressive distinction develops in a child's history between what he can see, feel, smell, touch, hear, and taste and what others perceive with their own senses. For example, a child might stand in front of the TV, which prevents his little brother from seeing the screen. His mother then takes his hand and says, "Don't stay here. Your brother can't see from there." Words are taught, such as up and down, or in front and behind, or over and under, and require a frame of reference (as seen from a particular point of view). Multiple experiences like this occur as the child interacts with others, which over time allow him to make the distinction between things that happen from his point of view (perceptions of sensations, movements of his body) and what others perceive from their own points of view. Further, the child is exposed to multiple verbal interactions involving relations of perspective between *I* and *you*, *here* and *there*, and *now* and *then*. The child may be asked, for example, "How do you feel now?"; "What did you see yesterday?"; "What do you think your brother would like to have for his birthday? What about you?" Each of us goes through this multiple exemplar training in interpersonal, spatial, and temporal perspective taking. As these dimensions begin to come together, a sense emerges that experience is normally perceived from I/here/now, but that other points of view are possible. In other words, a sense of perspective taking emerges.

When the Self Becomes a Concept

In order to notice that experiences are perceived from a point of view, we first need to notice experiences themselves. Perspective taking is applied to the things we sense, feel, think, or do. Inner knowledge is just an extension of external knowledge, despite the illusion that these dimensions are radically different. We started this book with learning to say "apple" given an apple, but it would have been just as correct to say learning to say "apple" given the sight of an apple, or even learning to say "apple" given particular forms of retinal stimulation. Learning to say what we feel is a bit more complicated only because the community that trains us has a bit harder time discriminating when we are, say, hungry, than when an apple is likely being seen. The relational framing skills are identical.

Learning to note our own experiences is extremely useful because, with time, we become able to explain why we feel the way we feel, to predict how we are going to feel, and to communicate this useful information to others. For example, if a person feels pleasant emotions when she is around her friends, she knows she is likely to feel this way again by spending more time with them. If she tells her friends that seeing them makes her feel good, they will know that she likes being around them and that inviting her more often would be appreciated. We learn about ourselves in part by *noticing* our experiences, which in turn allows us to inform the social community about how to be of use to us.

For humans, because we have relational framing skills, anything we notice inevitably enters our relational networks. Once it is there, a wide variety of derived relations tend to occur. Experiences we perceive are quickly evaluated and categorized. If you notice a sensation of pain in your stomach, you may soon generate a possible explanation for it and try to find out what you should do about it. For example, you may think that you ate something spoiled or that you are sick and need medication, or that you are hungry and need to eat again. Thus, not only do we take perspective on our experiences, and notice these experiences, but we also build and derive networks around these experiences.

If talking in front of an audience makes you feel painful sensations of anxiety, you may evaluate this activity as bad for you. If it makes you feel good instead, it becomes something categorized as "pleasant." Thus, you engage in three relational activities with regard to your self: you take perspective (I/here/now), you notice (I feel pain), and you evaluate (public speaking is bad because it makes me feel anxious). Because all these activities happen almost simultaneously, and often more implicitly than explicitly, it is difficult to notice each as a different process. Furthermore, people around us reinforce us less for noticing perspective taking than for noticing the content of this experience and how we evaluate it. After giving the talk, a friend asks, "How did you feel? I thought *you were* good!" and you may respond, "Really? Oh I felt horrible. I don't like public speaking. *I am* a terrible speaker. . . ." In a sense, as the experience is evaluated and elaborated, we move from noticing an experience to *becoming* this experience as a quality of self (i.e., a frame of equivalence, or coordination, is built between the self and the experience). If we act with caution, we are labeled and label ourselves as cautious. If we worry often, we become "worriers." If we feel sadness, we are sad and perhaps "depressed," and so on. And since all these labels are themselves related to a number of other evaluative labels (e.g., worrying is stupid, it is a sign of weakness, it is not healthy, etc.), we become concepts evaluated like any other objects of our universe.

The Traps of the Self-Concept

Identifying ourselves with our actions and experiences would not necessarily be a problem if it didn't influence our behaviors in a narrowed, and often detrimental way. One main issue comes from our inability to identify with a multiplicity of labels. Contradicting experiences and actions appear as incoherent in our networks, so only a few are selected to qualify ourselves. Once you have started to see yourself as shy, it becomes difficult to notice when you are not. Clients who say, "I have always been anxious" or "I am passive" will tend to forget times when they were different and dismiss new instances where they show an alternative pattern. They may say, "Well, I am not anxious right now, but that is only because . . . " or "Sure, I do decide things on my own, but only when I feel really self-confident." Our identity is thus reduced to a limited number of facets while the richness and the potential of our experiences and actions are actually far greater. Symbolic relations transform the function of the events of our environment and prevent us from responding to other functions (e.g., a sensation is "unbearable," so we avoid it even though it is not intrinsically impossible to bear). Similarly, when the self becomes a label, we engage in behaviors coherent with this label, or we distort what we do so that the label fits.

It is easy to see how behavioral problems can arise from excessive attachment to self-concepts. Clients avoid engaging in activities that could bring lasting satisfaction because these actions don't fit the image they have of themselves. A client may see himself as too depressed to ever find a job. Another may think she is too immature to have children. As a result, life satisfaction is inhibited because the gap between what matters and what is being done remains large in order to maintain the coherence of self-concepts. Even positive labels applied to the self can lead to a narrowing of clients' behavioral repertoire. If a client thinks of himself as self-confident, he may avoid situations where he would not appear that way (e.g., accepting a job offer that requires taking more responsibilities); he may avoid sharing vulnerabilities, thus limiting the intimacy of relationships; he may insist that others reflect back his self-concept even when his actions would not lead to this evaluation; he may compare himself to others and secretly enter into a prideful and lonely world in which he is "better than" others. Even positive labels can therefore put us on the path to a narrowed and unsatisfying life when we buy into them.

If a life experience contradicting the self-concept can't be ignored because it is too big, the incoherence it creates is often perceived as deeply disturbing. People can become angry or even violent when self-concepts are threatened, particularly among those who are overly attached to their self-concepts (Bushman et al., 2009). This process of entanglement is seen in the clinic all the time. For example, a client may see himself as "broken" after a traumatic event. Another may feel "worthless" after losing her job. They will likely also derive rules such as "I can't be around people if I am broken now" or "I won't be able to find another job because I am worthless now." In this case also, even a positive event can be experienced as a disturbance of the self-concept. For example, although moving to another country for a new job may be a very good thing, it can also lead to a deep change in the way a client perceives herself. She doesn't feel as confident in her interactions with others, she starts doubting her skills at work, and she keeps seeing herself as fundamentally different from the people around her. As a result, she may withdraw and avoid situations where she feels like she doesn't fit, even though those situations may bring satisfaction in the long run. If self-concepts are readjusted to fit the new event, then future actions will be programmed in coherence with the new label.

From an RFT perspective, rigidity, instability, emptiness, defensiveness, self-criticism, or hopelessness can all arise from attachment to labels and evaluations derived from these labels. However, self-concepts also bring some symbolic stability to people's lives, which is probably why it is so difficult to let go of labels even when holding onto them is harmful. Many of us, including our clients, strive to know who and what we are in order to feel grounded. How can we find a balance between stability in the self and variability in the behavioral repertoire?

THE FLEXIBLE SELF

The Goal

It is natural to want to have a concept of "who we are." Language naturally seeks coherence due to the centrality of derived relations in symbolic behavior, but finding coherence in the elimination of any contradictions among self-concepts can happen only if we deny certain experiences, or if we distort these experiences symbolically (remember what we saw in Chapter 3 about essential coherence). The goal is to find a more flexible form of self-coherence that can empower people to be more open experientially, to be more honest with themselves, and to form a foundation that can allow them to act more energetically in their own interests.

Why This Is Important, from an RFT Point of View

Because looking for stability in narrow self-concepts leads to rigidity in our behaviors and limits the variety of experiences we are willing to contact, stability must be found in a different way. RFT suggests that building a flexible sense of self is possible by means of three ways of using relational framing: (1) Observing, describing and tracking experiences (using different kinds of frames as seen in Chapter 5, while avoiding frames of coordination between the self and these experiences); (2) observing the activity of perspective taking (using *deictic framing*); and (3) conceptualizing the self as a container or context of all psychological experiences (using *hierarchical framing*). The active integrated sense of self that results is both stable and variable; coherent and open; integrated and empowering; compassionate and responsible.

The flexible self begins with ongoing self-awareness: noticing experiences in the moment, not with the goal of self-management or self-manipulation but merely with the goal of awareness. Now I'm feeling this; now I'm thinking that; now this sensation occurred. Ongoing experience is grist for the mill—it is the substance of life as it flows through our moments of living. By learning to notice experiences and their contexts, and to move on, it is possible to increase contact with a variety of experiences and see the variation of our behaviors in the contexts we are in. This level of knowledge in turn sets up a more reflective self-awareness that is extended in time or across settings—such as noticing how what is felt now differs from what was felt an hour ago, or a month ago; or noticing that urges to act in one context differ from those in other contexts.

We bring perspective-taking skills to these experiences. We don't just see—we see that we see, and we do so from a particular point of view in time, place, and person. Flexibility in perspective taking is also possible and it is essential to empathy and social awareness, but once a sense of "I/here/now" fully forms, it anchors our experience. I can imagine being somewhere else, but yet I'm here. I can view myself in imagination from the distant past or the far-flung future, but yet I am imagining in the now. I can imagine what it might be like to be you looking back at me, but *I* am doing that act of imagination. When this skill is at strength, we can continuously expand perspective taking across time, place, and person and then come back to the "I/here/now" constellation, which means that perspective taking is both individualistic and social; both limited in time and place, and expansive across time and space. There is stability in that skill: stability is found in perspective taking itself, and variability is preserved in our experiences and actions.

This kind of contemplative and nonjudgmental process of perspective taking tends to come and go inside the evaluative relations that inevitably build around the self, but perspective taking contains within it another symbolic relation that can also be consistently applied to the unavoidable evaluations, judgments, contradiction, and labels about ourselves. Experiences are contained within awareness, and "contained within" is a hierarchical relation. By consciously including experiences, behaviors, and evaluations as part of a hierarchical network, variability in actions and experiences can be preserved, while still establishing a sense of stability in the self. This is not just abstract theory. An RFT study found with high-risk adolescents that adding hierarchical framing to perspective taking helped participants deal with difficult thoughts more effectively (Luciano et al., 2011; see also Foody, Barnes-Holmes, Barnes-Holmes, & Luciano, 2013).

Finally, from an RFT point of view, it is worth remembering that "self" is not a thing—it is a set of symbolic actions. People learn to "self" much as one learns to talk, think, or dance. Viewed this way, the self is not an entity that fully controls or is fully controlled; rather, it is a set of symbolic interactions between an organism and the context. A flexible sense of responsibility can be developed upon this interaction, by helping clients perceive the mutual influence between themselves and the context.

How This Method Touches on Various Clinical Traditions

Issues of self are dominant in many clinical traditions, including humanistic, existential, and analytic approaches. An example is Kohut's "self-psychology" approach to psychoanalytic psychotherapy (1971/2009). In Kohut's approach, the generation of a cohesive self is thwarted due in part to a failure of parents and others to put themselves in the child's shoes, and the child's resulting inability to let go of grandiose visions of omnipotence. Although some details of this approach may not translate beyond the boundaries of psychoanalysis, the centrality of perspective taking in therapy and its role in leading to a different kind of self-coherence is resonant with RFT.

Another example that is perhaps even more resonant is Carl Rogers's approach (1951) in which consistency with the structure of the self determines the degree to which experiences can be known symbolically without distortion. If a self-structure is rigid or narrow, experiences are closed off, and a sense of incongruence develops as the person tries to maintain a fiction. Psychological health is defined in part by the degree to which experiences can be assimilated symbolically into the self-structure. Greater self-acceptance (fostered in therapy through unconditional positive regard and empathy) leads to a diminishment of an unhealthy gap between the "real self" and a self-defensive "ideal self." As that gap diminishes, a great sense of congruence emerges with greater potential for self-actualization. Rogers's approach is largely in agreement with the approach taken here, but RFT adds a bottom-up process-based explanation that leads to more specific forms of assessment, analysis, and intervention.

How to Do It

The flexible self is built on four features: an ongoing and reflective awareness of changing self-experiences; an awareness of continuous perspective taking; a coherent and contextual sense of self; and the interactive nature of "self" as an action. None of these can stand fully apart from the others, and thus as these components translate into interactions in the therapy room, we will draw upon multiple features.

Finding Variability in Awareness of Experiences

Developing a greater sense of awareness of experiences through an ongoing and reflective process helps clients recognize that their psychological experiences—thoughts, sensations, emotions, or actions—are more various than what they generally think. Even if it made sense to define ourselves by the content of experiences, there would not be just a few, but a wide variety of experiences. For example, a client who is mostly influenced by limited labels such as "I am selfish" can be led to notice instances where his experiences don't match this definition (e.g., feeling worried about someone else's well-being). Awareness of experiences and their variability brings useful incoherence into the self-network since the client can't be just "a selfish person" anymore. He is in fact a lot of things, some of which contradict each other.

It is difficult to notice the variety of our experiences because derivation processes are often driven by essential coherence, which tends to narrow our perception. Once we notice an experience and label it, it begins to hide other experiences, especially if we identify with this label. We already saw in Chapter 5 how to help clients observe, describe, and track their experiences with greater precision, thus improving the awareness that these experiences are various and changing. All these techniques can be used to increase variability in the sense of self, but in this chapter, we will focus on the use of perspective taking because in our experience, it often helps clients transition toward other dimensions of the flexible self (in particular, the awareness of perspective taking itself).

Stabilizing Perspective Taking. To be able to notice the process of derivation and the constant change and flow of experiences, you need a stable point of view. You need to stop moving with the experiences and stay still. Metaphorically, this is as if you were watching a multicolor train slowly passing by in front of you. If you walk at the same pace as the train while staring at a red wagon in front of you, it will feel like the whole train is red. But if you stop moving and keep looking at the train as it passes in front of you, you will now see that there are many wagons with different colors. In the same way, stabilizing perspective taking on our experiences can allow us to witness the flow of those experiences.

A variety of techniques can be used to stabilize perspective taking on our experiences. This skill is often trained through formal practice (e.g., meditation exercises), but in this section we will focus only on methods that can be used in natural verbal interactions.

A simple approach is to repeatedly direct clients' attention to what they can perceive in the present moment. As the session goes on, you can ask them what they feel and you can emphasize cues that help them notice what is immediately available to their perception. In particular, using adverbial phrases of time such as "now," "right now," "in this moment," and phrases of place such as "here," "right here," "from where you are" helps ground the client in a here/now point of view. Slowing down your speech and using gestures that increase the salience of a fixed point as you talk can also help the client "stop moving." At the same time, using gestures that emphasize changes in perceptions helps them notice the flow of experiences. Observe this technique in the following exchange:

CLIENT: I am really stressed out.

THERAPIST: Right now?

CLIENT: Yeah, it's been going on all day. It's constant.

THERAPIST: I see. . . . What are you feeling exactly?

CLIENT: I don't know . . . I am edgy, jumpy . . . easily irritable today.

THERAPIST: Right now (*pointing to the floor with his finger*), as you are telling me about it, are you feeling irritated and worried?

CLIENT: (*sighs*). . . . Well, yeah,. . . . It's just that even talking about it makes me feel anxious.

THERAPIST: I see. Is there a specific sensation that you can notice right now in your body? (*Shows his own body with his open hand against his chest.*)

The therapist orients the client's observation toward sensations in order to help him notice changes (in contrast, sticking with self labels like "anxious" tends to prevent flexible observation because it maintains coordination between the self and the experience).

CLIENT: Some kind of contraction in my belly.

THERAPIST: Are you feeling it just now?

CLIENT: Yeah . . . Uh . . . No, I don't know, I think it's gone now.

THERAPIST: Ah okay, interesting. So what are you feeling now?

CLIENT: You are going to think I'm crazy. . . . I feel the contraction again now.

THERAPIST: (*gently playful*) Ah, it's back! It seems like this sensation is playing tricks on you, uh?

CLIENT: (*smiling*) Yeah.

THERAPIST: How does that feel to smile a bit now?

CLIENT: It feels good.

THERAPIST: Is the contraction still there? (*Points at the client's belly.*)

CLIENT: Mmm . . . Yeah, a little.

THERAPIST: Is that like ups and downs? (*Mimics the movement of a wave.*)

CLIENT: Yeah, exactly. I feel okay, and then I feel stressed again. It's been like that all day long.

THERAPIST: Ah, okay. All day long, it has been changing back and forth? (*Moves his hand back and forth in front of him.*)

CLIENT: Yeah.

In this exchange you can see that the client originally reports his feelings with little attention to the variety of his sensations. He even says, "It's constant" and happening "all day"—which is extraordinarily unlikely at the experiential level. It is "true" only at the symbolic level, and then only by not noticing. As the therapist helps him pay attention to the present moment and to specific parts of his body, he starts noticing the fluctuation of these experiences. The generalization the client began with is never challenged verbally; rather, the client's own experience challenges the generalization.

A similar approach can be applied to the process of thinking itself. In this case, the therapist helps the client notice the stream of derived relations moment by moment. Observe this method in the following vignette:

THERAPIST: You just stopped talking. Did you start thinking of something?

CLIENT: Yes. I just realized that I am not going to be able to get my work done tonight.

THERAPIST: And what about now? What's on your mind?

CLIENT: I'm concerned about spending time talking with you here while I barely have the time to finish my work these days.

THERAPIST: How does it feel to tell me about this?

CLIENT: I feel a bit embarrassed.

THERAPIST: It feels embarrassing to tell me about your concerns?

The therapist reformulates the client's observation by avoiding frames of coordination between the self and the experience (from "I feel embarrassed" to "it feels embarrassing").

CLIENT: Yes, because I know it is important that I do this work with you, or else I won't get anything done in any parts of my life.

THERAPIST: Your concerns seem to have shifted to your whole life now. Did you notice? It seems like one thought is leading you to the next. Is that what you are experiencing right now?

CLIENT: I have a lot on my mind, yes.

THERAPIST: Does it feel like thoughts are racing? Or maybe like a lot of thoughts are there at the same time?

CLIENT: I think of one thing, then another very quickly. That's why I stopped talking earlier. I really have a hard time focusing these days.

THERAPIST: How about right now?

CLIENT: What about now?

THERAPIST: Are you focusing on what we are talking about?

CLIENT: Yes, it is better. When you ask me these questions, it helps me refocus on what we are doing.

THERAPIST: What is on your mind right now?

CLIENT: I am a bit confused.

THERAPIST: Yeah? Thoughts racing again?

Again, the therapist orients the client's observation toward her experiences as a way of undermining frames of coordination between the self and the experiences (e.g., from "I am a bit confused" to "thoughts are racing").

CLIENT: More like a dilemma.

THERAPIST: Like several contradicting thoughts at the same time?

CLIENT: Yes. Exactly.

In this exchange, the therapist doesn't discuss the content of the client's thoughts. Although dealing with content can be useful for other purposes (e.g., see Chapter 5 and Chapter 7), the goal here is to help the client detach herself a bit from evaluations of the content of self-concepts in order to notice the process of evaluating itself. Repeatedly asking the client what she perceived in the moment leads her to notice how her thoughts are constantly changing. This way, the client also notices the variety, and often the contradiction of the evaluations she derives from her experiences.

Shifting Perspective Taking. A second approach that can be used to enhance the perception that experiences are richer than they seem is to evoke *shifts* in perspective taking. Following the metaphor of the train, this would be like looking in different directions to notice that there is not just one wagon but there are many wagons of different colors. Asking a client to remember different situations and moments of his life and to notice the changes in self-experiences is much like that. Depending on situations and times, we can contact a variety of experiences and label ourselves in very different ways. Clients easily forget this variability when they are attached to the content of a specific self-concept.

Observe an example of this approach in the following vignette with a client suffering from social anxiety:

CLIENT: I tried to start conversations with colleagues, but there is nothing really interesting in my life. I am just not this kind of person, you know, who always has interesting things to say.

THERAPIST: What kind of person are you?

CLIENT: I am reserved. I prefer listening to people. I guess I am passive and boring. But that's what I am. I have always been like that, so I guess I should not try to be someone else. I feel like I am embarrassing myself trying to engage in conversations like that.

THERAPIST: Are you this kind of person with your family? You said you often have long conversations with your sister. . . .

The therapist evokes a first perspective taking shift.

CLIENT: Oh yeah, but that's completely different. I have known her for my whole life. It's easy to talk to her.

THERAPIST: What kind of person are you with her?

CLIENT: You mean how do I talk to her? What do I do with her?

THERAPIST: Yeah. Are you reserved, passive, and boring?

CLIENT: No . . . I don't think so! No, I think I am very different with my sister because I feel comfortable with her. I talk more, I can make jokes.

THERAPIST: That sounds like a different you.

CLIENT: Yeah. But in general, I am very shy. Very passive.

THERAPIST: In what other situations are you this version of you?

The therapist evokes new perspective taking shifts.

CLIENT: Where I am passive and shy?

THERAPIST: Yeah.

CLIENT: I am very shy when I don't know people. At work, because we have professional relationships it is very difficult for me to feel comfortable. It's like we know each other but not really. Although . . . My colleagues seem to get along well together. . . . But for me, it takes too much time to feel comfortable enough so I stay behind, excluded.

THERAPIST: How about here? What kind of person are you with me?

The therapist evokes another perspective taking shift.

CLIENT: Hmm . . . I don't know! I guess . . . I am not as passive as at work. . . . I talk a lot with you because I need to tell you what is going on in my life.

THERAPIST: So, you are not reserved?

CLIENT: I guess not.

THERAPIST: How about shy? Are you shy when you are here?

CLIENT: I don't think so. Not so much.

THERAPIST: What kind of person are you here with me then?

CLIENT: I guess I am . . . normal. Not too reserved but not friendly either because it is therapy. I talk with my sister about my life too, but it is different.

THERAPIST: Would you say that the versions of you, the kinds of person you are, are different at work, with your sister, and with me?

The therapist evokes observation of the various self experiences.

CLIENT: Hmm . . . Yeah, definitely. I guess we are all different depending on where we are and who is around us.

In this exchange, the therapist asks the client what perception she has of herself in a variety of situations. Note that she doesn't explicitly challenge the labels in order to lead the client to adopt another definition of herself. Rather, she helps her see that these definitions are highly dependent on the context and can thus be extremely various. While the exchange starts with the client defining herself as passive, boring, or shy in a quite absolute way, she ends up with three different "selves" that are all legitimate in describing who she is. When conducting an exchange like this, it is easy to fall into the trap of trying to convince clients that they are not really what they think they are. Here, you see that the therapist gently and playfully challenges the client by simply exploring what she experiences in a variety of situations. It shows curiosity for the richness of the client's life and avoids a priori conclusions about what she actually experiences. Exploring multiple situations with openness allows the client to show different facets of her personality and to start seeing beyond labels, which currently restrain the variability of her actions. Eventually, labels might even be abandoned altogether by focusing on describing experiences instead. In fact, if the attachment to a self-definition is strong, the therapist will tend to prefer exploring experiences rather than self-definitions (e.g., "What do your <u>interactions</u> with your sister look like? And what about your interactions *with me?"). This way, the client feels less need to defend any particular definition and is more likely to let go of self-definitions altogether (i.e., framing the self in coordination with experiences is undermined).*

Finding Stability in Perspective Taking

If we were to only notice the constant change of experiences but still believed that we *are* these experiences, our sense of self would probably feel extremely unstable because at the content level, evaluations and judgments can feel essentially contradictory. A sense of instability can be useful as a step to shake the rigid foundations of an ossified self-concept, but it is not a viable position in the long term. There is a source of stability, however, in the very act of noticing—namely, that we are noticing from a point of view defined by time, place, and person. An I/here/now point of view may not be continuously evident, but it is continuously *available*. Using the train metaphor again, it means that as we stop moving to observe the wagons passing by, we can also notice that we are not moving. The ground under our feet remains the same while we watch the wagons. An infinite number of wagons could pass, at various speeds and in both directions, and our feet would still be at the same place, here and now. If we look in the direction of different wagons or walk along the train and look at different wagons, we can also notice that each time, our feet are under us. As soon as we move there, there becomes here. Thus everywhere we go, an I/here/now point of view goes with us.

While a dramatic change in our experiences can threaten self-concepts, nothing, either bad or good, can threaten perspective taking as long as consciousness itself survives. Thus, the sense of stability and continuity of the self can be improved with no need to feel attached, threatened by, or defensive of any of the labels of the self-concept. We can feel whole and stable across time and situations, regardless of how we feel or what we think.

In development, perspective taking emerges alongside the awareness of experiences. Both arise together, which is often the case in formal contemplative practice as well. Nevertheless, it is important to notice the *distinction* between experiences and perspective taking. This distinction is abstracted by the client as she observes the variety of her experiences and notices what is common across these experiences. This is sometimes felt as a strange, fleeting, transcendent experience: like a person noticing she is talking, then noticing that she is noticing that she is talking, and then noticing that she is noticing that she is noticing that she is talking. Because the symbolic relations that give rise to perspective taking expand across time, place, and person, there may be a sense of oneness, or merging with others, or timelessness. In these "spiritual" moments, it is as if all derivation processes except for perspective taking are shut down, leaving a sense of self independent from any other experiences (Hayes, 1984; Villatte, Villatte, & Hayes, 2012).

Noticing the Common Perspective Taking Activity across Experiences. In the more day-to-day world of psychotherapy, "ah ha" moments of this kind are perhaps less important than are techniques you can use through natural verbal interactions (we will explore more formal practice exercises in Chapter 9). Often, noticing the common perspective-taking activity across all experiences begins with the observation of a variety of experiences, as we addressed in the previous section. For example, as the client is encouraged to notice his feelings, thoughts, and sensations in the present moment and compare those in different situations and different times, he is led to notice the common perspective-taking activity that is present as all these experiences occur. Observe this technique in the following vignette:

> CLIENT: Since my girlfriend left me, I am like a shadow. I feel ashamed and I don't want to see anybody. I'm the guy who has been left by his girlfriend, and I don't want people to see me like that.
>
> THERAPIST: Right now, you are seeing yourself as a shadow, as the guy who was left by his girlfriend . . . I am curious about how you saw yourself before she left you.

The therapist reformulates the client's definition of himself as taking perspective on this definition ("you are seeing yourself as"). He then leads the client to notice different definitions in different contexts.

> CLIENT: I was very self-confident. I didn't doubt anything. I was very popular in my group of friends because everybody saw me as attractive, with a great sense of humor . . . not afraid of anything. Now the picture is torn apart.
>
> THERAPIST: Were you also seeing yourself as attractive, with a great sense of humor, not afraid of anything?
>
> CLIENT: I think so. I mean, that is what people told me, so that is what I thought of myself, I guess.
>
> THERAPIST: How would you see yourself if she came back?
>
> CLIENT: I wouldn't let her come back.
>
> THERAPIST: Why?
>
> CLIENT: I am not a guy you can leave and take back like that. I am not an object. I would have no respect for myself if I let her come back.
>
> THERAPIST: I see. So you would see yourself as an object if you let her come back, something like that?
>
> CLIENT: Yeah, exactly.
>
> THERAPIST: Okay. But tell me something. . . . You would see yourself

like an object if you let her come back. You are seeing yourself as a shadow right now. You used to see yourself as self-confident, with a great sense of humor . . . But who is seeing all of that?

The therapist leads the client to notice the common perspective-taking activity on all definitions of himself.

CLIENT: What do you mean?

THERAPIST: The way you are seeing yourself changes across these different situations, right?

CLIENT: Yeah.

THERAPIST: Who is noticing these changes?

The therapist starts to underline the distinction between the labels and perspective taking.

CLIENT: Me.

THERAPIST: Which you?

CLIENT: What do you mean, which me?

THERAPIST: It seems like there is a "you" that changes, that becomes a shadow or a torn-apart picture, and a "you" that can see these changes.

CLIENT: It is the same me, no?

THERAPIST: Is it? Can a picture see itself?

CLIENT: Hmm . . . I guess not. But I don't see where you are going.

THERAPIST: What I mean is, is it possible that a part of you changes and another part doesn't?

CLIENT: I guess. My body hasn't changed since my girlfriend left me, but what I think of myself has.

THERAPIST: Across all your life experiences, hasn't your body changed? Will it not change again?

CLIENT: Sure. So everything changes?

THERAPIST: What do you think?

CLIENT: I am confused.

THERAPIST: I can understand that. It is a strange feeling to notice that how we see ourselves changes and at the same time something remains the same. Like right now, you have become confused. And yet, there is a part of you, or another you, which sees that you are confused, right?

CLIENT: Hmm. Yeah!

Noticing perspective taking is not an easy thing to do; it often brings up confusion. It is important not to harm the relationship by making the client feel like the therapist is playing with him. For this reason, it is tempting to explain the concept of perspective taking rather than leading the client to experience it. The difficulty is that if the client doesn't contact perspective taking himself, the explanation is likely to feel arbitrary. Thus, a good balance needs to be found between helping the client observe his experience and helping him abstract useful conclusions. This is possible by letting the client be confused for a short moment and then giving him a clue to move forward in understanding the distinction between perspective taking and all the other experiences.

THERAPIST: What would happen to the you that can see yourself as a shadow if you let her come back?

CLIENT: Nothing?

THERAPIST: What if nothing had happened and your girlfriend had not left?

CLIENT: I would feel better.

THERAPIST: Who would notice that?

CLIENT: The part of me that doesn't change. Is that what you mean? Why is it important to make that difference?

THERAPIST: The way you see yourself has changed and may change again, right?

CLIENT: Yeah.

THERAPIST: This is the part that is painful right now?

CLIENT: Yes. I hate seeing myself this way. I want to feel self-confident again.

THERAPIST: Is there a "you" that can see that and that is not affected by what you think of yourself?

CLIENT: I see . . . You mean, nothing can happen to that part of me?

THERAPIST: Whatever happened, you were always there, right? Don't just reason to it—I'm not asking for a belief or an opinion. Look at your experience.

CLIENT: Deep down I'm always me. Yes.

A good way to wrap up interactions such as these is to help the client perceive the advantages of approaching himself as a point of view on all his experiences (i.e., moving toward functional coherence). Note that at no point did the therapist argue with the client about the accuracy of what he thinks about himself, nor did he try to change the conceptual definition of himself. What is targeted here is the experience of perspective taking that doesn't depend on any specific conceptual definition.

Noticing the Common Perspective-Taking Activity across Points of View. Another way of contacting continuous perspective taking is to invite the client to look at an experience from different points of view. This is like looking at a stationary train while walking alongside it or even going to the other side of the train to see how the wagons look from this location. The wagons will look different, not because the train is different, but because the perspective is different. In practice, this consists of shifting deictic relations of time, place, or person. This can be done using verbal interactions that include perspective-taking cues such as "How would you see yourself if it was tomorrow, and you were thinking about what is happening to you right now?" or "How would you see yourself if you were sitting over there, listening to yourself talk about you like this?" or "If you were your wife hearing this right now, what would you be feeling?" (Note that these three examples change time, place, or person, respectively.) The impact of shifting perspective like this is twofold: variability in experiences may be noticed (and thus this technique is also relevant to the previous section), and there is a greater sense of standing back and observing, increasing a sense of stability that can be found in perspective taking itself.

As dimensions of perspective change, the client can be asked to notice the common perspective-taking activity across these changes of experience. The therapist can also use physical cues that materialize the client's experience and allow distant observing. For example, the therapist may raise her hand in front of herself and, while looking at it, say, "So you are thinking that you are hopeless there" or "There is the you that feels scared right there. Can you see him from where you are?" Observe this technique in the following vignette:

THERAPIST: How do you feel about this new job?

CLIENT: Pretty weird. I have never led a group, and it is weird to be seen as the boss by my colleagues.

THERAPIST: Are you saying that it has changed something about you?

CLIENT: Yeah. I am not the same person at work anymore. It scares me. You know, I have lots of responsibilities now. Plus, I am a woman. No woman has ever had this position in the company, so I have to be different, not just like any woman in the company. I don't like that.

THERAPIST: What is it that you don't like about being different?

CLIENT: I am not really sure. It feels . . . weird. Like I am losing a part of myself. I don't like that I am not myself anymore.

THERAPIST: Imagine that in a year, you were remembering how you are feeling right now. How do you think you would see yourself?

The therapist leads the client to engage in an initial perspective taking shift.

CLIENT: You mean, how I will see myself a year from now?

THERAPIST: More precisely, how you will see yourself as you look back in time.

CLIENT: Ah . . . Well, I guess . . . I guess I will be a very different person by then. So looking back, it might feel like another life, really.

THERAPIST: Like another person?

The therapist underlines the change of perception as the client adopts a different point of view.

CLIENT: Yeah, really. I already feel like a very different person than what I was last week . . .

THERAPIST: Last week, how were you thinking of the person you would be one week later?

The therapist evokes a second perspective taking shift.

CLIENT: I was imagining . . . I don't know . . . I thought I would manage these changes better.

THERAPIST: A very different way of seeing yourself right now, huh?

CLIENT: Yeah . . . I guess I was naïve to think that everything could remain the same.

THERAPIST: This is how you see the you of last week?

CLIENT: Yeah . . . A pretty naïve person indeed. . . .

THERAPIST: And then, you were seeing the you of today as . . .

CLIENT: More self-confident. More stable.

THERAPIST: And the you of next year will see the you of today as . . .

CLIENT: I don't know . . . As lost, probably.

THERAPIST: It seems like when you look at the you of today from different points of view, you have a very different perception each time (*showing his left hand open in front of him and circling it with his right hand to materialize the different points of views adopted by the client*).

The therapist helps the client notice how the way she sees herself changes across different points of view.

CLIENT: I know. That is what feels scary. I feel unsettled these days.

THERAPIST: Every time you look at yourself from another point of view, there is a part of you that changes?

CLIENT: Yes. I have a hard time recognizing myself. Feeling whole. I don't like that I am not myself anymore.

THERAPIST: Does the "you" that sees these transformations change too?

The therapist helps the client notice the part of her that is the same across the multiple exemplars of perspective taking.

CLIENT: I am not sure I understand.

THERAPIST: Every time you look at yourself, it seems like you are changing, and that is disturbing, right?

CLIENT: Yes.

THERAPIST: And yet, you are seeing that with the same eyes, no?

CLIENT: Yeah . . . I mean, I know not everything is different.

THERAPIST: What is not different?

CLIENT: I mean. I am still me but . . .

THERAPIST: What is still you, exactly?

CLIENT: I . . . I am aware of these changes. I would rather not be, actually. It would be less disturbing!

THERAPIST: Are you saying that the part that is aware of these changes is still you?

CLIENT: Yes, probably. I can see what is happening. It is like I see myself from the outside sometimes. Like a character on a comic strip.

The client uses a metaphor that suggests the beginning of awareness of perspective taking on her experiences. The therapist will use this metaphor in the following exchanges to help her notice which part of her remains stable across changing experiences.

THERAPIST: The character on the comic strip changes, but the reader doesn't?

CLIENT: Yes. And the reader doesn't like the character anymore.

THERAPIST: Who sees that the reader doesn't like the character?

CLIENT: I don't know . . . I do.

THERAPIST: The reader is only reading.

CLIENT: I can see what is happening to me or in me . . . but there is still a me.

THERAPIST: You've been you your whole life, no? Ever since you showed up as an aware person.

CLIENT: There is something deep down that never changes.

As you can again see in this vignette, working on a sense of perspective taking can bring up some confusion in the client. It is important to maintain a strong relationship during this process so that confusion doesn't become unnecessarily aversive. The therapist thus emphasizes the playful dimension of this work and shows interest and curiosity all along the process. Wrapping up in a way that helps the client see the potential benefit of finding stability in perspective taking also helps her see this process as a beneficial approach rather than just a pointless thought experiment. However, it is more effective not to overexplain the perspective-taking experience if you want the client to observe the benefits she can take from it by herself.

Finding Coherence in the Context

In the previous sections, we noted that greater awareness of experience allows for contact with a greater variety of experiences and that perspective-taking skills afford a greater sense of stability of self. However, processes of symbolic derivation prevent us from limiting our language activity to noticing our experiences and our perspective-taking activity. Before we have the time to realize it, we are back into self-concepts. This is not a bad thing per se. Conceptualizing oneself allows for owning our personal stories and distinguishing ourselves from others in a symbolic fashion. As verbal social beings, we need to be able to talk *about* ourselves. But we need to be able to build and listen to self-narratives integrating the sum of our experiences *without identifying with these narratives (i.e., without framing ourselves in equivalence with our experiences)*. Thus, additional steps are needed to find a balance in the self between the needs of variability, stability, and symbolic coherence.

A helpful step is the deliberate use of hierarchical framing to create a more expansive symbolic network that contains the awareness of experiential processes and perspective taking but is one in which self is the *context* of all experiences. This type of framing is present in the many mindfulness metaphors that point to a different sense of self that is open and aware: the sky contains clouds passing by; a chessboard contains the pieces of a chess game; a house contains furniture and people. In these metaphors, self is a container—a context—not the content of what is contained.

This type of conceptualization has the advantage of maintaining a distinction between the self and psychological experiences, while affording the normal use of language that occurs at the base of the hierarchy. For example, evaluations can be deliberately used without harming the flexibility of self because what happens at the base of the hierarchy doesn't fundamentally change the top of the hierarchy. Conceptualizing the self as a context can be seen as a form of essential coherence (there is almost a sense that the self is intrinsically a context which grounds it in the continuous perspective taking experience), but because hierarchical, rather than coordination, framing is used here, variability remains possible (i.e., the self is not just "that"; it is this and that and many other things).

As an analogy, we often conceptualize humankind as a hierarchy in which all humans are equally placed at the base and the name of our species is at the top. Even when one or even several people do something bad, humankind remains humankind. We may not like what they did, but it doesn't change that these people are still humans. They still belong to the same group because something beyond their actions remains the same. Similarly, by approaching the self as the context of all experiences in a hierarchical network, no matter what happens in these experiences (actions, feelings, definitions, evaluations), the self remains stable and beyond the content.

The combination of perspective-taking relations and hierarchical relations is important in dealing with issues of self-order to avoid a downside of hierarchy when it is used alone. Just as observing a human doing something we judge terribly wrong might change the way we see humankind in general (e.g., Hitler's crimes might alter our view of humanity in general), we often end up judging the self negatively because one thing we did was wrong. For this reason, framing the self in a hierarchy with the experiences is safer if it is done through relations of containment rather than summation—the metaphor of a container versus a totality of content—as the transfer between these two parts is less likely to occur. A sense of "I/here/now" fits with this form of hierarchical relation (consciousness contains what we are conscious of, rather than being the sum of conscious content), and thus the combination seems especially helpful. Self as a relation of containment can help decrease self-stigmatization without removing responsibility (e.g., "I *did* something bad" vs. "I *am* bad"). The recent RFT literature on hierarchical relations has begun to address these various delineations (e.g., Slattery & Stewart, 2014); more definite recommendations as to the utility of one or other pattern of hierarchical relational responding awaits the results of further empirical research.

The idea of self as a context is much easier to embrace in a healthy way after developing a greater awareness of experiences and a richer sense of perspective taking. A hierarchical sense of self could be just another story about the self, but if it is built on process knowledge and the experience of taking perspective, it more directly matches what the client was able to observe by herself. Done this way, conceptualizing the self as a context can function as a cue to remind the client of what it was like to observe self-experiences and to observe the perspective-taking activity on these experiences. Having various experiences and remaining stable at the same time can thereby feed a sense of functional coherence.

Emphasizing the Hierarchical Dimension of the Self. In practice, several methods can be used to help the client conceptualize his self as a context. These techniques use hierarchical framing in various ways, and given the metaphorical nature of this conceptualization, they generally take the form of images or figures. We will talk about the formal use of metaphors in Chapter 8; for now we will only focus on natural metaphorical verbal interactions that convey a sense of a contextual self. For example, leading the client to formulate his experiences as something he *has* rather than something he *is* is a good and simple way to build hierarchical relations. Many other metaphorical forms of language that evoke the relationship between a container, or a context, and its content can be used in natural speech to progressively shape this sense of self. Observe this approach in the following vignette:

CLIENT: I am not sure what I want to do with my life anymore. I am dragged in all directions. I don't know how to integrate all the people I am in my life. I have a family, I have a great job, I have everything. But I don't feel like a normal person anymore. I feel split. It is like I am a different person in every area of my life, and it feels fake because nobody knows who I really am.

THERAPIST: You see yourself as split in different directions right now. Is it a bit like my hand there (*showing his open hand, fingers spread, between the client and himself*) with each finger going in a different direction?

The therapist uses a physical metaphor to help the client conceptualize herself through hierarchical framing.

CLIENT: Yeah, it is literally like going in all directions and each finger is a different person, a different me. It doesn't feel right.

THERAPIST: Each finger is part of the same hand, though.

CLIENT: Yeah.

THERAPIST: The different roles you have in your life, are they part of a same thing?

The therapist uses "having" rather than "being" forms. While the client said earlier that she was different people, the therapist reformulated by saying that she has different roles.

CLIENT: They are parts of me. But they feel split. That is what is disturbing right now.

THERAPIST: Imagine for a second that you didn't have five different fingers, able to go in different directions, but that they were all attached to each other, like one big flat finger. What would be different? What could you do and not do with your hand?

CLIENT: Ha. That is funny to imagine! Well . . . I guess it would be hard to get dressed. It would be impossible to play the guitar (laughing). I definitely could not put make up on or fix my hair in the morning.

THERAPIST: Is there anything you could do better if they were attached?

CLIENT: No, I don't think so.

THERAPIST: If there was only one way you could be, would you be able to do all the things you want to do in your life?

The therapist emphasizes the utility of having variable experiences.

CLIENT: I have never thought about it that way. Probably not. I have to be different with my family and at work. It is two completely different universes! But that is what I don't like. I feel like I am not myself. Split into different people like that.

THERAPIST: What if you were the hand rather than the fingers?

The therapist leads the client to approach herself as the top of a hierarchy including all her roles.

CLIENT: But I feel like the fingers . . .

THERAPIST: Exactly. That is how you feel. And what difference would that make if you were the hand instead of the fingers going in every direction?

CLIENT: I would feel whole.

THERAPIST: It would not be a problem if you had different roles, because they would only be parts of a bigger you, right?

CLIENT: No. That would not be a problem. You mean that I could see these roles as all parts of me? I had not thought about it that way.

Emphasizing the Distinction between the Self and the Experiences. Another technique to improve a contextual sense of self is to redirect evaluations about the self toward the actions, thereby using distinction framing between the self and psychological experiences. When evaluations of actions merge with the self, the risk is that the self becomes the target of change if the evaluations are unsatisfying. Even if the client does something she is happy with and as a result, she qualifies herself as "good," such evaluation about the self may strengthen the idea that when things go wrong, the self needs to be fixed. Instead, a conceptualization of the self as the context containing a variety of actions suggests that no matter what is done, the self is above these actions. Observe this technique in the following exchange:

CLIENT: I feel horrible. I can't believe I was so stupid to trust him again. I guess I must be a really naïve person. I always have been . . .

THERAPIST: You feel like it was stupid to trust him again?

The therapist redirects the evaluation toward the action.

CLIENT: Yeah. I wanted to give him another chance but I am just too naïve.

THERAPIST: What is naïve in what you do?

The therapist redirects the evaluation toward the action again.

CLIENT: That I still think he can change.

THERAPIST: What did you do because you thought he could change?

The therapist directs the client's attention toward her actions.

CLIENT: I prepared a weekend together. He had said that he would be done with his work by Friday night and we could leave early Saturday. But when he came back from work on Friday night, he said he would still have to work on Saturday morning and we would have to leave in the afternoon. I just couldn't see the point of going out for the weekend if we arrived late on Saturday. So I said we should cancel.

THERAPIST: I hear that you really wanted to spend this weekend together. That must have been really disappointing.

CLIENT: Yeah. I am disappointed by him and by myself for being so stupid.

THERAPIST: What do think you could do to avoid having a weekend together be ruined again?

The therapist helps the client target actions rather than the self to change outcomes.

CLIENT: I need to stop being naïve.

THERAPIST: What would you do differently that would not be naïve?

The therapist redirects the evaluation toward actions again.

CLIENT: I would have to tell him that I don't think he can get his work done by Friday night if he doesn't arrange his schedule better during the week.

Finding Responsibility in the Interaction

The last component of building a flexible self is to develop a balanced sense of responsibility. Two typical opposite positions often lead clients to dead ends when considering their role in the relationship between causes and consequences. Often, they see themselves as excessively responsible for their actions and for the results of their actions; conversely, they may think that they have no control over their actions and that outcomes are independent of what they do. In the first case, we find clients who experience a lot of shame, who self-criticize, and who beat themselves up for not being able to change and obtain what they want. They spend a fair amount of time trying to change a self seen as the primary or even unique cause of their difficulties. In the second case, we find clients who feel hopeless, out of control, or insignificant and think that they can't do anything to change their condition. They see their self at most as a mere outcome of external variables, which they can't ever reach to make a difference in their lives.

Developing a balanced sense of responsibility consists instead of approaching the self as a situated action; that is, as an interaction between an organism and the contextual variables of its environment. In this view, the self is neither a primary cause nor a final consequence. Self is both a consequence and a set of actions that impact other actions; it is influenced by contextual variables and able to influence these variables in return. From a functional contextual perspective, the influence exerted by the self on contextual variables is itself influenced by contextual variables. However, just as all operant behaviors impact the environment and are produced by the environment, these forms of influence are not linear and unidirectional but are multidirectional.

This way of approaching the self has two advantages. On the one hand, it undermines the responsibility of the self when the client feels excessively responsible for what is happening to him. It helps him consider other variables, which may have a more decisive impact on his behaviors and on the production of more desirable outcomes. On the other hand, it increases the client's willingness to change contextual variables that are behaviorally important, which helps the client engage in new actions, allowing desirable outcomes to occur.

Obviously, it would be a very rare day that any of these technical terms would be used with clients; we would not usually use terms such as *self-concept* or *hierarchy* either, and the reader will search in vain for technical terms of this kind in the previous vignettes. Developing an interactive sense of self occurs through natural verbal interactions, which, as with the other components of the flexible self, emphasize concrete observation. Given the bidirectional nature of the relationship between the organism and the contextual variables, the techniques you can use go in reversed directions. Some techniques consist of drawing the client's attention to the influence of contextual variables, whereas other techniques improve awareness that the client's actions can have an impact on these variables.

Noticing the Impact of the Context. It is possible to help the client notice the influence of contextual variables by asking questions about a variety of current and past elements that may contribute to the client's ineffective actions. The use of conditional framing is particularly helpful to identify functional relationships between behaviors and elements of the context (in a similar approach to evoking tracking, as we saw in Chapter

5). For example, the clinician may say, "I can see that you are feeling very guilty for getting mad at your wife. Can you think of things that characterized that day that might have led you to act this way?" (e.g., pointing to the client's lack of sleep) or "You are unhappy because you didn't do as well as you were hoping. Do you think parts of your past help explain why you are not comfortable in this situation yet?" (e.g., pointing to the client's history of trauma). The goal here is not to remove the client's sense of responsibility but to underline other variables that may *also* play an important role. Identifying these variables can then lead either to direct modification (e.g., the client getting more sleep) or to the alteration of their influence if they can't be removed or replaced (e.g., the client shows greater self-compassion).

Contextual variables are often difficult to notice, especially if the client is excessively controlled by a rigid sense of self seen as the cause of his actions. Fortunately, it is possible to use deictic relations here also, this time to improve the awareness of the other variables at play. Following the same principle as in previous sections, the clinician helps the client to adopt different points of views on his current situation, such as the point of view of other people. This is helpful because other people often have different interpretations of the client's situation. Although the client often knows that this is the case, he is not necessarily in touch with these different points of view. Temporarily looking at his situation through the eyes of others therefore leads him to see other, potentially crucial, elements of the context. Given that, in this context, the aim is to decrease shame and self-criticism, it is naturally better to involve the point of view of someone who is more likely to have a kind attitude toward the client. Similarly, the therapist can invite the client to imagine that a person he appreciates is in his situation or did the same thing as he did, and how he perceives this experience from the outside. Observe an example of this perspective-taking technique in the following vignette:

CLIENT: I feel ashamed. I almost didn't come today because I didn't do what I had committed to do the last time I saw you.

THERAPIST: So you didn't start exercising like you had planned to?

CLIENT: No. And I feel like a failure. I know it was a simple thing to do. Just getting up and going to the gym. Not that hard. But no . . . I couldn't do it. I don't know what is wrong with me. What seems easy to everybody, I can't do it because I am too weak.

THERAPIST: What do you think happened?

The therapist draws the client's attention to the situation in order to explore contextual variables influencing the client's behavior.

CLIENT: I don't know. I am not motivated enough. I say I am going to do things, but I never do them.

THERAPIST: You said you almost didn't come. What did you think I would think about this?

CLIENT: I didn't want to disappoint you.

THERAPIST: I understand. But what did you think I would think?

CLIENT: Maybe that I am not worth all your efforts.

THERAPIST: If you were me right now, how would you see this situation?

The therapist leads the client to observe her situation from his point of view in order to help her notice other variables influencing her behavior.

CLIENT: I guess I would think I need more work. I doubt you would think I am a failure.

THERAPIST: How come?

CLIENT: You said it might take time to learn a new skill. It might be hard to change my habits.

THERAPIST: Yeah, that's true, I said that. What can make it hard?

CLIENT: My lack of motivation.

THERAPIST: What have you noticed about motivation coming and going? It seems clear here and then later on it is not clear.

The therapist redirects the client's attention toward contextual variables each time she looks for the cause of her behavior inside herself (e.g., a lack of motivation).

CLIENT: I don't know. It's like I don't see the point anymore when it is time to get up and exercise.

THERAPIST: So when the point is not visible enough you lose motivation. What would make it more visible?

The therapist reformulates the client's statement in a way that transfers the causal role to the contextual variable (from "the client doesn't see the point" to "the point is not visible").

CLIENT: I need to remember why I want to exercise, but in the morning I have a hard time thinking right.

THERAPIST: What could you do to connect with why exercising matters to you?

The therapist encourages the client to explore actions she could do to influence her motivation.

CLIENT: I don't know . . . If I push myself maybe?

THERAPIST: (*smiling*) Isn't that what you have been doing this week?

CLIENT: (*sighing*) Yeah. But I am weak so I guess I need to push myself more!

THERAPIST: Like what?

CLIENT: I need something to motivate myself.

THERAPIST: What have you noticed lifts you up? What bring you down?

In these last exchanges, the client keeps looking for a change inside herself, so the therapist continues to encourage her to target contextual variables that may improve her motivation.

CLIENT: Beating myself up is probably the biggest downer.

THERAPIST: Neat. So perhaps we could not do that in here either. . . . What if we looked at what lifts you up?

CLIENT: Music—sometimes anyway. Maybe I could listen to some music when I wake up.

THERAPIST: Yeah? What kind of music?

CLIENT: Sometimes I just dance around the house when I put on trance music. I think they even call it "dance music."

THERAPIST: Could that connect you with why exercising matters to you?

CLIENT: I think so. I think that could help. It puts me back in my body. I actually like to exercise. I just sort of forget.

As you can see in this vignette, by adopting the point of view of another we can also change the way we treat ourselves. While the client was judging herself very harshly at the beginning of the exchange, she progressively adopted a different tone toward herself. Once again, the aim of this approach is not to lead the client to some kind of self-indulgence but to decrease the influence exerted by useless evaluations about the self. Thus, the client can focus on the contextual variables that she can modify to increase the chance that she will engage in the desired behavior.

Noticing the Impact of Behaviors. Increasing the awareness of the client's own influence follows a similar approach in that it consists of helping the client notice the conditional relationships that link causes and consequences. This time, however, an emphasis is put on the client's role. This is also similar to our previous discussions of assessment (Chapter 4) and tracking (Chapter 5), except that the sense of responsibility is more specifically targeted here. The typical techniques used in this context include conditional and temporal framing (to evoke tracking of consequences) and comparison/distinction framing (to evoke observation of changes).

Concretely, the therapist asks the client about specific actions and underlines the connection with their impact whether it is positive or negative. Observe this technique in the following vignette:

CLIENT: What I need is a new job. And then I could move to another place. That would change everything. But I can't find a job. Nobody is interested in a guy like me. There is nothing I can do about that. I can't become another person at my age, so it's hopeless!

THERAPIST: What has changed since we have started this work together?

The therapist draws the client's attention to changes that have followed his actions (distinction framing).

CLIENT: Nothing! Nothing . . .

THERAPIST: I remember that a few weeks ago, you said you would not even consider working again. Do you remember?

The client is so stuck in his position that the therapist brings some elements to his attention, but without trying to convince him.

CLIENT: Yes, I remember. And I was right because after spending hours on the phone, I didn't get any interviews for a job.

THERAPIST: What happened when you decided to make those calls?

The therapist helps the client observe more directly the consequences of his actions in order to undermine the influence of overgeneralized evaluations (temporal framing).

CLIENT: I called several places to see if they had open positions, but there was nothing for me.

THERAPIST: What were you doing before you decided to make those calls?

The therapist helps the client notice the changes that have occurred since he started to engage in his job search (temporal framing).

CLIENT: Nothing. What do you mean?

THERAPIST: When you started therapy with me. You said you couldn't imagine working again. And like you just said, you were not doing anything, right?

CLIENT: Yeah. I was spending all day in bed . . .

THERAPIST: So, I am wondering if something has changed since you have made the decision to look for a job . . .

CLIENT: I feel like I am in the same place, except that I am more active. But I still feel hopeless. I can't see how things are going to change.

THERAPIST: How has your wife reacted to you being more active?

The therapist helps him consider different areas that may have been impacted by his new behavior (conditional framing).

CLIENT: She was happy. . . . She had been asking me to do that for months. I understand her. I have not been very useful in the house either this past year.

THERAPIST: What impact would you say your decision to look for a job has had on your relationship with her?

CLIENT: I see what you mean. . . . Yeah, sure, our relationship is better now. That's true. It is.

THERAPIST: Is it something important to you?

CLIENT: Yes, of course. She is the reason I'm trying to find a job. So we can move to another place.

In these last exchanges, the client notices elements of his life that have changed in a desired direction. Although not everything is working as he wishes, being more aware of the influence he can have on what matters in his life was useful to strengthen his commitment to effective actions.

CLINICAL EXAMPLE

Given the richness of the interventions discussed in this chapter, it is impossible to show a brief exchange between a therapist and a client where all components of the flexible self are developed in depth. However, you will see in the following vignette that we can still make a variety of moves, sometimes subtle, in a relatively short exchange that contribute to fostering all flexible self skills.

This exchange involves an 18-year-old female client who self-harms by cutting herself.

THERAPIST: When do you cut?

CLIENT: When I can't stand the way I feel.

THERAPIST: What kind of feeling?

CLIENT: I feel empty. When I talk to people, it is like I am transparent. I go through days like a ghost. I don't feel anything.

THERAPIST: It must be really painful to see yourself as a ghost, is it?

The therapist helps the client to notice possible feelings that appear <u>in reaction</u> to feeling empty, in order to bring more awareness to various experiences.

CLIENT: I don't know. I don't really care. That is the problem.

THERAPIST: It is a problem?

CLIENT: Yeah. Who wants to feel empty?

THERAPIST: I probably would not like that.

CLIENT: Exactly. It is the worse feeling you can imagine.

THERAPIST: Do you think you could tell me more about it?

CLIENT: You feel numb, like your body's not even yours. I hate that.

THERAPIST: That seems like a really painful feeling.

CLIENT: Yes it is.

THERAPIST: Can you notice that you have at least those two feelings, the feeling that you are empty and the feeling that it is painful to feel empty?

In this exchange, although the client first says she doesn't feel anything about feeling empty, the therapist helps her notice that she is actually bothered by this experience and that this, in and of itself, is a feeling different from emptiness (i.e., amplifying the awareness of experiences).

CLIENT: Hmm. Yeah, I guess. But I can tell you that what it really feels like is *nothing* at all. Sometimes I think I am an empty shell.

THERAPIST: Like a shell you would find on the beach, brought by the sea?

CLIENT: Yeah, exactly.

THERAPIST: Imagine that you find that empty shell on the beach and take it in your hand. You look at it and see that it is empty.

CLIENT: Yeah?

THERAPIST: Who would you be?

CLIENT: What do you mean? I am me, with the shell in my hand.

THERAPIST: So you are not the shell.

CLIENT: Not in this case.

THERAPIST: What is different?

CLIENT: I think I am an empty shell because I feel empty.

THERAPIST: Okay. But who is seeing that?

CLIENT: Me.

THERAPIST: From where?

CLIENT: From where I am, what do you mean?

THERAPIST: From where you are, okay. So where are you? Are you the empty shell or the one holding the empty shell?

CLIENT: It is weird.

THERAPIST: Yeah, it is. It is strange to feel something and see that you are feeling it at the same time, right?

CLIENT: It's just that I don't usually think about it that way.

In this last exchange, the therapist uses the metaphor of the empty shell brought up by the client to help her change her perspective on herself. The client is then led to notice the distinction between the experience of feeling empty and the perspective-taking activity on this experience.

THERAPIST: What difference would that make if you did?

CLIENT: If I didn't think I am a shell?

THERAPIST: If you saw yourself as the one holding the shell, which may be empty, or filled with pain because of the feeling of emptiness.

CLIENT: I don't know.

THERAPIST: What if you could hold this shell no matter what is inside? Even if it is empty, that wouldn't change anything about you.

CLIENT: But I care about what is and what is not in the shell!

THERAPIST: Of course. That is why you are holding it in your hand, right? And that is why you are looking at what is inside . . .

In this last exchange, the therapist keeps using the shell metaphor to encourage the client to approach herself and her experiences as a hierarchical network. The advantage of this approach is emphasized by the distinction between what happens at the base (the experience of feeling empty) and the top of the hierarchy (the self). Notice how the therapist acknowledges that the content matters too but that it can't alter the contextual self.

CLIENT: I know I shouldn't cut myself. I know it makes things worse but I am crazy. I am crazy so I cut myself.

THERAPIST: If you were me, what would you say to a client who is telling you that she is crazy?

CLIENT: I would probably tell her that she is not crazy, I would try to reassure her, but that is because I would not know what it is like to be crazy.

THERAPIST: What else would you know?

CLIENT: I would know lots of stuff about psychology, I guess.

THERAPIST: What else would you see if you were me?

CLIENT: Someone who is suffering, who is feeling empty and needs to cut herself to feel better.

THERAPIST: If you were me, would you see a girl who is crazy or a girl who is suffering?

CLIENT: If I were you, I would not say "crazy."

THERAPIST: Why?

CLIENT: Because you are nice. I know you don't want to hurt me.

THERAPIST: So if you were me, you wouldn't want to hurt the you who is right there in this chair, right?

CLIENT: No.

In this last exchange, the client expresses harsh self-criticisms. The therapist leads her to adopt his point of view as a way of opening her up to other variables that may also contribute to her behavior— exploring an interactive sense of self. As she adopts this different point of view, she begins to see the suffering instead of thinking that she is cutting herself just "because she is crazy."

In a short exchange like this, the therapist obviously doesn't immediately expect a complete transformation in the way the client approaches herself. But seeds were sown that will help her develop flexibility in the self as these types of exchanges are reproduced across sessions. Together with formal practice exercises (see Chapter 9), significant changes can begin to appear and lead to more effective behavior.

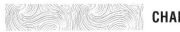 **CHAPTER SUMMARY**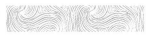

In this chapter, you learned to use verbal interactions to help clients develop a flexible sense of self that fosters variability, stability, coherence, and a balanced sense of responsibility. Here are the main principles to remember:

- Fostering greater awareness of experiences decreases rigidity by allowing the client to notice the variety of his experiences and notice that if he *was* these experiences, he could not be completely defined by just a few of them. Developing these self-awareness skills consists of:
  - Stabilizing perspective taking by repeatedly directing the client's attention to the present, so as to help him notice the changes in his experiences.
  - Shifting perspective taking by exploring a variety of contexts to help the client notice the changes in experiences and self-labels across contexts.
  - Observing experience from different points of view defined by time, place, and person, which increases awareness of the variability of experience itself.
- Fostering a sense of perspective taking increases stability by allowing the client to notice what is common to all his experiences. Developing a sense of perspective taking consists of:
  - Helping the client notice the common perspective-taking activity across all experiences, actions, and labels. Helping him notice that there is something he does ("a part of himself") that is stable: the activity of noticing from I/here/now.
  - Helping the client notice the common perspective-taking activity across points of view defined by time, place, and person. By noticing the changes in the perception of experience, it is easier to notice the I/here/now aspect of awareness.
- Fostering a contextual sense of self that integrates the qualities of self-awareness and perspective taking into a coherent network based on hierarchical relations. Developing these skills consists of:
  - Emphasizing the hierarchical dimension of the self by using metaphorical forms of language that replicate the relation between a context, or a container, and a content.
  - Emphasizing the distinction between the self and the experiences by redirecting evaluations about the self toward the experiences.
- Fostering an interactive sense of self that encourages approaching responsibility with flexibility, which prevents unnecessary self-criticisms and hopelessness. Developing this interactive sense of self consists of:
  - Helping the client be more aware of the influence of the context on his actions.
  - Directing the client's attention toward the impact of his actions on the context.

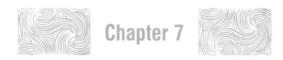

Chapter 7

Fostering Meaning and Motivation

In the last two chapters, we explored how to alter clients' sensitivity to sources of influence as a means of reconnecting them to a greater sense of effectiveness and flexibility. However, increasing contact with what works and allowing a variety of experiences to occur make sense only if these serve a meaningful purpose. Behaviors are problematic or ineffective only insofar as their consequences interfere with achieving such a purpose. Thus, behavior change needs guidance to ensure that it will bring sustainable satisfaction in clients' lives. In this chapter, we explore how to use RFT principles to help clients draw meaningful life directions and establish strong motivation to move in these directions.

THE LANGUAGE OF MEANING AND MOTIVATION

Virtually all clients we meet in therapy have, in one way or another, difficulties related to motivation or to finding meaning in their lives. They perceive a discrepancy between how things currently are in their lives and how they wish things were. To reduce that discrepancy, actions generally need to change. In many cases, this is obvious to the client. For example, people who come to therapy to quit an addiction or to stop obsessive rituals usually know that their actions are problematic. In other cases, clients complain about their situations or the results of their actions, and they hope for changes rather than exploring ways to change their own actions (e.g., clients who struggle with depression or relationship difficulties). Although it may be true that changes in a client's situation would lead to a dramatic improvement in his life (e.g., having a new job, having a partner who shows more affection), it is only through new behavior that these changes are likely to occur.

Behavior change needs a direction that ensures lasting satisfaction. Clients may be willing to change and able to stay engaged in new activities, but sometimes they have no idea what to do for their lives to be worth living. In other cases, clients are already doing many things that might lead to satisfying lives but are deriving no satisfaction from them. Building a sense of life meaning will help them find this kind of lasting satisfaction, sometimes without having to change their actions much (what changes in that case is mostly how they symbolically relate to their actions and experiences).

Of course, even when clients know what matters in their lives, and know what they could do to achieve what matters, they can still have great difficulties with actually engaging in and persevering with needed actions. Sadly enough, many clients struggle with both meaning *and* motivation. They don't know what matters in their lives, they don't know what to do in order to find sustainable satisfaction, and they seem unable to sustain engagement in effective action.

Meaning, and motivation to engage in meaningful actions, are not gifts people receive at birth, and very little progress can be made if we limit our understanding of clients' issues to the observation that they don't know, and don't do, what could bring them a lasting sense of life satisfaction. To help clients who lack motivation, or who have no clear sense of what matters most to them, we need to identify and target the sources of influence that are likely to move the client in a useful direction. RFT principles can be applied to guide verbal interactions in the therapy room and lead the client to elaborate useful relational networks. Turned to the clients' advantage, language processes can give meaning to their actions and strengthen their ability to perform these actions even when no concrete satisfaction is immediately present.

Meaning as Hierarchical Networks

The Goal

When we find meaning in our actions, this is generally because we are able to tell what purpose they serve. For example, if we asked you what the purpose of reading this book is for you, you would probably say you want to learn more about RFT and how it can be used to improve your skills as a clinician. However, a purpose is not enough to find meaning. If we ask clients the purpose of engaging in obsessive rituals, abusing alcohol, or staying home all day long, they will often have answers: that they are working to decrease anxiety, to feel better about themselves, to wait for depression to go away. Such answers identify a purpose to some extent, but they don't really convey meaning, a difference we will elaborate upon later.

The clinical goal is to discover, or more precisely to construct, the abstract symbolic purposes of action that both bring a client satisfaction now and extend forward in time as guides to action. Constructing such abstract purposes requires going beyond the specific consequence clients expect from their action to qualities of action (e.g., with compassion, honesty, integrity, love, precision) and overarching goals (e.g., in order to learn, protect, teach, connect). In acceptance and commitment therapy, these qualities of action and overarching goals are termed "values," but we have deliberately avoided the term here in part to help connect our present approach to broader and older clinical traditions.

Why This Is Important, from an RFT Point of View

From an RFT perspective, we find meaning when we are able to link our actions to *intrinsic*[1] and *inexhaustible* sources of satisfaction that project into the present moment but that remain present even once the action is over. Meaning can be thought of as a kind of psychological catalyst, which causes an interaction to occur but that is not used up in the processes. We will use the term "reinforcement" here for these sources of satisfaction because they meet the technical requirements of that behavioral term. From an RFT perspective, however, these reinforcers are dependent in part on the symbolic actions of clients, and thus they are neither primary reinforcers nor conditioned reinforcers in a classic behavioral sense. They are symbolic (relational) reinforcers, or "sources of meaning," and are not to be found purely in the external environment or in mere associations between primary reinforcers and symbolic events. What RFT adds are details of the conditions under which meaning and purpose can be successfully constructed and the conditions under which they can influence other actions.

Let's assume you are reading this book because you care about delivering the best treatment possible to your clients. In this case, improving your language skills in therapy is only one means of doing that, among many others. Once you have read this book, there are still ways to serve the overarching purpose of delivering the best treatment possible to your clients. And even if this book was not helpful in the end, having read it would still be meaningful if you saw this action as part of your efforts to deliver the best treatment possible to your clients. The attempt itself was meaningful, even if the hoped-for consequences never occurred. In contrast, when clients don't find meaning in their current or potential actions, that is because they are not able to link these actions to overarching and inexhaustible sources of satisfaction.

---

[1] As we will see throughout this chapter, here we are not using the term "intrinsic" as a synonym of "nonsymbolic," as we do in the rest of this book. By "intrinsic" source of satisfaction, we mean "independent of external reinforcement in the direct context."

Our ability to relate things through language not only allows us to establish connections among them, but also leads to a transformation of their functions. An isolated action such as going to work, although it has the capacity to bring satisfaction in a client's life, can acquire attractive or aversive qualities, depending on how this action is situated in the client's relational network or, in more everyday language, to the larger scheme of things. If it is connected to such things as what he can do to improve the quality of his family's life, going to work has meaning. However, if it is just considered part of what people are obliged to do, it is unlikely that he will find much meaning in going to work. Although the action remains strictly the same, the way the client relates it to other events dramatically changes its reinforcing qualities. Thus, when adequately applied, language processes can improve the satisfaction we find in our actions sometimes even without needing to change the actions themselves.

How This Method Touches on Various Clinical Traditions

The humanistic and existential traditions have been especially clear about the importance of meaning to human functioning, but in broad terms it is an issue vital to many forms of depth-oriented psychotherapy, from psychodynamic work to Gestalt therapy. Perhaps no one more forcefully and clearly stated the essential human need for meaning than the existential therapist Viktor Frankl. In his book *Man's Search for Meaning* (1984), Frankl wrote about the centrality of meaning in his surviving the Holocaust:

> A thought transfixed me: for the first time in my life I saw the truth as it is set into song by so many poets, proclaimed as the final wisdom by so many thinkers. The truth—that love is the ultimate and the highest goal to which Man can aspire. Then I grasped the meaning of the greatest secret that human poetry and human thought and belief have to impart: The salvation of Man is through love and in love. I understood how a man who has nothing left in this world still may know bliss, be it only for a brief moment, in the contemplation of his beloved. In a position of utter desolation, when Man cannot express himself in positive action, when his only achievement may consist in enduring his sufferings in the right way—an honorable way—in such a position Man can, through loving contemplation of the image he carries of his beloved, achieve fulfillment. (p. 38)

The features of meaning as we have described it can be found in Frankl's ideas and in those of existential therapists generally such as Irvin Yalom, Rollo May, or R. D. Laing. The meaning of life is not in our experiences per se, but in the way we symbolically transform them. With RFT, we can clarify how to help clients "develop freedom and grow between stimuli and responses": by targeting contextual variables influencing language processes.

How to Do It

From a relational frame point of view, the primary way to bring meaning to actions that is present, intrinsic, and inexhaustible is to link those actions into *hierarchical* networks that put both a positive overarching goal (e.g., contributing to the community's growth) and a quality of action (e.g., with compassion) at the top, and actions and specific goals at the base (e.g., working 2 hours a week at a local charity). When actions are framed in a hierarchy with overarching goals and qualities of action, satisfaction and motivation become continuously available.

An overarching goal is one that does not end. Consider the overarching goal of delivering the best treatment to people in psychological need. This is a goal that is never finished. Even when you are retired, it will still be possible to contribute to mental health improvement in your community without seeing clients. But it is also a goal that is relevant now, in this very moment of reading this book.

It is important that a client's overarching goals be positive. Although *avoiding* aversive consequences (a negative goal) can be a powerful source of motivation (e.g., looking for a job to avoid money issues, quitting smoking to avoid cancer), it doesn't bring the same sense of vitality that positive goals offer. More than relief, we want our clients to find satisfaction in their lives. Thus, meaning is best cast in terms of positive overarching goals.

Qualities of action can be simply defined as the ways we pursue a given goal. Often, they are identified in our language by adverbs (e.g., gently, thoroughly, attentively) or qualitative complements (e.g., with caution, with humor). For example, someone who values integrity can find satisfaction in an infinite number of actions as long as they are done with integrity. Qualities of action have the ability to make positive consequences for action available at any time because such consequences are contained within the actions themselves.

The advantage of hierarchical networks of this kind is that they provide intrinsic and inexhaustible reinforcement. Overarching goals and qualities of action are symbolically constructed consequences that can guide action across time and situations. They are reinforcing independent of additional consequences, almost like primary reinforcers (e.g., eating food). While conditional relations focusing on specific goals only allow contact with satisfaction if the goal is met (e.g., "I need to work to get my degree to make a lot of money and *then* I will be happy," "I need to listen to others *so* I can be accepted by them"), hierarchical relations make *the process of engaging in the action reinforcing in and of itself* (e.g., "I am happy to work on my degree because it is *part of* my overarching goal always to be learning more"; "Listening to others contributes to being respectful, which is one of my valued qualities of action").

Through hierarchical networks, not only is satisfaction no longer dependent on the external result of an action, but it can also be reached through a wide range of actions, some of which can be very small and still meaningful. For example, a person who values acting with compassion may find meaning in smiling to a stranger on the street, or complimenting a waiter, or allowing someone at the grocery store to cut in line. The overarching goal of always learning more can be served by reading a lengthy book as well as by having a short conversation or reading the news. Thus, it is possible to find satisfaction in any given action, and even when one specific action can't be executed, it is always possible to engage in another action to contact overarching and inexhaustible sources of reinforcement.

Motivation through Augmenting

The Goal

While meaning gives direction to our actions, motivation helps us perform these actions by overcoming the limitations of the direct context. Even when we clearly know why we want to go in a certain direction, we don't always feel like it in the moment. If the gap between what we want to pursue and what we actually do keeps growing, we often feel frustrated, discouraged, and even ashamed. For example, a lot of people decide at the beginning of every year to exercise more often, clearly knowing the purpose of their choice (e.g., improving health, bringing more vitality to everyday activities). Yet, when the time comes to go back to the gym or to run the first mile, many give up right away. It is not necessarily that the meaning of exercising has disappeared, but the connection with this overarching and inexhaustible source of satisfaction is too weak *in the moment*. If other sources of influence are also involved such as needing to rest or spending time on other activities, the probability of exercising is even smaller.

Note that these types of problems rarely occur with activities that are naturally and immediately reinforcing. How often have you decided to eat a slice of chocolate cake and, when the moment came to actually do it, you didn't feel like eating it anymore? Even if it happened, because you were not hungry, for example, not having done what you had originally decided probably didn't bother you afterward. When activities are naturally and immediately satisfying, motivation to engage in them is not much of a problem because we can easily contact their reinforcing consequences. Unfortunately, many meaningful activities are not sustained in this way, and if we don't engage in an activity after deciding to do so, we feel disappointed because that activity mattered, and still matters. So, what we need to do is build effective connections, in the moment, with what matters to us so that the chances increase that we engage in meaningful activities and find satisfaction. The goal is to build motivation by building positive symbolic connections to distant or abstract goals.

Why This Is Important, from an RFT Point of View

You may remember from Chapter 2 that symbolic relations can help us connect to distant consequences because they transform the function of cues contacted in the current context. When you wake up in the morning, most of the time, you still feel a bit tired. It is only because you are able to contact the distant consequences of getting up and not getting up that you are able to leave your bed. In the immediate context, the fatigue you feel is not a source of motivation. However, as you look at the time, relations quickly build, such as, "If I don't get up, I will be late and disappoint my coworkers" or "If I get up, I can take a nice hot shower and have a good breakfast." As a result, getting up becomes reinforcing through the anticipation and imagination of consequences that will occur later.

Fortunately, the skill of actively engaging in a symbolic transformation of the consequences of actions can be trained to increase our motivation. This skill in turn helps strengthen actions that can supply intrinsic and inexhaustible sources of satisfaction.

From an RFT perspective, motivation can be approached through the process of augmenting, which consists of building symbolic bridges between actions and distant, probabilistic, abstract, or hidden consequences. Through this process, some of the functions of these consequences are brought into the present moment and made more salient. Symbolic motivation overcomes the vagaries of time, probability, and confusion.

The advertising adage "Sell the sizzle, not the steak" helps explain how symbolic motivation works. We cannot actually eat a steak through symbolic processes, but we can imagine smelling it and tasting it. When advertisers are, say, using the chance of winning a car to motivate subscribing to a magazine, they will demand that raffle entrants specify the color of the car. The color can just as well be picked later, after the car is won. Why demand such a silly thing? Because a low-probability event is not motivating (you may know you have more chance of being struck by lightning than of winning the car) until you imagine in concrete detail what you would do with the prize. Picturing yourself driving down the street in a *silver* convertible is much more motivating than thinking about a car in the abstract.

There is a long research tradition showing that nonsymbolic processes can motivate action. What is unique about language is not so much the motivational process itself but how it comes into human psychology. For example, if a dog has a history of doing tricks to earn doggie treats, one of the quickest ways to get him in the mood for tricks is to give him a little taste of a doggie treat. If one of Pavlov's dogs knew how to do tricks, a quick way to get him in the mood and doing tricks would be to ring a bell (in fact, B. F. Skinner once did an experiment exactly like that early in his career, and that is precisely what he found). These motivational processes work because *contact with reinforcing consequences motivates actions that give rise to these consequences.* The dog tasting a doggy treat is making that contact directly; a dog who has been exposed to pairings of a bell with food can do so through classical conditioning. People have another way: through language and the changes in functions that symbolically guided imagination can provide.

When immediate features of the context don't sufficiently influence an effective behavior, symbolic connections between the action and its consequences bring the reinforcing qualities of meaningful purposes into the present, thus making the action almost intrinsically[2] reinforcing (almost like a piece of chocolate cake!). Clients suffering from depression experience profound difficulties with reengaging in activities that are no longer pleasurable. We can help them persist by building hierarchical connections that overcome the current lack of reinforcement (e.g., by asking, "What could going back to work contribute to in your life?"). When clients with anxiety try to engage in activities they have been avoiding so as to stay away from painful emotions and sensations, building hierarchical connections can help increase the influence exerted by the meaning of these activities (e.g., "What if doing that scary thing was the stone of a house you are trying to build?"). When clients suffering from addiction have a hard time letting go of urges, building hierarchical connections can change the function of these uncomfortable feelings and increase the willingness to stay away from harmful activities (e.g., "What if urges were signs that you can do something that matters instead of using drugs?").

How This Method Touches on Various Clinical Traditions

Psychodynamic therapists often deal with the ways that motivation is hidden from view. Sometimes this motivation is negative (e.g., avoiding losing weight due to an unconscious fear of sexuality), but whether it is or is not, the analyst is interested in expanding awareness and in contacting feelings, urges, and motives in the present, so that the person can take ownership of them.

Humanistic therapists (e.g., Maslow, 1966; Rogers, 1951) have emphasized the key role of intrinsic motivation, very much as we have described in this chapter. Intrinsic motivation is driven by enjoyment in the task itself

---

[2]The action is not intrinsically reinforcing in a literal sense given that we still need to engage in the augmenting process, but reinforcement doesn't depend on additional consequences.

and its direct properties rather than in the outcome, and is based on choices by the individual rather than compliance, external pressure, or arbitrary external consequences.

A modern extension of humanistic therapies is motivational interviewing (Miller & Rollnick, 1991), which emphasizes the importance of the client himself examining the consequences of his actions and envisioning a different future, with the clinician helping the client to see what is true for him without imposing her views on the client. The therapist engages the client, helps him focus, and evokes responses, through the use of open-ended questions, and summaries. As motivation becomes clearer, practical change steps are designed. An RFT perspective on the clinical conversation generally aligns with these points of view, but with a functional contextual model of how and why such issues might be addressed and with a detailed basic process account of how to do so.

How to Do It

The key use of language in motivation is to overcome the vagaries of time, probability, and confusion by clearly contacting the satisfying properties of actions: their meaning. These properties are brought out by hierarchical framing questions that delve into their direct effects (e.g., Why is doing this action important? What is it part of? What does it contribute to?). In effect, therapists are helping the client taste and smell the steak of overarching goals and qualities of action—to see themselves in their silver car of meaning and purpose. As that happens, motivation increases quite naturally, not due to arbitrary pats on the back or M&Ms, but by making the motivational properties of meaning clear, direct, sensory, and present.

LIFE MEANING AND MOTIVATION IN PRACTICE

Together, symbolic processes of meaning and motivation constitute the engine of behavior change by ensuring that the client's efforts to adopt more flexible behavioral repertoires are connected to lasting satisfaction. Let's now explore the ways to build meaning and motivation in therapy with RFT principles.

Building Life Meaning

In practice, RFT principles involved in life meaning consist of two main aspects: first, the client is led to identify or build positive overarching goals and qualities of action; second, he is encouraged to identify broad patterns of various actions that help him engage in the direction of his overarching goals and qualities of action.

Often, at least some positive overarching goals and qualities of action are already relatively well established in the client's life, but not enough attention is given to them. The culture and other elements of the client's external world are often of little help because various commercial and other interests are constantly pushing her to formulate meaning in ways that serve their own selfish interests, but not hers. For a long time, cigarette producers seemed to have little shame in casting smoking as a meaningful action. As a result of this confusion and inattention, the client experiences little or no satisfaction, even when she performs meaningful actions. Helping her to formulate what matters in her life in ways that ensure lasting satisfaction will help her contact and notice the reinforcing qualities of her current or potential actions. In other cases, it seems that no source of lasting satisfaction is present in the client's life. Then, therapeutic interactions will aim at building positive overarching goals and qualities of action, based for example on the satisfaction the client was able to find in past actions, on the exploration of various domains of life, or on the inspiration she finds in other people's actions and to link actions to these goals and qualities.

It is important to formulate meaning in ways that translate into actions that are in the client's control (i.e., things to do, rather than things to have or to be). Consider the difference between saying, "I want to be a good mother. When my children grow up, I want them to be grateful for what I have done for them," and "I want to give my children the best chances to succeed in life by showing them unconditional love and respect for their own choices." In the first statement, satisfaction depends on evaluations about the self[3] and on social approval. In the second statement, satisfaction depends on doing things that serve an overarching goal (increasing the chance of children's success) through a quality of action (unconditional love and respect).

Helping the client identify actions that are consistent with sources of lasting satisfaction involves two main steps. First, the clinician helps the client position the actions he or she chooses in a hierarchical, rather than merely conditional, network in order to ensure that they become intrinsically and widely reinforcing. For example, if a client chooses to look for a new job so as to get a better salary, the therapist can encourage the client to connect this action to an overarching positive goal such as improving the well-being of his family. This way, the action of looking for a job becomes part of a more general process, and not only a means to reach a specific outcome (which may or may not happen). In addition, even if a greater salary is not available, other options may exist that will serve the ultimate positive

---

[3] However, talking about evaluations of the self can be a step toward identifying ways of being that correspond to qualities of actions (e.g., "I want to be a good mother" might be defined as being loving and respectful, and eventually as acting with love and respect).

purposes of that salary. Thus, the clinician can lead the client to identify a variety of behaviors that serve the same positive overarching goal or quality of action. Doing this makes lasting satisfaction always available while protecting the client from potential future limitations. For example, a client who values living a life that is challenging may identify actions to serve this value that require physical health (e.g., taking part in a sports competition) as well as actions that are less physically demanding (e.g., learning a new language). Keeping a wide variety of behavioral options open is like subscribing to "life satisfaction insurance" that will allow the client to consistently engage in challenging behaviors, regardless of his physical condition or difficulties in his life situation.

Note that hierarchical framing is added to, but doesn't eliminate, conditional framing that links actions to specific goals. When an action is *part of* an overarching goal or quality of action, it is satisfying regardless of the outcome, but outcomes are important. Imagine, for example, a student in medical school preparing for a test. Passing tests is a necessary outcome in order to move on to professional life. Thus, assessing the effectiveness of this preparation work is important because if the student passes, he might want to prepare the next test the same way, but if he fails, he might want to make some changes. If he connected his preparation only to the overarching goal of "contributing to the well-being of others" and reacted to failing at tests by thinking "I am consistent with what I care about. It doesn't matter whether I fail or succeed," he would be insensitive to useful contingencies and wouldn't change his preparation even if it were not effective. As we saw in Chapter 5, tracking requires conditional framing. When hierarchical framing is added, satisfaction can be found even in case of failure, but it doesn't hide the fact that behavior changes could, and at times should, be made to improve outcomes.

Identifying and Building Sources of Meaning

Therapists can conduct verbal interactions that help clients identify and build intrinsic and inexhaustible sources of reinforcement. Although this type of work will benefit greatly from using formal exercises (see Chapter 9), for now we will only focus on informal exchanges that happen with clients in the therapy room.

Finding or Creating Sources of Meaning. Often, sources of reinforcement come up spontaneously in the course of natural conversations. For example, a client who wants to be less socially anxious may say his goal is to have a job or a romantic relationship. Another client who wants to get rid of obsessive thoughts and rituals may hope that she will have more time for her family. Those are certainly legitimate sources of motivation, but they are formulated as specific goals rather than positive overarching goals and qualities of action—and thus, they don't guarantee lasting satisfaction. In order to identify the positive overarching goal or the quality of action, the clinician must help the client extract the *higher function* from these specific goals, which enables the key hierarchical relationship to be established cognitively as related to action. An adequate source of lasting satisfaction is found when it defines a goal that can never be finished, linked to a quality that together characterize a high number of actions. For example, if a client says that she wants to be able to go to work, the therapist can explore with her what higher function going to work serves (e.g., providing for her family, interacting with other people), as well as the way she wants to engage in this activity (e.g., with diligence, with reliability, with kindness). We know we can stop the process of exploration once there is an overarching goal and/or a quality of action at the top of the hierarchical network. However, it is generally possible to keep exploring further if necessary. This can be done typically when there is a values conflict between two persons. In this case, the clinician can help them identify the higher function of what they care about in order to find commonality at another level (e.g., a parent cares about authority, and the other cares about compassion in the way they raise their children; they can meet each other at a higher point by identifying that they both care about raising their children with love). Ultimately, all human beings can meet each other on most basic sources of motivation (exploration, safety, attachment, etc.). Thus, it is probably always possible to find commonality if the elaboration of the hierarchical network is pushed far enough. Linking overarching goals and qualities of actions to nonsymbolic sources of motivation (i.e., basic needs) can also help give them an essential dimension, which is particularly useful when contacting the arbitrariness of symbolic experiences has led to meaninglessness (e.g., after a trauma).

Conditional framing and hierarchical framing are two primary language tools used to identify higher functions of specific goals through verbal interactions. For example, a therapist might ask, "And if you had a job, what difference would that make in your life?" If the client answers, "I would have money," the therapist keeps using conditional and hierarchical cues until a positive overarching goal or a quality of action is identified (e.g., "What would you be able to do if you had money?"; "What would getting a job be part of in your life?"; "What would this mean to you?").

Comparison and distinction framing can also be used to extract overarching goals and qualities of action because they encourage clients to identify their preferences (i.e., "Why this action more than that one?"; "Why this goal and not that goal?"). Even when clients have very little sense of what is important in their lives, they are generally able to state that one thing is better than the other, or at least not as bad. For example, a clinician might ask a client who spends all day on the couch watching sports on television, "Why do you watch sport channels rather than the news or a movie?" The client might respond, "It is less boring," and from there, the therapist could help him identify what makes sports less boring, until a quality of action is formulated (e.g., challenge, uncertainty).

Once the higher function is identified, it is useful to explore if different actions, perhaps even in different domains, can serve the same purpose. This ensures its hierarchical quality and maintains a variety of ways to access it (i.e., it can potentially include a range of actions). This can be done both by exploring other specific actions within the hierarchy (e.g., "Are there other things you might do that would have that same goal and quality?") or by using analogical framing (e.g., "Are there other things you do that have the same purpose?" Or as a metaphor "If a job like that was like a film, what film would it remind you of? Are there other things you might do that would be like that film?").

Often, clients have difficulty seeing beyond the psychological experience that they want to get rid of. If asked what they care about or what they would like to change in their lives, they respond that they don't want to suffer anymore, or they don't want to remember past traumas. It might be that they have focused so much on this problem that they have completely lost contact with a sense of higher purpose. In these cases, using distinction or opposition framing can help clients explore what might be on the other side of this barrier. For example, to a client saying, "I don't want to be bothered by thoughts anymore," the clinician might ask, "What would you be able to do if you were not bothered by your thoughts?" Sometimes, this process requires a series of questions before identifying the potential source of satisfaction, which might be at first formulated as a specific goal. If this happens, the therapist goes on with conditional and hierarchical framing to identify the higher function as explained above.

Observe the use of distinction/opposition, conditional, and hierarchical framing in the following exchange with a client suffering from generalized anxiety:

CLIENT: What I want is to be less anxious.

THERAPIST: What would be different in your life if feeling anxious was not a problem?

The therapist uses distinction framing to delink the client from his problem.

CLIENT: I would be more productive at work. Right now, I waste a lot of time second-guessing myself, so I am not very productive. And I end up doing a lot of work at home.

THERAPIST: What difference would it make in your life if you were more productive at work?

The therapist uses conditional framing to explore higher function.

CLIENT: I would have more time with my family.

THERAPIST: Would this contribute to something that matters to you?

The therapist uses hierarchical framing to identify a positive overarching goal or quality of action.

CLIENT: I would be more involved in my husband's and my kids' lives. I would share more things with them. I could support them, not just with money like right now, I would be there for them.

The client identifies a positive overarching goal and begins to identify qualities of action.

THERAPIST: Are there other reasons why you would like to be more productive at work? What other impact would this have to be more productive?

The therapist uses conditional framing again to explore other sources of reinforcement.

CLIENT: Well, it was hard to get this job, you know. When I applied for this job, I told them I would do really great, but right now, I am not nearly as productive as my colleagues. It makes me feel like . . .

THERAPIST: Like?

CLIENT: Like I am not performing up to my boss's expectations.

THERAPIST: It is important for you to meet her expectations?

CLIENT: Yes. I will lose my job if I don't.

THERAPIST: I understand. Do you feel like how you are at work is also part of something you care about in your life in general?

The therapist uses hierarchical framing to identify a positive overarching goal or quality of action and moves it away from pliance in a specific area.

CLIENT: I want to be reliable. When I say I will do something, I want to do what I said.

The client identifies a quality of action.

THERAPIST: Is reliability something you care about in your life in general?

The therapist uses hierarchical framing to explore if this quality of action functions as an overarching reinforcer.

CLIENT: Yes, definitely. I don't necessarily think about it all the time, but it is something I care about in many areas.

THERAPIST: What are other things you do or want to do in your life that are also in the service of reliability?

The therapist inverts the hierarchy to further explore other actions encompassed by reliability.

CLIENT: In my relationships, I try to make sure that people can count on me.

THERAPIST: I've sensed that in here, almost as if you are wanting to lay a foundation for your family.

The therapist uses analogical framing to broaden the hierarchy.

CLIENT: Exactly. I've even used that word before. Reliability is like a foundation.

THERAPIST: Where else does that desire to lay down a strong foundation show up?

The therapist uses analogical framing again to broaden the hierarchy.

Sometimes even specific goals are difficult to identify. It often happens when clients are depressed or when they have focused so much on the behaviors and psychological experiences they *don't* want that they don't know what matters to them anymore. In these cases, using perspective taking (deictic framing) to review past or potential future actions and enhancing the observation of the feelings that these actions once brought up (or could bring up) can help build or rebuild new sources of lasting satisfaction. Evoking observation and descriptions of feelings connected to meaningful moments is important in order not to leave the exploration of sources of meaning at an intellectual level. If this exploration skips what is experienced by the client at a deeper, more intrinsic level, then there is a higher risk of taking arbitrary directions. Concretely, the clinician can ask questions such as "When you were 15, what did you hope your life would be like?"; "Was there a time when you knew quite well what you cared about in your life? Could we try to go back there for a moment?"; "Imagine that we are 10 years from now. As you look back to this decade, what do you think you would like to have stood for in your life?" Then the therapist asks questions evoking observation and description of experiences associated with these meaningful moments (e.g., "What were you feeling in that moment?"; "How does that make you feel to reconnect with this moment of your life?"). As connection with sources of satisfaction is strengthened, not only does meaning increase—so too does motivation. Observe this approach in the following exchange:

CLIENT: I don't know what to say; there is nothing I care about anymore.

THERAPIST: Did you have the hope you would care about something again when you decided to come see me?

CLIENT: Yeah. I don't want to stay like that forever.

THERAPIST: What did you care about in the past?

The therapist evokes memories of former sources of meaning.

CLIENT: It is hard to say. I mean I can think of things I used to care about, but they seem so uninteresting now that I am not even sure it mattered that much at the time. Maybe I was just trying to convince myself that it was important.

THERAPIST: Could you try to give me an example?

CLIENT: I used to spend a lot of time reading.

THERAPIST: What kind of books?

CLIENT: Novels, mostly.

THERAPIST: What did you like about reading?

The therapist evokes the client's observation and description of the satisfaction he used to get from this reading.

CLIENT: I don't know . . . I am not sure anymore.

THERAPIST: Can you remember a book that you enjoyed reading?

CLIENT: Sure.

THERAPIST: Can you picture in your mind a moment when you were reading it, and imagine that you are back then?

The therapist evokes the client's change of perspective to facilitate the observation of what he used to enjoy.

CLIENT: I can easily recall that. It was during a holiday.

THERAPIST: Okay, great. Can you try to describe to me what was going through your mind as you were reading the pages?

CLIENT: I was completely absorbed. I generally was when I used to read.

THERAPIST: Absorbed. Okay, that is interesting. Like something that grabs all your attention?

CLIENT: Yes, exactly.

THERAPIST: What is grabbing your attention so much in this book?

The therapist intentionally uses the present tense to help the client stay in touch with the memory as vividly as possible.

CLIENT: The story was compelling, I guess.

THERAPIST: What is the story about?

CLIENT: About a guy who tries to find his wife's murderers.

THERAPIST: What is compelling about this story?

CLIENT: There is something powerful about this guy remembering the good times he had with his wife. It is moving to see him try to find out what happened, as a kind of way of reconnecting with her because they were separated just before she died.

THERAPIST: This seems like a beautiful story.

CLIENT: Yes, it is.

THERAPIST: And you remember being moved by the character's attempt to reconnect with his deceased wife. . . .

CLIENT: Yes.

In these exchanges, the therapist helps the client observe and describe with precision the satisfaction experienced while reading the book, thus increasing the salience of reinforcing qualities.

THERAPIST: What about now? Does this sense of connection means something to you?

CLIENT: I don't know. I feel disconnected from everybody right now.

THERAPIST: Does that bother you?

CLIENT: Yes and no. I don't really like being like that, but at the same time, it doesn't really touch me. I know it is weird. I just don't feel much right now.

THERAPIST: As you were talking about the story, you seemed moved earlier. Is that right?

CLIENT: I guess I was remembering that time, when I was much better. . . . And yes, that story was moving. I guess it still is.

The therapist evokes the client's observation and description of his current experience as he recalled the story of the book in order to explore positive overarching goals and qualities of action that may still be meaningful, such as connection with others.

THERAPIST: Have you ever felt closely connected to someone in your life? Can you think of a specific instance or time?

The therapist begins to explore sources of meaning more directly in the client's life.

When nothing seems to be reinforcing in the client's life, conditional framing can also be a powerful tool to create sources of meaning. For example, the clinician can say, "If you had a billion dollars to donate or invest, where would you put your money?"; "If everything was possible, what would you want to change in the world?" Sometimes the client will answer in a way that indicates that she is still more focused on her difficulties than on positive sources of meaning. For example, an inpatient in a hospital might say, "I would buy this hospital and fire everybody!" Although this response doesn't immediately seem to indicate that the client cares about something meaningful, the additional use of conditional and distinction framing can help progress toward a higher and more positive function, as in the following example:

> THERAPIST: If all these people were fired, what would you do with this hospital?
>
> *The therapist uses conditional framing.*
>
> CLIENT: I would hire people who are not so careless and judgmental.
>
> THERAPIST: If they were not careless, how would they be instead?
>
> *The therapist uses distinction framing.*
>
> CLIENT: They would be attentive to patients' needs. They would care about how we feel. They would realize how hard it is for us to be here.
>
> THERAPIST: They would show compassion?
>
> *The therapist reformulates what the client said as quality of action.*
>
> CLIENT: Yes.
>
> THERAPIST: Is compassion something important for you?
>
> *The therapist explores if compassion is a quality of action that the client cares about.*
>
> CLIENT: Yes.

As these types of exchanges are repeated with a variety of material and across multiple situations, the seeds of a positive overarching goal and qualities of action begin to be sown. At no point does the therapist try to *convince* the client to seek a particular source of meaning. That would shift the focus to pliance, which is very different from tracking intrinsic consequences that the person holds dear. The task is to help the client find what brings satisfaction and formulate these sources as positive overarching goals and qualities of action. This work requires patience if the clinician wants the client to fully endorse new life directions and genuinely find meaning in his actions.

Distinguishing Sources of Meaning from Pliance. The importance of limiting pliance in the process of identifying and building lasting sources of reinforcement pertains not only to the therapeutic relationship, but also to other social sources of influence. There are few sources of meaning that are not influenced at least in part by a social community. A quality of action such as altruism, for example, is likely to be approved by the members of a community. Pursuing the overarching goal of always learning more will probably be well perceived in many social groups. The vast majority of positive overarching goals and qualities of action people settle on have a clear social dimension. But pliance is more than social caring—it moves the goals and qualities of action from the person and their choices into the choices and reactions of others. When that happens, actions cannot be intrinsically reinforced: the consequences are not in qualities of action and overarching goals but instead are in the qualities of ultimate reactions and others' goals.

The empirical work on meaning shows that goals and qualities have little positive impact if they are avoidant, compliant, or psychologically coerced (Sheldon, Ryan, Deci, & Kasser, 2004). If a person volunteers for a charity because he feels that it is what others expect from him, little meaning will be found in this activity. Thus, when the client's formulation of overarching goals and qualities of action shows excessive attachment to social rules (if they have a quality of "must" or "have to" without a clear purpose), they predict poor outcomes. In these cases, the therapist can use distinction/opposition framing to help her assess the satisfaction she would find in following these life directions if nobody approved or knew about it. If this thought experiment leads to a significant decrease in satisfaction, the client is encouraged to explore the higher function of her actions. Virtually removing social influence is generally more appropriate when we suspect that the client is afraid of others' judgment. In contrast, if the client seems to be *positively* reinforced by social approval, it might be wiser to conduct the thought experiment in a reversed direction. For example, a client could be asked what she would do if everybody liked her, or approved what she did regardless of her actions.

Sometimes, attachment to social rules can reflect a strong interest in connection with others. For example, it is possible that a person would still volunteer for a charity after realizing that his overarching goal is to take part in social activities, but knowing so would now convey greater meaning to his actions. Observe in the following short exchange how the therapist helps the client find meaning beyond social influence:

CLIENT: I have to be there for my kids. This is what a mother does.

THERAPIST: I think most people would agree with you. Yet, I am interested to hear why it is important to you.

The therapist orients the client to potential sources of intrinsic reinforcement.

CLIENT: I want to be a good mother, to be there for my children. Can you imagine what people would think if I didn't take care for them properly?

THERAPIST: How about we approach this in a slightly different way? For example, I wonder what *you* would think if you were there for your children but nobody knew or cared about it.

Since the client seems to focus mainly on social consequences, the therapist encourages her to assess the meaning of being there for her kids, regardless of what other people think (opposition framing).

CLIENT: Well . . . Hum . . . It is a very strange question!

THERAPIST: You think?

CLIENT: Yeah . . . I mean . . . Of course I would still be there for my children, I would take care of them even if people told me it is wrong.

THERAPIST: Or just didn't care?

CLIENT: Yeah, absolutely. It is not just about what people think.

THERAPIST: Okay, this is really interesting. Would you like to explore a little further what would be a more meaningful reason to be there for your children other than doing what people think you should do?

The therapist encourages the client to further explore what is intrinsically meaningful about being there for her children, beyond social approval.

CLIENT: I love my children. They are everything to me.

THERAPIST: I can see that. How does that fit with the need to be there for them?

CLIENT: It is a way of showing them that I love them.

Distinguishing Sources of Meaning from External Consequences or Self-Concepts. Building intrinsic reinforcement is not only about ensuring a relative independence from social compliance. More generally, it consists of formulating positive overarching goals and qualities of action in ways that suggest actions rather than external consequences or qualities of the self-concept. This way, engaging in an action connected to intrinsic meaningful directions will become reinforcing, regardless of the external result of this action or of evaluations about the self.

In therapy, we often see clients who express what matters in their lives as things they want to have or to be. This is not surprising given our culture's tendency to encourage us to focus on these ways of describing what we hold as important. The cultural limitations of our language tend to favor evaluations about the self, which can make it hard to use formulations as qualities of action instead (e.g., one might say that they care about being thoughtful, which is more usual than saying "acting with thoughtfulness").

Such evaluations about the self are to some degree unavoidable, but it makes sense from an RFT perspective to point as much as possible to what matters in terms of concrete actions (e.g., listening to others, paying attention to their needs) in order to maintain intrinsic motivational qualities. In this way, rather than contradicting the client, we are gradually helping him expand his relational network toward higher functions of specific goals and qualities of action. Observe this approach in the following exchange:

CLIENT: I want to have a normal life. A job, a partner, friends . . . You know . . . a normal life.

THERAPIST: When you say normal life, do you mean like everybody else?

CLIENT: Yeah, I guess.

THERAPIST: Why do you think people want this kind of life?

CLIENT: It makes them happy.

THERAPIST: Okay, let's take a concrete example. Let's say you get a job tomorrow. Would that make you happy?

CLIENT: Yes, of course.

THERAPIST: What difference would that make in your life?

CLIENT: I would have more money. It is already important. I would feel like I am a real person.

The sources of meaning were expressed as external consequences and self-evaluations (things to have: more money; things to be: a real person).

THERAPIST: Okay, there are two things in there. Let's start with money if it is okay. What would it change in your life if you had more money?

The therapist uses conditional framing to explore the higher function of getting more money.

CLIENT: I would be able to go out with my friends, for example. I can never go out with them right now. It is too expensive, even to just have drinks.

THERAPIST: You like spending time with your friends?

CLIENT: Yes, I do.

THERAPIST: What do you like about it?

CLIENT: It makes me feel connected, like I can share things. Right now, I feel isolated.

THERAPIST: Would you say that getting a job is important to you because it would help you connect with your friends?

CLIENT: Yes, sure. This is one reason for sure.

In this exchange, the therapist helps the client formulate his source of satisfaction as an overarching goal that is within his control— connecting with friends—rather than an external consequence.

THERAPIST: You also said that you would feel like a real person. What does *real* mean to you in practice?

CLIENT: I don't like feeling assisted. I want to be active. I feel like a zombie without a job. I am nothing.

THERAPIST: So you want to live your life actively?

Client: Yes, I want to contribute . . . you know . . . to society.

In this last exchange, the therapist invites the client to define what "real" means in more practical terms so as to turn the self-evaluation into a quality of action.

Exploring Positive Sources of Meaning. If aversive control is excessively at play when clients identify or build meaning in their lives, they will lack a sense of vitality. Consider the difference between quitting smoking either to avoid dying young or to live a longer, healthier life. These goals are similar in appearance, but their impact in terms of vitality will differ. Thinking of health will softly draw the person toward a wide variety of healthy action; avoiding dying will prod the person with fear, which can be escaped in many ways other than stopping smoking (e.g., drinking enough alcohol will remove that fear; thought suppression will temporarily remove that fear).

For this reason, as much as possible, clients are encouraged to formulate their overarching goals and qualities of action positively rather than negatively. This can be done by exploring what will be *added* (even symbolically) rather than what will be *removed*. The following exchange illustrates this approach:

CLIENT: I am going to ruin my relationship if I keep having these anger bursts. I really need to do something about it.

THERAPIST: Your relationship seems important to you.

The therapist orients the client to positive reinforcing consequences.

CLIENT: Yes it is! I love my husband, and I know I am horrible right now. I complain about everything, I break stuff. I can't keep going like this or I will lose him. I would understand if he left me. But I don't want that!

THERAPIST: If you changed the way you interact with him, how would that make your relationship better?

The therapist orients again to positive consequences.

CLIENT: We would not fight all the time.

THERAPIST: I am sure this would be a relief. Are there other things that would change and not only remove what is problematic in your relationship but also bring something you care about?

The therapist orients again to positive consequences, seeking a positive overarching goal and qualities of action.

CLIENT: Well . . . Maybe that could help us get closer again. . . . We barely talk to each other right now. I miss feeling close to him, having good conversations. It would be nice to feel closer physically too.

THERAPIST: Can you tell me about a time you felt especially close to your husband?

The therapist explores qualities of overarching goals in specific actions.

CLIENT: I remember one time when his mother died, we just talked hours about what she meant to him and it kind of spilled over into what we felt about each other. It was strange because it was such a sad day, but yet it was so sweet to be together.

THERAPIST: So when you share your deeper feelings—including your feelings about each other—you feel closer.

The therapist clarifies goals and qualities.

CLIENT: It doesn't happen that often I guess, but the times I can think of are all like that.

THERAPIST: Are there feelings you have that you would kind of like to talk about with your husband but don't?

The therapist redirects toward specific examples underneath the hierarchy.

Building Patterns of Meaningful Actions

The second step of building meaning is to help the client identify and choose a variety of actions consistent with her positive overarching goals and qualities of action. Using natural verbal interactions, the clinician targets two main processes. First, she must ensure that the client connects her actions to overarching goals and qualities of action situated at the top of the hierarchical network. Then, a variety of actions targeting the same function (i.e., serving a given overarching goal or quality of action or both) ought to be identified in order to maximize the availability of these sources of meaning.

Connecting Actions to the Top of the Hierarchy. To help the client establish a connection between actions and her sources of meaning, the therapist can use hierarchical, conditional, and deictic framing. Although these types of framing were already involved in the identification of overarching goals and qualities of action, they now target the identification of patterns of actions. Metaphorically, we could say that instead of climbing the hierarchical network to the top, we now descend it to the base. An example of hierarchical framing might be asking, "What are the things you could do that would be part of/contribute to/in the service of _____ [quality of action or overarching goal]?" Conditional framing in this context generally requires the use of a specific intermediate goal. For example, the clinician might ask, "What do you want to do in order to have more money [specific goal] and support your kids' well-being [overarching goal]?"An example of deictic framing might be, "A year from now, looking back at what you have done since today, what would you like to have accomplished in the service of _____ [overarching goal or quality of action]?" Or using interpersonal deictic framing, "Do you know someone in your acquaintances, or even a famous person, who shares the same _____ [overarching goal or quality of action]? What are the things they do in the service of _____? Are there things they do you could imagine doing too?" When possible, the therapist encourages the client to find an action that is connected to both an overarching goal and a quality of action so as to increase its reinforcing properties. Observe this approach in the following exchange:

THERAPIST: You said that what is important to you is to build a socially rich life. What could you do to contribute to this purpose?

The therapist uses hierarchical framing to explore actions serving the overarching goal "building a socially rich life."

CLIENT: I don't really know right now. I am kind of lost to be honest.

THERAPIST: That's understandable. Imagine that we are one week from now, at our next session. Imagine that we talk about what you have done during this week. What do you think you may like to have accomplished since our last session?

Since the client is a bit stuck, the therapist uses deictic framing to help the client identify meaningful actions.

CLIENT: I could call my friends. It would bring me closer to them. And I think they would appreciate that too.

THERAPIST: You told me before that you like to be thoughtful in your relationships.

The therapist brings up another source of meaning: the quality of action "thoughtfulness."

CLIENT: Yes, I care a lot about that. I like to make sure my friends are well and to do things for them. I feel really bad because I haven't done that much in the past few months.

THERAPIST: If you called your friends, would it also be an opportunity to be more thoughtful in your relationship with them?

The therapist uses conditional framing to explore the connection between the action and the quality of action.

CLIENT: Hmm . . . I think that if I took the time to listen instead of having short conversations, I could be more thoughtful with my friends, yes.

THERAPIST: Okay, so calling your friends is one action that can help you make your social life richer, and at the same time, you can be thoughtful when you do that. Is this something you want to do?

The therapist helps the client notice that calling friends can serve both an overarching goal and a quality of action.

CLIENT: Yes, absolutely. As we talk about it, I definitely feel like I want to do that.

Note that certain actions are not always identified as satisfying even if they help access sources of meaning. This is often the case when one needs to engage in an intermediate action in order to access more satisfying activities later. For example, people who want to adopt a child need to go through a number of steps, which can be time consuming and frustrating, before they can build their family. Even though these intermediate actions are understandably less reinforcing than finally having a child, the more strongly related they are to the higher purpose, the more satisfying they will be. Observe how the therapist helps the client make this type of connection through hierarchical framing in the following exchange:

THERAPIST: What could you do to be more involved in your children's life?

CLIENT: I know they would like me to spend more time with them on weekends, but I would need to change my work schedule, and I would probably have to work with a different partner. I have been working with the same colleague for 4 years. It would be a lot of work to build a new team.

THERAPIST: I see. It would bring more work and it would not be easy for you. Would that contribute to involving you more in your children's lives in the end?

The therapist uses hierarchical framing to help the client connect his action to the overarching goal.

CLIENT: If I did that, I could probably have more time on weekends, yes. I could spend more time with them, and they would like that.

The client identifies a specific intermediate goal connected to being involved in his children's lives.

THERAPIST: Is it something you want to do?

CLIENT: If it can help me be more involved, I think I could do that, yes. It will be hard but it is worth the price.

Often a single action can serve different functions. For example, in this last vignette, it is possible that the client wants to spend more time with his children as a way of avoiding arguments with his wife or because spending time with children on weekends is generally approved by the social community. This means that the action is also influenced by aversive consequences (avoidance) and social approval (pliance). That is not necessarily a problem as long as the action is not chosen solely for those reasons and if a more positive and intrinsic function is clearly identified. As when identifying overarching goals and qualities of action, the clinician can help the client make sure that the actions he identifies are intrinsically and positively reinforcing, regardless of other functions. This can be done using distinction/opposition framing (e.g., "If nobody knew about you doing this, would you still want to do it?") and conditional/hierarchical framing (e.g., "Would this still contribute to something meaningful if you were to do this?") Observe this approach in the following exchange:

CLIENT: I think it would be good if I tried to get more interested in new things, like going to museums maybe, reading more books.

THERAPIST: Would this be part of something important to you?

The therapist uses hierarchical framing to explore if the action is connected to a source of meaning.

CLIENT: Most of my friends do these kinds of things. I think it might be good for me to do that too.

THERAPIST: Just as a thought experiment, do you think that you would still consider these new activities if your friends didn't care about museums and books?

The therapist uses distinction framing to explore if the action is at least partially intrinsically reinforcing.

CLIENT: Hmm. Probably not. But I would like to be more like my friends. I feel a bit excluded from our conversations right now. They don't think I am as smart as they are. I should probably make an effort if I don't want them to think that way about me.

THERAPIST: So, as I hear you, going to museums and reading books have a lot to do with improving your social relationships; is it the case?

The therapist invites the client to explore other sources of meaning connected to reading books and going to museums.

CLIENT: Yes, that's true.

THERAPIST: You say that you don't want them to think you are not as smart as they are. Is there something positive that may also come if you were to read books and go to museums?

The therapist uses coordination framing to connect the action to positive consequences (i.e., what would also come).

CLIENT: What do you mean?

THERAPIST: I mean, not only something that doesn't happen such as your friends thinking that you are not smart, but also something that does happen and that is satisfying to you; perhaps something that would enrich your life, not just prevent something unpleasant from happening.

CLIENT: I see . . . I think I would be more included in the group, and I would be more able to share interests with them, probably. And maybe I will find these activities interesting if I try. I have always found that these kinds of things are not for me, but I like listening to my friends when they talk about their experiences. Maybe I was just not ready to make the effort until now.

THERAPIST: You think it would be worth it now?

CLIENT: I think so, yeah. I mean, there is no risk in trying, right? And at least I will better understand what my friends are talking about. I will feel like I can share more things with them.

Building Variability at the Base of the Hierarchy. The second main aspect of building broad patterns of meaningful actions consists of developing variability at the base of the hierarchical network. The more variety there is in the actions serving a direction, the greater chance the clients will have of finding something to do in any kind of situation. This is particularly useful when some barriers to actions are impossible or difficult to bypass (e.g., exercising when one is hospitalized or spending time with children when they live far away). If the client had only one way to serve an overarching goal or to honor a quality of action, she would be at risk of giving up on these sources of meaning when this very specific action can't be performed. In contrast, having multiple possible actions to choose from makes satisfaction always available.

In order to ensure variability in the actions directed toward lasting satisfaction, the therapist helps the client identify a range of activities sharing a common function. In essence, this identification process is either analogical (what network is like this network?) or hierarchical (what other things are part of this category?); and thus includes coordination among similar actions. For example, the clinician might ask, "What other things could you do that serve the same purpose?" or "What other actions share the same quality in your life?" The client is also encouraged to identify actions of various amplitudes, using comparative framing (e.g., "Are there other activities that have the same meaning to you, even if they take less time or less effort?"; "What smallest and what biggest action could you do in this direction?"). Although talking about certain actions will seem to yield more significant progress than others toward an overarching goal or a quality of action, the functional similarity that characterizes all the actions at the base of a hierarchical network gives them all a genuine meaning. With this approach, the client can find satisfaction not only in great accomplishments but also in casual moments of everyday life.

Opposition and distinction framing can also be employed to create variability through the identification of alternative actions. For example, the therapist might ask, "Imagine that you could not do this activity anymore. What else could you do that would contribute to _____ [overarching goal]?", or "If for some reason, this action was not as satisfying anymore, what else would you do with _____ [quality of action]?"

Observe this approach in the following exchange:

THERAPIST: What could help you connect with your wife?

CLIENT: We could take some vacations together. We haven't done that in a long time. We could go on a trip maybe.

THERAPIST: How would that be an opportunity to connect?

The therapist checks the hierarchical connection with the overarching goal.

CLIENT: It would be just the two of us, and we would do things together.

THERAPIST: So it would be meaningful to you?

The therapist strengthens again the hierarchical connection with the overarching goal.

CLIENT: Yes, I think so. Although . . . Maybe I am dreaming. I am not sure it will be possible. We are a little short on money. You see, this is exactly the problem we have. We don't have the luxury to spend time together, to go on vacations like other people.

The action chosen by the client is difficult to do, which increases the risk that he will give up on connecting with his wife.

THERAPIST: Yeah, this is hard. I understand. So, going on vacations would be really great, and you don't know if it is possible right now. If this was not possible, what else could you do that would also help you connect with your wife?

The therapist uses distinction and analogical framing to explore alternative actions serving the same function.

CLIENT: We could go out more often maybe.

THERAPIST: What kinds of things would you do out together?

CLIENT: See a movie. Go to dinner.

THERAPIST: These would be opportunities to connect with her?

The therapist checks hierarchical connection with overarching goal.

CLIENT: It could work. We used to like doing that together, so yes, it is possible.

THERAPIST: What else? Are there things you could even do at home, that don't need you to spend money or to plan anything?

The therapist uses coordination framing ("What else?") and distinction framing again to further expand the range of actions, including small activities that are easily accessible, regardless of the situation.

CLIENT: We could listen to some music together.

THERAPIST: Okay. Is that something you could easily do?

CLIENT: Yes. All we have to do is put the radio on. We never do it, I guess, because we are too busy and we have been spending too much time on our own. We could do that, I think.

Variability at the base of the hierarchical network of meaning also includes unsuccessful attempts to reach a specific goal. For example, a client may choose to go on a date as a way to develop intimacy with a partner. Obviously, there is no guarantee that this specific action will lead to finding the ideal person with whom she will want to build an intimate relationship. However, it can be recognized as part of the actions serving intimacy.

This way, whether or not this exact action allows her to reach the specific goal of finding a partner doesn't remove its meaning. To this end, instead of focusing on the conditional relation between the action and the specific goal, the therapist helps the client strengthen the hierarchical relation with the source of meaning. Observe this approach in the following vignette:

> THERAPIST: What could you do to show more appreciation to your colleagues?
>
> CLIENT: I could tell them that I think they do a great job.
>
> THERAPIST: Okay. Is this something you think you could do tomorrow, for example?
>
> CLIENT: Well, I could. But you know, I am afraid that with the reputation I have at work now, they won't think it is genuine. It is not that I don't appreciate their contribution, but I am very perfectionistic. I know that. So I tend to be very critical. I think they won't think I am being honest with them. They are not used to hearing me say nice things about their work!

The client worries that her action won't be successful at meeting a specific goal—being well received by her colleagues.

> THERAPIST: I hear you. So you mean there is no guarantee that showing your appreciation will be well received, right?
>
> CLIENT: Yeah.
>
> THERAPIST: I can understand that you would like your words to be well received. But what is the purpose of telling them that they did a good job? Why is it meaningful to you in the first place?

The therapist uses hierarchical framing to help the client connect her action to the quality she is trying to develop.

> CLIENT: I want to be more appreciative of other people. I want to leave the critical spiral I am in right now.
>
> THERAPIST: If you tell them that they are doing a good job, will it be a way of being more appreciative?

The therapist again strengthens the hierarchical connection with the quality of action.

> CLIENT: Yes. But I don't think they will believe me.
>
> THERAPIST: Yeah, it is possible. If that happens, will it mean that you were not being appreciative?

The therapist uses distinction framing to explore if being appreciative is a quality intrinsically connected to what the client plans to do.

If the action is still meaningful regardless of its specific result, it may still bring satisfaction.

CLIENT: No. I really appreciate their work.

THERAPIST: If they don't believe you, will you regret that you said that?

The therapist uses distinction framing again.

CLIENT: Hmm . . . I don't know. I guess I might be disappointed. But I know it might take time for them to see the change. And at least, I will have made an effort to show more appreciation. And *I* will know that it is sincere, even if they don't.

In certain cases, clients might choose actions that are connected to a source of meaning but are also problematic because they negatively impact their general functioning or the well-being of other people. For example, a client who lost his beloved partner might spend a significant amount of time at her grave or reading letters they exchanged and looking at pictures of her. These actions may be considered to serve the overarching goal of "honoring his partner's memory" or the quality of action "with fidelity." However, if it leads this client to disconnect from other important areas of his life, it can become problematic (e.g., not seeing friends anymore, not investing in his work and leisure, not taking care of his children, etc.).

These are the kinds of situations often discussed as "values conflicts." In fact, there is usually no conflict per se—it is more a matter of accepting the finite limits of life. In these types of situations, the therapist helps the client expand the variety of actions serving the overarching goal or quality of action so that he can engage in activities that are more compatible with the other areas of his life and the well-being of other people. Observe this approach in the following exchange:

THERAPIST: What are the things that you do with creativity?

CLIENT: I paint. I love painting. I spend hours on weekends on my paintings. I feel like I can do anything I want, but I never know in advance what is going to happen. This is what I like. It is a constant process of creation. My wife would like me to do other things too, so we could spend more time together. It is true that I spend too much time on my own, but I don't find the same interest in the things he likes.

THERAPIST: What kinds of things does she like?

CLIENT: She likes cooking and doing outdoor stuff, like hiking. Not really my thing.

THERAPIST: If you could find an interest in doing some of the things your wife appreciates, would it be easier for you to spend more time with her?

CLIENT: Yeah, if I could like what she likes, at least a bit, I could maybe leave my paintings from time to time.

THERAPIST: Painting seems like a great way to be creative for you. Do you think you could find this in cooking, for example?

In these first few exchanges, the therapist invites the client to explore if she could hierarchically frame her wife's activity with the quality of action she cares about.

CLIENT: Hmm. I never saw it that way. I am not a good cook at all though. When I cook, all I do is follow a recipe. This is hardly creative!

THERAPIST: What do you do that reflects being creative in your painting?

CLIENT: Doing something different. When I paint, I try to do something I have never seen before.

THERAPIST: Could you do that when cooking?

The therapist encourages the client to explore concrete actions serving the quality of action she cares about in her wife's activity.

CLIENT: Maybe I could look at new recipes. Maybe my husband would have ideas on how to improve them. He is creative too. We just have different ways of expressing our creativity.

THERAPIST: Not that you won't miss your painting. . . .

CLIENT: No, I love painting. But I love my wife too, and I guess it could be fun to try cooking with her, if it is a way of being creative. I will probably not be great at it, but maybe it would be fun.

Fostering Sustainable Motivation

Working on motivation in therapy with RFT principles consists of helping the client build symbolic bridges between an action and its distant, probabilistic, abstract, or hidden consequences, so as to increase rich contact with these consequences. Although some actions are immediately attractive enough to be performed, others (not less meaningful) require connecting oneself to things that are not yet present in the environment. For example, a client who decides to go out with her partner in order to strengthen their relationship may be easily motivated to do so. The identification of this action as a way to find lasting satisfaction and the pleasure she usually finds quickly in going out may be sufficient. However, if this action is likely to trigger difficult memories of being mugged, for example, the motivation to engage in this activity may be impaired even if it is genuinely meaningful. In another case, a client suffering from depression may have identified this activity as meaningful to her but may not have experienced the satisfaction she can get from it in a long time. As a result, when the time comes to actually go out, she doesn't feel like it and has a hard time engaging in the direction that matters to her. By leading clients to elaborate symbolic connections, it is possible to transform the function of an action so that it becomes immediately, intrinsically reinforcing. Consequently, the chances that they will actually commit to this action, do it, and find satisfaction during and after the action significantly increase.

In practice, developing motivation is divided into three main phases: preparing the action, performing the action, and debriefing the action. At every step, the clinician helps the client build and strengthen the parts of his symbolic relational network that convey intrinsic reinforcing properties to the action. Particular attention is given to the process of being or moving *in the direction* of positive overarching goals and qualities of action in order to limit the influence of extrinsic consequences per se. This is useful because extrinsic consequences often depend on a number of factors external to the action itself. For example, a client suffering from social anxiety who decides to give a talk may not be satisfied with her performance if what motivates her is praise from her audience. Although there is nothing wrong with aiming for positive feedback from other people, limiting her expectation to this extrinsic reinforcement does not provide a reliable guide to action. For one thing, initially her talk may not reach the standards that elicit praise from her audience, due to her lack of practice. As a result, she may not enjoy giving the talk or want to do it again. In contrast, symbolic relations that bridge the action to a source of meaning at the top of a hierarchical network will help make the performance satisfying regardless of what the audience thinks, which in turn will build larger patterns of meaningful action. For example, if the client thinks, "I know I am not giving the best talk but I am expressing my opinion, which is important to me," she will be more likely to give the talk and do it again. Eventually the external reinforcers will likely follow, but in the meantime the person is growing. In the following sections, we will explore the techniques you can use in verbal interactions during the three phases of fostering and sustaining motivation.

Preparing Actions

Building motivation during the preparation of an action consists of two main principles. On the one hand, the therapist encourages the client to *augment reinforcement*, that is, to connect the action to the positive overarching goals and qualities of action. On the other hand, he helps the client consider potential barriers to action and risks of failure.

Augmenting can be accomplished through many ways since multiple types of symbolic relations can transform an event (see Chapter 5). For example, a client may say, "I will look for a job so I can be independent" (coordination framing); "I will look for a job so I won't be dependent" (distinction framing); or "I will look for a job so I won't be as dependent as my sister" (comparison framing). All these statements may increase the chances that the client actually looks for a job, but notice that the first statement emphasizes positive reinforcement whereas the two others foster actions that seem more like escaping. As with identifying actions (see the previous section on meaning), the way augmenting is elaborated in our language matters. For this reason, the clinician should help the client state his intentions to engage in an action in a manner that increases contact with lasting satisfaction rather than avoidance or escape from undesirable consequences. It is important to try to word augmenting interventions in ways that are concrete and felt. Motivators that can be sensed and felt are closer to what it is like to touch the consequences being sought. For example, if an action is meaningful because it is loving, augmenting should focus on what it feels like to love and be loved; to be touched, held, seen, and valued. Staying at a purely intellectual or abstract level is almost always less motivating.

Formulating intentions to perform an action is also a means to use coherence in an effective way. Remember that in Chapters 5 and 6, we used coherence to help clients aim for effectiveness rather than essential truth when assessing their thoughts, and flexibility rather than rigidity when approaching their sense of self. In motivation work too, the tendency to behave in ways that are consistent with existing relational networks can be used to the client's benefit. If a client says, "I will take my children to school every morning," doing so maintains the coherence of the relational network while failing leads to aversive feelings associated with incoherence. This effect of commitment to an action can therefore improve motivation to engage in an action that is not sufficiently appealing at the moment. It is useful for most clients because actions they have been neglecting so far are generally impacted by competing sources of influence. A client who commits to stop smoking usually knows that he will experience painful withdrawal sensations. However, stating his intention to engage in this new action and connecting it to a meaningful purpose may decrease the impact of detrimental sources of influence. Observe how the therapist helps the client augment reinforcement in preparation for an action interfering with his obsessive rituals:

THERAPIST: So, what are you going to do in order to be present with your family?

CLIENT: Well, I would really like to start with sitting with my wife and my kids when we have dinner. But I am really nervous about doing that because I know I will need to check the news on my computer to make sure nothing bad has happened.

THERAPIST: Okay. So, there will be two different actions competing with each other?

CLIENT: Yeah. I am not sure I can sit still for a whole dinner without checking the news.

THERAPIST: If you actually stayed at the table for the whole dinner, what would that mean to you?

The therapist evokes augmenting through hierarchical framing.

CLIENT: It would be huge. I can't remember the last time I was able to have dinner with my family without leaving to check the news every 2 minutes.

THERAPIST: Huge is a big word, and it makes me think that there is something important there. Could you tell me more about what it means to you?

The therapist evokes further elaboration of augmenting to identify the source of meaning more clearly.

CLIENT: It would mean that I am with my kids, with my wife. It would mean we are a family and we are sharing something.

THERAPIST: So sharing is important to you. Can you tell me what it feels like when you share moments with your family and they are with you? Try to express it in a way that is as physical or emotional as you can.

CLIENT: What it feels like? I guess the thing that comes to mind is that I feel almost like I am being held, or like I'm holding someone. It is like a hug.

THERAPIST: So you want a dinner hug.

CLIENT: (laughs) I'd love that. It may not be the biggest thing, but I know my wife would be very happy. I would really like to show her that I am making a real effort to be more present. And I'd just like to feel her presence again—to be with her. And the kids too. Group hug!

THERAPIST: (laughs) So what is more important/more vital/more uplifting: checking the news or a group "dinner hug" with your family?

The therapist uses comparative framing to assess the meaning of competing actions and deliberately uses sensory language drawn from a metaphor to focus on the qualities of being close.

CLIENT: Well, stated that way, for sure it is my family. Holding them in my mind and heart. Being with them. But in the moments when dinner is happening, you know, it is hard to resist checking the news.

THERAPIST: I can understand that it is hard to do something different. Perhaps you can spend a few moments almost to taste these
  alternative options. Do you know what I mean? It would be as
  if you were given two different things to eat and you could taste
  them both before choosing. Where is there more life for you in
  this situation? What is most tasty?

*The therapist reorients the client toward the hierarchical connections
with the source of meaning and again uses a sensory metaphor to
orient toward deeper feelings.*

CLIENT: Being with my family. Loving my family. Showing them I
  care. Checking the news—it is just because I have to.

THERAPIST: So, as you sit here, what are you going to do? You've
  tasted the alternative options. What are you going to do?

*The therapist invites the client to state the action he intends to do,
using the positive effect of coherence and a sensory metaphor to
increase motivation.*

CLIENT: I will do everything I can to stay with them. . . . Group hug!

In this last vignette, you can notice that the client is concerned about
failing to perform the action he has chosen. Anticipating possible failures
is an important part of preparing an action. In some cases, clients are
reluctant to commit to an action because they are afraid of failing, and in
other cases, they think they can perform the action, but they don't take
potential barriers into account. This can be a problem because unrealistic
commitments will turn the action into an aversive experience, while the
original purpose was to contact more satisfaction. For this reason, it is
useful to gently challenge the client and make sure that he is prepared to
deal with what might get in his way. To this end, we can use techniques
from Chapter 5 aimed at noticing and overcoming detrimental sources
of influence (i.e., observation/description/tracking, functional sense making through normalization and effectiveness, and response flexibility).
Observe this approach in the following exchange with a client suffering
from depression:

THERAPIST: What do you plan to do this week?

CLIENT: I really want to get back on track, so I will get up early every
  day and go back to the gym again, and then I will go to work on
  time. I think this would be a good start.

THERAPIST: This would be consistent with what you care about?

CLIENT: Yes, I want to go back to my usual schedule and try to enjoy
  what I do again.

THERAPIST: Ok, great! I understand this is what you want to do, but you told me that in the past, it was often difficult to actually do what you had planned to do, right?

The therapist evokes the observation of potential barriers.

CLIENT: Yeah, but I think I am really motivated this time.

THERAPIST: This will certainly be helpful. I would like to suggest something though. How about taking a moment to think about the difficulties that might come up as you go back to the gym and to work?

CLIENT: Okay.

THERAPIST: What could get in your way?

The therapist evokes the description of potential barrier and tracking of responses.

CLIENT: There is a risk that I will be too tired when I wake up and that I won't be motivated to go to the gym anymore.

THERAPIST: Okay. What else?

The therapist evokes a further description of potential barriers and tracking of responses.

CLIENT: Maybe I will try to go to the gym the first day, but if I arrive late at work, I might not want to exercise the second day because I don't think I have the time.

THERAPIST: Okay, let's pause on these two potential difficulties. It seems like at some point, there might be a competition between two things that drag you in different directions, right? On the one hand you want to go to the gym, and on the other hand. . . .

The therapist evokes the observation of alternative actions.

CLIENT: I want to stay in bed! I can already predict that this is going to happen. . . .

THERAPIST: What could make a difference in this case? What could make you go to the gym instead of sleeping longer?

The therapist evokes augmenting.

CLIENT: I guess if I can motivate myself enough.

THERAPIST: How can you do that?

The therapist helps the client be more concrete to strengthen augmenting.

CLIENT: If I can think of why it is important. It is hard in the moment though. I know I will feel tired . . . .

THERAPIST: So, it will be more difficult to hear the voice that tells you to go to the gym, huh?

CLIENT: Yeah . . . I guess I was a bit naïve to plan to go back to the gym.

Augmenting is decreasing, and detrimental sources of influence start to take over the client's decision.

THERAPIST: Why do you say that?

CLIENT: Well, I think it is going to be harder than just saying that I want to go back to the gym.

THERAPIST: So you are tempted to change your plans now?

CLIENT: Yeah . . .

THERAPIST: This is interesting because in a way, you are now in the exact same situation as when you will wake up. You want to plan to go to the gym, but on the other hand, there is a voice that tells you that you can't make it, right?

The therapist uses analogical framing to help the client notice the functional similarity between the present situation and what will happen when he tries to engage in the chosen activity. This is an opportunity to shape an effective behavior in the therapy room—see Chapter 5).

CLIENT: Yes, exactly.

THERAPIST: Spend a little time to feel how you would feel an hour after you chose to go to the gym or an hour after you changed your plans to stay in bed. See if you can picture those two moments, one after the other, and take a little time to allow feelings to percolate up.

The therapist evokes further augmenting of reinforcement through comparative framing.

CLIENT: I'd feel satisfied and in my body if I went to the gym. I'd feel defeated and in my head if I slept instead—my head would be filled with judgmental thoughts and self-criticism. Been there. Done that. It is time to do something else.

THERAPIST: Well the "gym voice" and "bed voice" will both be persuasive, but your experience seems to suggest that one might be closer to what you care about. Which is more important?

The therapist evokes tracking of alternative experiences resulting from the two options.

CLIENT: Ha! My experience has been pretty consistent if I stand back and look at it. Going to the gym is what I really want.

THERAPIST: Okay, so when you will wake up tomorrow, what do you think will happen?

The therapist evokes functional generalization to the client's life outside the room.

CLIENT: It will be hard. I probably won't hear the gym voice anymore, and my experience might be far away.

THERAPIST: What can you do to touch what you care about?

The therapist evokes a strategy to augment reinforcement outside the therapy session.

CLIENT: I need to remember why it is important. I need to trust my gut sense.

THERAPIST: What is your gut sense? Why does it matter?

The therapist evokes further elaboration of hierarchical connections with source of meaning to strengthen augmenting.

CLIENT: I do want to live more healthily. I want to be in better shape. I want to feel my body again. I want to feel alive.

THERAPIST: Is there a way for you to connect with that when the time comes to go to the gym?

The therapist evokes again a strategy to augment outside of the therapy session.

CLIENT: I am not sure . . .

THERAPIST: Is there a way to remind yourself of the importance of this when you are getting up in the morning? Something you can do or say or see?

The therapist helps the client explore augmenting strategies in a nondirective fashion.

CLIENT: Perhaps I could write a note on my bed table.

THERAPIST: Yeah? What can you write?

CLIENT: What I care about. Why it is important that I go to the gym. I could write myself a note from the heart.

The client comes up with a strategy using a cue connected to his overarching goal and easy to notice. This is often a good step before being able to augment without external cues.

In this vignette, it is interesting to notice the difficulty in helping the client stay on the track of his sources of meaning without telling him what he should choose to do. At some point, the client is tempted to give up and the therapist helps him go back to his original decision, but only through questions about the meaning of this action. Ultimately, the client is the only one who can tell what is meaningful to him.

Performing Actions

Helping clients develop motivation while performing an action partly overlaps with the work done during the preparation of the action, since meaningful activities are mostly available outside the therapy room. As we saw at the end of the previous section, this work consists in particular of preparing clients to build and contact overarching goals and qualities of action when the time comes to engage in the chosen action. However, it is also possible to practice these skills in the therapy room on actions that genuinely serve the source of meaning. For example, a client who wants to develop more intimacy in her relationships may choose to share her feelings more with other people. This action can be performed in the context of the therapeutic relationship, thus providing an opportunity to train useful motivation processes.

During the execution of an action, two main processes can be targeted to help the client find immediate satisfaction and stay engaged. First, the clinician helps the client connect her current engagement to the positive overarching goals and desired qualities of action using similar techniques as in identifying broad patterns of meaningful actions (see above in this chapter). Second, she can help her notice the actual experiences (physical sensations, thoughts, emotions) that come up while acting in coherence with this meaningful life direction.

Although augmenting was already part of the preparation phase, the aim is a bit different while performing the action because the client is now making concrete efforts, and competing sources of influence are more tangible. The key is thus to help the client strengthen the symbolic relations that give the current action its intrinsic reinforcing quality. This way, urges to disengage are seen for what they are even when the action is difficult to perform.

Sometimes, during the execution of an action, clients are more focused on extrinsic than intrinsic motivation. Extrinsic sources of motivation can be useful, but it is important to also contact the intrinsic source of satisfaction to ensure that staying engaged in the action doesn't depend solely on external variables. In this case, the therapist gently draws the client's attention to the top of the hierarchical network, without diminishing the satisfaction that is also brought by external consequences. Observe this approach in the following short example:

THERAPIST: It seems like you have been listening and asking about what I think more than usual.

CLIENT: Yes, I think I am getting better at interacting with others. I have been trying to listen more, to pay attention to what you say today. It is difficult for me, but I am happy because I think that this way, my wife will see that I can change.

The client is focusing on an external consequence (his wife's reaction).

THERAPIST: I know it is important for you to show your wife that you can change. I can imagine how satisfying it must be to make progress. Why is it important to you, to listen more to others in particular?

The therapist evokes hierarchical connections with intrinsic source of meaning.

CLIENT: I want to develop better interactions, with mutual connection and understanding.

The client connects the action to an overarching goal and qualities of action.

THERAPIST: And would you say that the way you are interacting with me today serves mutual connection and understanding?

The therapist evokes the strengthening of the connection between the client's action and its meaningful purpose.

CLIENT: I feel like I'm making progress. It feels good. It is difficult to change, you know.[4]

In addition to augmenting, clients can be encouraged to observe and describe experiences associated with performing an action, in particular, those reflecting the satisfaction of engaging in a meaningful direction. Doing so increases the intrinsically reinforcing properties of the action and helps the client stay engaged. Observe this technique in the next exchange that directly follows the previous vignette:

THERAPIST: How are you feeling now, as we are talking about this progress you are making?

The therapist evokes the observation/description of experiences linked to meaningful action.

---

[4]The therapist can also share his own impression about the quality of their interaction, but in this very context, the goal is to increase the client's capacity to connect with his own appreciation of what matters. Thus, it makes sense to refrain from adding external reinforcement in this moment.

CLIENT: Well, you know it is difficult because I am not used to listening. I have always talked a lot. So, I feel urges to interrupt you, to finish your sentences myself.

THERAPIST: And when you don't, how do you feel?

The therapist evokes further observation/description.

CLIENT: At first I feel a little edgy because I always want to move on faster than you do, I guess. (*pauses*)

THERAPIST: And just now, you waited before continuing, right?

The therapist evokes tracking.

CLIENT: Yes, I was trying to give you a chance to answer, or else I could talk for hours!

THERAPIST: Ah thanks for the space! (*pauses*) So how do you feel now?

The therapist evokes observation of experience linked to meaningful action.

CLIENT: Kind of self-conscious, but sort of happy, you know.

THERAPIST: Yeah? How is it to feel happy right now?

The therapist evokes further observation/description.

CLIENT: It is sort of exciting. . . . Like I can actually do what I said is important. It feels really good to know I'm in charge of me.

Debriefing Actions

The last component of the therapeutic work on motivation consists of debriefing an action after it has been performed by the client. In this phase also, particular attention is given to connecting the action to positive overarching goals and qualities of action. The purpose of debriefing is more specifically to ensure that the action makes contact with the desired outcomes in order to increase the probability that the client will do it again—in other words, in order to produce a reinforcement effect. This is a critical moment because the completion of an effective action is not in and of itself sufficient to ensure that an action contacts important consequences when those consequences are built by the client's relational framing (i.e., language). Depending on the type of symbolic connections one develops, very similar actions can be considered either satisfying or disappointing. For example, clients prone to self-criticism can easily dismiss the progress they have made and thus lower the functional impact of positive consequences that have actually been produced.

As in the previous sections of this chapter, the RFT therapeutic strategy adopted here consists of connecting the action to the positive overarching goals and qualities of action. The therapist doesn't attempt to eliminate current evaluations made by the client, but instead, she encourages him to move toward augmenting that creates a symbolic bridge above otherwise detrimental sources of influence. Observe this approach in the following exchange:

THERAPIST: So, how did it go?

CLIENT: Well, it was good. I made that phone call, like I had planned to, so it was good.

THERAPIST: When you made this decision last week, it seemed like it was a big move for you.

The therapist evokes the connection between the action and the source of meaning.

CLIENT: Yeah . . . That's right. I am not sure it was such a big move in the end. I mean, making a phone call really isn't such a big deal for most people. It is just for people like me, who are so scared of everything that it is difficult. I'm glad I did it, but I am not going to celebrate either, you know . . .

THERAPIST: Whether it is a big move or a small step, I am curious about the direction you were taking when you made that phone call.

The therapist emphasizes hierarchical framing that conveys meaning even to small actions.

CLIENT: I was trying to be more in charge of my life.

The client begins to connect the action with an overarching goal.

THERAPIST: It is interesting that you say "trying." Did you actually make this phone call?

CLIENT: Yeah! I was very nervous. My voice was shaking, and I could barely say two words without humming. This was not a great experience, I can tell you. I definitely did it, but it doesn't make me particularly happy.

THERAPIST: I am quite impressed that you were able to make this phone call while you were having such difficult experiences. It must have been hard, yet somehow you persisted.

For the client, having difficult experiences during the phone call can diminish the potentially reinforcing qualities of his own action. Thus, the therapist frames the difficult experience lived by the client as a sign of an important performance.

CLIENT: Yeah, I had to motivate myself because I was really tempted not to do it.

THERAPIST: So not only was your voice shaking and you were humming, but you also had urges to give up?

CLIENT: Yeah . . . Not a very good experience.

THERAPIST: In a way I'm even more impressed though. I'm curious about what motivated you to do it despite that it was difficult.

The therapist evokes augmenting.

CLIENT: I was thinking about how I want things to change.

THERAPIST: About being more in charge of your life?

CLIENT: Yes, more independent. More in charge.

THERAPIST: And making this call was part of a set of actions that makes you more independent?

The therapist uses hierarchical framing to evoke a more elaborated form of augmenting.

CLIENT: Yes. It is small, but honestly I have never really taken care of these kinds of things by myself.

THERAPIST: How does it feel to be more in charge?

The therapist evokes the observation/description of feelings of experience linked to meaningful action.

CLIENT: It's huh . . . It's different. It's scary.

The client is still not in touch with the reinforcing qualities of the action.

THERAPIST: Do you still want that in your life?

Since the client still seems to be mainly influenced by evaluations that take him away from contacting reinforcement, the therapist keeps encouraging him to formulate the meaning of this action.

CLIENT: Yes. I just wish it was easier.

THERAPIST: Yeah, I can understand that. It must be difficult to look at other people and think "Wow, it seems so easy to them! Why is it so hard for me?" Huh?

The therapist normalizes the difficult experience.

CLIENT: Exactly!

THERAPIST: Like you said, for them, it's no big deal.

CLIENT: No.

THERAPIST: And for you, is it hard but important?

The therapist again evokes hierarchical connections with the source of meaning.

CLIENT: It is the most important right now.

THERAPIST: How does it feel to do something hard but important in your life?

The therapist evokes the observation/ description of the experience linked to meaningful action.

CLIENT: It's huh . . . It's good. It feels right.

In these last exchanges, the therapist once again attempts to transform the function of evaluations that, so far, have prevented the client from contacting lasting satisfaction. The client still has difficulties finding his action satisfying, but progress is being made as he recognizes how much this phone call means to him. Through further exchanges of this kind that follow actions directed toward sources of meaning, the client will become more able to appreciate the small steps he is making.

In other cases, clients are satisfied after performing an action, but they link their action mostly to specific goals (e.g., having a new job, getting married, or completing a degree). As explained before, the risk is then that clients may exhaust these sources of motivation because specific goals often can't be reached again, or they don't bring the same satisfaction once they have already been accomplished. Similarly, clients may mostly connect the completion of an action to the removal of aversive experiences or to other people's approval, thus altering their deeper meaning. When this happens, the therapist helps the client elaborate hierarchical connections between her action and the intrinsic source of meaning. Observe this approach in the following exchange:

CLIENT: I am really happy that I was able to go to work this week. It was nice to show my boss that I can be relied upon, and I think he really appreciated that.

The client connects her action to her boss's approval. Although this can legitimately be a desirable consequence, it is a limited source of satisfaction because her boss will likely not show appreciation every time she goes to work. Thus, motivation might wear off once the excitement of the first week has passed.

THERAPIST: I am very happy for you that you were able to go to work. How meaningful is that to you? What is inside it that matters?

The therapist evokes hierarchical connections with the source of meaning.

CLIENT: It's very meaningful. I have been feeling horrible. Not going to work was like not existing.

This time, the client connects her action to the removal of an aversive experience. This can be a source of motivation, but it doesn't convey positive satisfaction.

THERAPIST: And what is meaningful about going to work, exactly? What is inside that?

The therapist evokes a more elaborated connection with the source of meaning.

CLIENT: I really care about this work. We can help a lot of people who have financial difficulties, and when I'm focused I do a pretty good job for them. I want to be there for them.

In many cases, a client comes to therapy reporting that she was not able to perform the action she had planned to do. This type of situation also requires a debriefing and actually constitutes an excellent opportunity to analyze what got in the way, using relevant assessment processes such as what we laid out in Chapters 4 and 5. If alternative sources of influence are excessively controlling the client's behavior (e.g., emotions or evaluations about the self leading to avoidance), the clinician can use techniques to alter their impact (see Chapters 5 and 6). If the client is not in contact enough with the source of satisfaction linked to his action, the therapist helps him augment reinforcement in order to increase motivation before and during the completion of the action, as seen in the two previous sections. The last vignette of this chapter will illustrate this process.

CLINICAL EXAMPLE

It is impossible to demonstrate in a single vignette the whole set of principles for building meaning and motivation, applied in depth. Instead, we want to show you a critical sequence during which a client reports that he was not able to perform the action he had committed to at the end of the previous session. In a moment like this, the therapist can use both processes of meaning and processes of motivation to strengthen the client's connection with sources of meaning and encourage him to recommit to an effective action. This vignette involves a 32-year-old woman suffering from depression.

THERAPIST: So, last week you decided to spend at least one evening with a friend. Where you able to do that?

CLIENT: No. It was a complete failure. I canceled at the last minute. But honestly, I think it was better this way.

THERAPIST: You seem disappointed and relieved at the same time. . . .

CLIENT: I guess so. I feel horrible because I didn't do it. . . . You know . . . I didn't keep my promise. But if I had not canceled, I would have probably felt even worse.

THERAPIST: It sounds as though you felt that either way it was not going to be a satisfying week. Yet, you had decided to spend an evening with your friend. Was it important to you?

The therapist evokes hierarchical connections with sources of meaning.

CLIENT: Yes, yes . . . But I didn't feel like it that night, so I don't think either of us would have been happy in the end.

THERAPIST: I can understand you would not want to spend a night with your friend if you didn't feel like it. But if you had gone, why would you have done it? What was the purpose?

The therapist normalizes experiences perceived as barriers and again evokes hierarchical connections with sources of meaning.

CLIENT: I wanted to connect with other people.

The client formulates an overarching goal.

THERAPIST: I know we have talked about this before, but I would be interested in hearing more about this again because sometimes, you know, what we want in our lives can change. So, would you say that it still matters to you to connect with other people?

The therapist explores if the overarching goal can still be a source of motivation.

CLIENT: Yes, yes. Absolutely. I don't want to stay by myself. I want to have something to share. I have been ruminating alone in my apartment for too long. I would like to hear other people talk. I would like to talk to other people.

THERAPIST: Can spending an evening with a friend be an opportunity to do that?

The therapist evokes augmenting to connect the action to the overarching goal.

CLIENT: Yes. For sure, yes.

THERAPIST: And yet, something gets in your way, huh?

The therapist evokes the observation of the experience perceived as a barrier to action.

CLIENT: Yeah . . . I am motivated to change when I leave this room, but when the time comes, it is not the same, you know. I think about dark things, I don't see the point of going out anymore.

THERAPIST: You lose contact with what matters to you?

CLIENT: Yeah.

THERAPIST: But it still matters?

CLIENT: Yes. I am just not motivated enough in the moment, I guess.

In these last exchanges, the client notices the lack of connection between her action and the overarching goal she is trying to pursue.

THERAPIST: What could help you be in touch with what matters? What could help you make this step, even when thoughts and feelings get in your way?

The therapist evokes strategies to augment reinforcement outside the therapy session.

CLIENT: If I could remember that it is better for me than staying home.

THERAPIST: How do you think you could remember that?

The therapist evokes more concrete ways to augment reinforcement.

CLIENT: I don't know. When the time comes to do something that is difficult, I tend to forget why it is important.

THERAPIST: It seems like you have two alternative options, where you can either do something difficult and meaningful, or something easier but . . .

CLIENT: But not what I really want. Yes.

THERAPIST: So when it starts to be difficult, what do you think it means?

CLIENT: You mean . . . If it is difficult, it means it is important?

THERAPIST: What do you think?

CLIENT: Well, if it was not difficult and important, I would not be talking about it I guess!

THERAPIST: Ah, this is very interesting. And you said earlier that you were relieved and disappointed because you got away from some-thing difficult and important at the same time, right?

CLIENT: Yeah.

In these last few exchanges, the therapist helps the client develop a relation of coordination between having difficult experiences and doing something meaningful. In Chapter 5, we saw how clients can learn to gain flexibility in contact with difficult psychological experiences. In the next exchange, the therapist will aim to transform the function of difficult psychological experiences so that they become <u>cues</u> to augment reinforcement and do the action.

THERAPIST: If you wanted to spend an evening with a friend this week, do you think you would have difficult thoughts and feelings again?

CLIENT: Probably, yeah.

THERAPIST: What if it was your cue to remember what is important to you?

CLIENT: Hmm . . . This is exactly the opposite of what I have been doing.

THERAPIST: Do you want to do something different?

CLIENT: Yeah. I want to be able to do something that matters.

THERAPIST: And it will probably be difficult . . .

CLIENT: And it could be a cue to remember that it is important. It could be. I guess it really is.

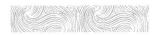 **CHAPTER SUMMARY**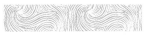

In this chapter, you learned to use verbal interactions to help your clients identify and build sources of meaning, and foster sustainable motivation to engage in meaningful actions. Here are the main principles to remember:

- Building life meaning consists of establishing hierarchical networks that put a positive overarching goal and/or desired qualities of action at the top and a broad pattern of various actions and specific goals at the base. This work consists of:
  - Identifying and building overarching goals and qualities of action by:
    - Extracting the higher function of actions and specific goals; extracting sources of meaning from problems; reconnecting to sources of meaning through perspective taking; and creating sources of meaning by exploring potential actions and goals.

- ▪ Encouraging formulation of intrinsic motivation in order to make sure that satisfaction doesn't depend solely on external consequences, social approval, or self-concepts.
- ▪ Encouraging formulation as positive motivation in order to make sure that satisfaction doesn't depend solely on avoidance of aversive experiences.
- ○ Building broad patterns of various meaningful actions by:
  - ▪ Choosing actions connected to an overarching goal or a quality of action.
  - ▪ Identifying a range of various actions (i.e., alternative actions and actions requiring various amounts of efforts, time, etc.) that serve the same source of meaning to ensure a wide and perpetual availability of satisfying actions.

- • Fostering sustainable motivation consists of helping clients connect their actions to sources of meaning (augmenting reinforcement) so that distant, probabilistic, abstract, or hidden consequences become more salient, present, and experientially rich, and of altering the impact of barriers and failures. This occurs during three main phases:
  - ○ Preparing the action:
    - ▪ Helping the client connect future actions to sources of meaning in order to encourage commitment.
    - ▪ Helping the client explore and overcome potential barriers and risks of failure.
  - ○ Performing the action:
    - ▪ Helping the client connect the current action to sources of meaning in order to encourage staying engaged in the action.
    - ▪ Helping the client notice natural reinforcing experiences that come up while acting in coherence with a meaningful life direction.
  - ○ Debriefing the action:
    - ▪ Helping the client connect the completed action to the source of meaning so that the probability of engaging in this action increases.
    - ▪ Drawing the client's attention to broad and intrinsic sources of meaning when there is excessive focus on extrinsic and specific consequences, or removal of aversive experiences, or social approval, or when the client didn't find satisfaction in the action at all.

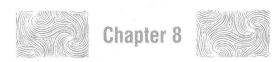

Chapter 8

Building and Delivering Experiential Metaphors

In this chapter, you will learn how to use RFT principles to choose, build, and deliver clinical metaphors. We will first explore how RFT approaches the use of metaphors in therapy, and then provide key elements for their successful application. Finally, we will analyze clinical vignettes step by step to illustrate alternative ways to present metaphors.

METAPHORS AS STORIES PROMOTING BEHAVIOR CHANGE

In some sense you are already using metaphors with your clients. It is unavoidable. The vast majority of our language is built on metaphors, especially in the areas psychotherapists normally address, such as satisfaction, emotion, intention, and expectation. These are not the issues of blood and bone that language originally evolved to deal with. The verbal community used metaphors to map out these territories probably long after the cultural supports for basic relational learning were well developed. Once these territories were mapped, the metaphors became frozen and were thereafter taught much more the way terms such as "apple" are taught: mostly by using frames of coordination understood by all. We no longer remember that it was hard for anyone to talk about an inclination to do something—and to express this idea you had to say that you felt something like a leaning object about to fall in a direction (literally "inclined"). We no longer remember that it was a cognitive stretch to talk about what we wanted—that to express this idea you had to say you felt like something was missing (as in phrases like "for want of food he died"). At best, we have only a vague sense of the metaphors underlying our use of almost all of our cognitive, emotional, dispositional, and intentional terms.

Metaphors are so useful in psychotherapy for the same reason they have been used by the culture at large in many areas: metaphors can rapidly extend existing symbolic knowledge into areas that are complex or subtle. The deliberate use of stories and analogies is common in most forms of psychotherapy. Consider the following metaphor used with a client who no longer drives after an accident due to his fears of what may happen on the road:

> "Developing a fear of driving after an accident is similar to accidentally putting hot sauce in soup that was not supposed to be spicy. You enjoyed the soup before, but you don't want to eat it anymore because now it has hot sauce in it. The problem is that you've been trying to get back to the old soup by somehow removing the hot sauce first. I suspect you came to me with that vision in mind, but practically speaking the only way to rebalance the taste is to add lots more soup that doesn't have hot sauce in it. In order to rebalance your fear of driving, you need lots of exposure to driving that doesn't involve similar accidents. This will rebalance the way you feel, just as it would rebalance the soup. At first, it will be unpleasant, like tasting the tainted soup after you've added just a little more mild soup and realizing that it is still too spicy. But as you expose yourself to driving more and more, you will eventually not be bothered anymore, even though you still remember the accident, exactly like eating soup with only a hint of the hot sauce that once spoiled it."

In a situation like this, the goal of the therapist is to educate the client about what needs to be done in therapy. By using a very simple everyday example that the client can readily understand, the therapist makes the technical processes underlying exposure much easier to grasp. As a result, the client has a better chance to accept the implications of these principles. The range of implications coming from this metaphor is quite large: Therapy will be about adding, not subtracting. It is natural just to want to get rid of fear, but it is impractical. What is needed will initially be hard but will gradually get easier. Success will require actual behavior change first, not emotional change first. Being afraid after an accident does not mean there is anything wrong with you. There is a way forward that makes sense even if it is not immediately, intuitively obvious. If these implications were simply stated without a well-crafted metaphor as a guide, the client might be confused, feel patronized or misunderstood.

Despite their everyday use, metaphors applied to clinical work can be poorly selected and constructed, and thus will fail to make a profound difference in understanding and motivation. It is easy to get metaphors wrong;

but we believe using RFT makes it much easier to get it right. Scores of RFT studies have worked through the key principles, and we now understand in some detail what a metaphor is, how it works, and why it can make a difference (see Foody et al., 2014). We can apply this knowledge to the deliberate use of stories and examples to promote behavior change, but as we will note later, we can even apply it to the more careful selection of the "frozen" metaphors in the everyday language we use in therapy.

SELECTING AND CREATING POWERFUL CLINICAL METAPHORS

Overview

The Goal

Clients who are stuck are nevertheless doing things to ameliorate their problems—they are simply applying solutions that to some degree do not work. Generally, these solutions *have* been helpful elsewhere or in the past, but in the current time or situation they are no longer fully helpful. Clients continue to apply failed solutions because they see no alternatives; they are not convinced they can or should implement alternatives if they do exist; and they are not sure alternatives will work in any case. The goal in the use of deliberate clinical stories or metaphors is to help clients see, in a new and more effective light, why they are stuck, how to move forward, why it is necessary, that it can be done, and what will happen if they do it. Building on the skills we have already addressed, clinicians need to be able to select, create, and deliver metaphors that produce powerful changes in behavior and motivation.

Why This Is Important, from an RFT Point of View

When a problem stems simply from a lack of knowledge, directly linear rules work fine. If you don't know how to get to a store, we can give you directions, and that is enough. But when knowledge that's called for depends on the context and is therefore subtle, complex, or counterintuitive, direct linear rules are often not enough. Carrying an entire set of knowledge from one domain to another through stories and analogies may be very helpful in such situations. When the issue is one of motivation, experience, or skill, simple "how to do it" rules often fail us. The emotional punch and felt sense of a good story may be a better guide. When it is important that rules not be based on compliance, we need to use language that does not readily lead to it. Stories can be interpreted in a variety of ways—if done well, the listener can bring their own experience to the story without excessive dictation by the speaker. When rules need to be used but held lightly, or need to be remembered for their overall gestalt, well-crafted stories use language in a way that is more experiential, sensory, and memorable than any simple verbal directive can provide.

We have proposed that language and cognition can be understood as the behaviors of building, understanding, and responding to symbolic relations among things (objects, events, and people). As this relatively simple definition has been unpacked into specific components, we have been able to analyze a number of clinical issues and build a variety of therapeutic techniques. From an RFT perspective, virtually any verbal or cognitive activity can be modeled in terms of symbolic relational responses.

That is demonstrably true of analogies and metaphors. We have used the term "analogical framing" in this book for ease of presentation, but in actuality metaphors are a composite or a collective of other relational frames. What is different is not the relation but *what* is related. Metaphorical reasoning is a matter of building, understanding, and responding to *relations among relations*.

Let's consider a simple example. Imagine a person who puts a lot of effort into collecting money for a charity that tries to alleviate poverty in developing nations. When asked about her motivation for working so hard for something that will have such a small impact when considered in the abstract, she says, "You may see my work as a drop in an ocean, but I prefer to see it as a brick in a wall." What she means is that while some believe that working so hard on a big problem is futile (a drop in an ocean), she believes that even a very small contribution can make a difference and be combined with similar things others are doing (a brick in a wall).

From an RFT perspective, metaphors usually (but not always, as we shall soon see) consist of establishing a frame of coordination (or more specifically, a frame of equivalence) between two sets of relations (see Figure 8.1). Depending on how we want to present the work done for this charity, a relation of equivalence can be established between either of the two metaphors. If we want it to be seen as a contribution that won't make any difference, then we can put it in equivalence with a drop in an ocean, but if we want to present it as a significant contribution, then we can put it in equivalence with a brick in a wall. Relations among relations change the functions of resulting symbolic networks.

RFT researchers have been able to reproduce the process of elaborating a metaphor in experimental laboratories (e.g., Lipkens & Hayes, 2009; Stewart, Barnes-Holmes, & Roche, 2004). As you can imagine, given the complexity of building a simple relational network from scratch (see Chapter 1), training participants to relate *two* sets of relations requires an even greater number of steps. Fortunately, going through these steps is not necessary to understand the RFT principles involved in metaphors. What will be useful is to understand the way a metaphor is organized: aspects of two relational networks are brought into a relation of equivalence, which leads to a change in the functions of some of the events in one of the networks. In

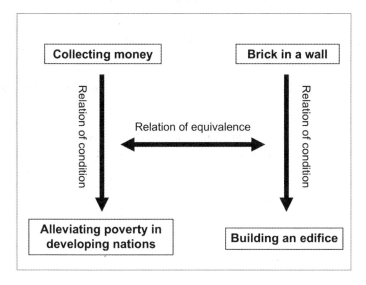

FIGURE 8.1

the previous example, saying that collecting money for a charity is a drop in the ocean transforms the function of collecting money: it becomes a futile activity. However, saying that collecting money for a charity is a brick in a wall transforms the function of this activity in the opposite direction: it is now useful.

The two relational networks are called the *target* and the *vehicle*. The target is the relational network including an element that will be transformed by the metaphor (i.e., collecting money for the charity). The vehicle is the relational network responsible for this transformation (e.g., a brick in the wall). In order to understand a metaphor, the person hearing it needs to be familiar with the vehicle and already know what kind of relations and functions it includes. The relation between the vehicle and the target sheds new light on the relations and functions in the target.

Apt metaphors are ones in which the set of relations in the target and vehicle map closely one to the other but with important differences. A key feature in the target has to connect in a powerful, almost sensory way to a related and dominant feature in the vehicle. The more concrete and visceral the connection in this area, the more it can be used and remembered (McCurry & Hayes, 1992). At the same time, the vehicle has to contain relations or functions that would otherwise be missing in the target, and these have to touch the very feature or features that draw together the vehicle and target.

The relations included in the networks that define the vehicle and the target can be of any kind (coordination, opposition, condition, hierarchy, perspective, and so on). For example, after buying a new, very powerful computer, you could say that "it is like night and day" compared to your old computer. In both the vehicle and the target, a relation of opposition links two stimuli. Night is to day as your old, slow computer is to your new one: the opposite. Furthermore, although in most cases the vehicle and the target are framed in equivalence, it is also possible to create metaphors using a relation of distinction or opposition between the two networks. In this case, functions included in the target are transformed through their difference or opposition with the functions included in the vehicle. For example, we say, "Life is not a fairytale," implying that, in *contrast* to stories told to children, life can bring many injustices and doesn't always end well.

Let's return to our example to see how all of this works. Both a drop in the ocean and a brick in the wall focus on a key feature of the charitable act: it is one small thing. What is different is the meaning of that smallness. The first metaphor, a drop in an ocean, implicitly contains a relation of condition between adding or removing a drop from an ocean and the insignificant effect it would have. One drop does not alter the other drops. The ocean exists only when all the drops are combined into the vast ocean, and that is a combination that is almost beyond imagination. A bucket or bathtub is not an ocean, and it is not really building toward an ocean except in some highly abstract sense; a lake or a stream is still infinitely far away from an ocean. A drop is insignificant, disconnected, and not progressive. It dissipates—disappears into the infinitely larger whole, and in that sense its very smallness shows it is functionally nothing. By putting the charitable act into a frame of equivalence with a drop, the conditional relation (*if* you add or remove a drop from an ocean, *then* it won't make any difference) now seemingly applies to the charitable act via a transformation of stimulus functions.

The second metaphor, a brick in a wall, also contains a relation of condition. If you add or remove a brick from a wall, there is a small but significant effect on the whole wall. Bricks interlock together and support each other. Yes, there may be thousands upon thousands upon thousands of bricks in a large wall, but any mason knows that even a *huge* wall is successfully constructed one brick at a time. If a brick is well placed, it strengthens the entire wall, and even when the wall is finished, it is identifiable. A brick is significant, connected, and progressive. It does not dissipate—it participates. Its very smallness shows that even very small things can successfully go together to make grand things if that small thing is solid and well placed. If you add or remove a brick from a wall, it makes a difference. If a charitable act is like a brick, then by the addition of relations and by a transformation of functions, it is meaningful and progressive even if many similar acts will be needed to address the entire need. It even suggests how that can best be done: make sure your charitable act is solid, well placed, and supports the similar acts of others.

Both of these metaphors are apt. They are sensory in their key connections (in this case, smallness and its relation to features like dissipation or interconnection), the vehicle is well known, and the response implications are rich. Both of these metaphors can make a difference. Thankfully for the charitable organization and the recipients in developing nations, our friend has chosen one that will support her prosocial actions.

What do metaphors add to other RFT-based techniques aimed at improving contextual sensitivity and functional coherence? First, they provide a concrete, easy, and often familiar situation that the client doesn't have to overanalyze in order to consider alternative actions. For example, in the "hot sauce" metaphor, the client can easily understand that when a soup is too spicy for him, the only way to eat it is to add more soup with no hot sauce. Otherwise he would have to throw the soup away. The situation is so concrete, and has such an obvious conclusion, that it should not trigger a battle of interpretations and counterarguments. No one would say you could "pick out" the hot sauce (even though the client likely has been trying to do exactly that with his painful memories). Most people would agree on the best way to solve the problem of the overly spicy soup (adding more soup or other ingredients), and it is obvious that it can be solved with enough effort. Thus, the metaphor allows the therapist to create a simple situation that he and the client can both agree on and to test out its plausibility mentally. There is a common-sense wisdom inside successful and well-crafted metaphors. This allows new ways to deal with the client's difficulties and for them to be mentally tested to a degree, based on their similarity with the metaphoric situation.

Metaphors are also a tool used to bring a variety of experiences to the therapy room. Using metaphors, the therapist and client can explore virtually any situation, observe together what happens, and extract new courses of action and perhaps more effective rules. This is a huge advantage for talk therapies that are conducted within a specific space and time, with limited access to the natural environment. For example, a client might follow a certain sequence of actions with success in one area and could apply the same strategy in more problematic areas of her life. She may be an excellent dancer, showing an impressive ability to pay attention to her partner's movement and to adapt her own steps in return. In social situations, however, she may have great difficulty paying attention to what others tell her and thus responds inappropriately, resulting in frustration with the poor quality of her relationships. Highlighting the functional parallel between these situations can therefore favor generalization of effective behaviors across areas that may seem very different. The therapist could say, for example, "Talking to people is like dancing with a partner. Paying attention to what your partner says can help you adjust your own words" (for an extended example of this kind with a competitive rock climber learning to face social anxiety, see Hildebrandt, Fletcher, & Hayes, 2007).

How This Method Touches on Various Clinical Traditions

Metaphors are at least implicitly in most clinicians' toolboxes, and they are used deliberately in many different approaches to psychotherapy. Therapeutic metaphors and stories are key to a variety of contextualistic approaches, including work that is foundational to psychotherapy, such as George Kelly's fixed role therapy (Kelly, 1955) or Milton Erickson's hypnotherapy (Rosen, 1991). Several modern approaches have continued in this vein, such as narrative therapy (White, 2007) or other constructivist therapies (Mahoney, 2005), including ACT. But the breadth of interest cannot be captured merely by listing specific brands of psychotherapy that openly embrace the key role of stories and narratives because virtually every book on psychotherapy tells stories—including stories about the stories told in psychotherapy. There are scores of books on metaphors and stories in psychotherapy.

How to Select or Create a Metaphor

In order to master the use of metaphors in clinical practice, it is helpful to see how RFT makes sense of this particular form of language. Although it will require that you increase your understanding of RFT principles a little bit, this will quickly prove to be rewarding as we demonstrate how to choose and build a metaphor with RFT.

A vast number of metaphors are already available and can be used effectively in therapy if they can be selected and delivered properly. However, in this section we will also describe the processes involved in creating new metaphors. This will allow you to go a step further in your understanding of how to use RFT principles.

The Metaphor Needs to Target the Appropriate Function

A key to developing powerful clinical metaphors is to focus carefully on the *function* in the target that needs to be changed and then to pick a vehicle that resonates powerfully with that function. To explain what we mean, we will use a metaphor drawn from ACT: struggling with anxiety is like struggling in quicksand—as you struggle to get out, it draws you in (Hayes et al., 1999). The purpose of this metaphor is to help clients recognize that attempts to avoid difficult emotions are often counterproductive. Imagine a client who tries not to feel anxious by engaging in dangerous and costly activities designed to reduce anxiety such as compulsive buying, binge drinking, or drug abuse. These strategies may work in the short term, but they generally lead to feeling even more anxious in the long term. Yet the client persists in acting this way as if he was blind to the actual consequences of his actions. From an RFT perspective, it is likely that the client, who is more sensitive to the short-term effects of his behavior, developed a rule such as "getting drunk is going to make me feel better."

Using the quicksand metaphor creates an opportunity to bring concrete but delayed consequences to the therapy room. In the most basic form of delivering the metaphor, the therapist could say, "When you feel anxious and go out drinking for hours in order to feel better, it seems to work the same as a person struggling to escape quicksand. The more you struggle, the more you sink." The client can see the conditional relation that links the action of struggling in quicksand and its consequence: sinking even more. Even if the client has never been directly confronted with such a situation, he probably knows the rule to follow here in order to avoid negative consequences: if you are sinking in quicksand, lay out flat upon it. This represents a useful rule that provides a guide for what might be more useful: explore anxiety itself. The therapist uses the metaphor with the goal of transforming the function of binge drinking and compulsive buying through the relation of equivalence linking the vehicle (struggling in quicksand) and the target (avoiding anxious feelings). Although those behaviors were previously considered to be the best way to escape and not to feel anxious, they may now be considered counterproductive strategies. The client can then explore new alternatives and may even formulate new, more accurate rules about anxious feelings that are metaphorical versions of lying out flat on quicksand, such as, "If I feel anxious, I need to stop and take time to feel what I'm feeling. I'm not going to make my feelings my enemy."

The quicksand metaphor is popular and widely useful in ACT, but it is important for metaphors to fit the client. A metaphor like struggling in quicksand has the advantage of being relatively easy to understand and applicable to many psychological problems involving experiential avoidance—particularly those in which active attempts at avoidance tend to amplify the avoided emotion. Not all problems are like that, however—not even all problems involving experiential avoidance. Imagine a client who is addicted to cocaine and uses this drug several nights a week when she goes out. Suppose a functional assessment reveals that she used cocaine to be part of a social group—without using cocaine, she feels as though her friends will reject her. This could indeed have an experiential avoidance aspect to it (e.g., a fear of rejection or anxiety may be linked to that fear), but cocaine is probably not a counterproductive strategy with regard to that anxiety in a way that is functionally similar to struggling in quicksand. In the metaphor, trying to escape quicksand will lead to more sinking. In the client's situation, cocaine use may not lead to more fear of rejection. Of course, the drug use may cause large problems—it may lead to health or legal problems, for example—but cocaine use trying to be part of a group leads to negative *side effects*, not counterproductive effects, so the quicksand metaphor is not an especially good fit. Hence, it may be more helpful to use a metaphor that more closely matches the particular sequence of action and consequence.

The blind writing exercise (Monestès & Villatte, 2011) is an example of a metaphor that targets the destructive side effects of avoidance. It is conducted as a genuine experiential exercise as follows. The client is asked to write a sentence on a board while the therapist blocks her vision with a barrier (e.g., a piece of cardboard). Because not being able to see what she writes is an uncomfortable situation, she is encouraged to do everything she can to push the barrier away in order to be able to see the board. However, the therapist keeps putting the barrier back in front of her eyes. Thus, as a result of using all of her effort on avoiding the barrier, she is unable to write a legible sentence on the board. In the second phase, the therapist invites her to leave the barrier where it is and focus on writing the sentence on the board even though she can't see what she is writing. This time, the client usually writes a legible sentence and without actually using much effort. This exercise demonstrates another feature of avoidance. Just as your sentence writing will suffer if you try to avoid the barrier, your health may suffer if you try to avoid anxiety and fear of rejection by using cocaine. This fits the key clinical function better and thus is more likely to be successful.

The Dominant Feature of the Vehicle Needs to Fit the Clinical Problem

Once the function you are targeting is clear, you need a vehicle in which the dominant feature of the network fits the key clinical issue. There are more dominant and less dominant aspects of any story or set of events. In any metaphor, the vehicle has to be connected to the target of course—but if the connection is dependent on a minor feature of the vehicle, the metaphor will feel thin. In clinical metaphors this provides a clear focus: the clinical problem in a functional sense has to have a deep and vivid parallel in the vehicle (Ruiz & Luciano, 2015).

Suppose you want to use a metaphor with a depressed person who has been leading a very restricted life focused on getting approval from others and meanwhile has been putting on hold the deeper desire she has for participation, play, and contribution. Her life has an obsessive, driven quality—she is worried about making the wrong life choices, she is perfectionistic, and she feels guilty if she makes even minor mistakes. She works very hard to gain social approval, but people sense the artificiality of her relationships, and as a result, she gets relatively little support and finds what does come her way to be unsatisfying and unfulfilling.

Any clinically useful vehicle will have to connect with that constellation of functions, ideally in a powerful and almost sensory fashion. Her endless, exhausting, and undignified effort to gain approval is the clinical focus; connection with these problems has to be the hook in the vehicle.

Suppose you use this metaphor: "I have the sense you've been living your life like a person who's been invited to a meal and is instead down on the floor on all fours, chewing on the table leg, occasionally getting a splinter or two and hoping that soon it will seem satisfying." This is not bad as a beginning. Chewing on a table leg on all fours would be hard work, and it is not likely to be much fun. The image of being down on all fours has a quality of desperation and a lack of self-care—as does the chase after social approval. Getting a splinter or two occasionally is a pretty unfulfilling yield for all the effort put in. The whole exercises sounds effortful, dry, difficult, and lifeless. If leading a very restricted life focused on getting approval from others is also experienced by the person in much the same way—effortful, dry, difficult, and lifeless—we have the beginnings of a good clinical metaphor. But we are not done. This metaphor is not yet ready for prime time.

The Missing Events or Functions Need to Be Dominant in the Vehicle

In the same way that the connection to the person's functional problem needs to be dominant in the vehicle, so too does what is missing in the target. There has to be a deep connection between what you want the person to see in her target problem area and what would be obvious in the situation described in the vehicle.

What is missing in this person's life is a connection with her own desire for participation, play, and contribution. She is bright and able. People like her when she gets out of her own way. She has a lot to contribute. Part of the work in therapy will be to help open her eyes to the amazingly wide range of wonderful life possibilities that can open up, once she realizes that she can make choices based on what she really wants, rather than what she has been told she has to have or do to pass muster.

It occurs to you that the idea of having a wide range of life choices is like having lots of food items to pick from, so you say, "I have the sense you've been living like a person who's been invited to a meal at McDonald's and is instead down on the floor on all fours, chewing on the table leg, occasionally getting a splinter or two and hoping that soon it will seem satisfying. Meanwhile, you are paying no attention at all to all the different food items on the menu, whether a Big Mac or a chocolate shake."

This is an improvement because instead of comparing leg chewing simply to a meal, now you've made the meal more concrete—which begins to flesh out metaphorically the alternative pathway you want the client to consider. You've even mentioned specific food items—and especially if you know the person likes chocolate shakes you are clearly ahead of version one. It's better—but the problem is that the dominant feature of McDonald's is not the range of wonderful food choices—it is the quick and inexpensive food. The shakes and burgers may be tasty, but they are not particularly nutritious over the long haul. McDonald's is just the wrong vehicle for what is otherwise a good approach.

A better way to craft that same metaphor would be: "I have the sense you've been living your life like a person who's been invited to a luxurious banquet at The Four Seasons and is instead down on the floor on all fours, chewing on the table leg, occasionally getting a splinter or two and hoping that soon it will seem satisfying. Meanwhile, you are paying no attention at all to all the incredible array of options just above your head. Wonderful steaks, beautifully made salads, incredible desserts, and there, as much as you want."

This is clearly better. The dominant feature of a "luxurious banquet" is the range and amount of amazing food choices. If you want the client to almost "taste" what a rich, full life would be like, it is a better vehicle.

But we may be able to do still better. We have not yet captured her perfectionism on the one hand, or her connection with a sense of play on the other. You decide to use the metaphor to build out these features:

> "I have the sense you've been living your life like a person who's been invited to a luxurious banquet at The Four Seasons and is instead down on the floor on all fours, trying to do the perfect job of chewing on the table leg. You work at it and work at it and occasionally get a splinter or two, which you hope will soon seem satisfying. Meanwhile, you are paying no attention at all to all the incredible array of options just above your head. Wonderful steaks, beautifully made salads, incredible desserts, and there, as much as you want. All of these choices— and they are free for the taking. You can take a little or a lot; you can try different things; just a taste here, or a full plate there. You can't get it wrong really—if you don't like one thing there are scores of others, and no one is keeping tabs. It's totally up to you."

Notice as we build the metaphor out that each step forward was dependent on a better vehicle or greater clarity about the target. Without these changes we could not have generated a metaphor that could carry the full clinical weight. If the McDonald's version of the metaphor had been used, for example, it might have been marginally workable for behavioral choices. At McDonald's people *are* keeping tabs, and options are *not* free for the taking. You can't just taste things or whimsically choose to have a lot or a little. That vehicle would not have worked because the missing events or functions were not dominant.

The Metaphor Needs to Fit the Client's Background

Before the client can see the similarity to his own situation (the target), he must be able to observe what is happening in the situation carried out by the vehicle as concretely as possible. For metaphors to work well, they must refer to situations that clients can easily picture in their minds, even if they have never directly experienced them. This is the case, for instance, in the quicksand metaphor. Although most of us have never stepped in quicksand, we have seen it happen multiple times in movies (parenthetically, many of the "facts" about quicksand we think we know turn out to be the case *only* in movies, but that is a story for another telling), which makes the experience quite familiar.

The problem is that individual and cultural differences can make metaphors very poor change agents if a client cannot readily picture and sense the vehicle being applied to a target. Like jokes or poems, if metaphors need to be explained to be useful, they have already failed. Common examples of metaphors sure to give inconsistent results unless you know a lot about the individual you are using the metaphor with are sports metaphors, metaphors based on file or popular media, literature metaphors, or political metaphors. Cautioning a client that if she is "swinging for the fences she is likely to strike out" will mean next to nothing if she is not a baseball fan.

One way around this is to use the client's experience directly. This way, instead of having to imagine the events in the vehicle, the client only has to remember them. Then, he can contact the function of these events using his own rather than others' experience. Let's look at an example of a client suffering from bipolar disorder who, among many hobbies, loves watching movies. Based on a functional assessment of his difficulties, the therapist concludes that the client's behaviors are influenced by certain emotions in ways that prevent him from engaging in activities bringing more sustainable satisfaction. Indeed, as is often the case in bipolar disorders, the client experiences rapid changes in his mood which leads to impulsive reactions, in particular when interacting with other people. Thus, a possible goal of the intervention could be to decrease the influence exerted by difficult emotions. One thing the therapist could do is help his client bring distant consequences to the present through augmenting (see Chapter 7). For instance, if the client didn't immediately react to his emotions, he could have more satisfying interactions with others. The influence from this augmenting process could then be strengthened using a metaphor that includes a similar relationship. That is, the metaphor should include a situation where not reacting to short-term events favors long-term consequences. Even if the only thing the therapist knows about the client's background is his passion for cinema, it would still be possible to use this personal experience to build a metaphor that appropriately matches his difficulties.

This is actually what we did for one of our clients who had similar social problems and also loved watching movies. In a summarized version, the metaphor was as follows:

THERAPIST: When you watch a movie, is the story sometimes so compelling that you desperately want to know what is going to happen next?

CLIENT: Yes, very often, especially when it is a good story, with a lot of suspense.

THERAPIST: At any moment in the movie, something really dramatic can happen. For instance, the hero could be wounded and fall into a hole where we don't know if he's dead or not. How do you feel in a moment like that?

CLIENT: Excited to know what is going to happen. If it is a good movie, the tension can be really high in a moment like that.

THERAPIST: But often, we don't immediately know if the hero is dead, right? There might be several scenes before the hero's friends find him in the hole and we finally know if he is still alive.

CLIENT: Yes, that is a classic technique for increasing suspense and tension.

THERAPIST: Do you feel like you want to know the answer right away?

CLIENT: Yes.

THERAPIST: So, do you skip the scenes in between and go directly to the one that reveals what happened?

CLIENT: No! That would ruin the thrill of watching the movie!

THERAPIST: How come? You said you really wanted to know . . .

CLIENT: But that's what makes the movie interesting to watch. If you skip these scenes, when the truth is revealed, it is not nearly as satisfying. I want to know right now, yes, but I prefer to let the story build up.

In this metaphor, the therapist uses a vehicle that contains a relation of condition similar to what the client is experiencing in social interactions. Responding to immediate impulses is satisfying in the short term, but it ruins greater satisfaction in the long term. Here, using the client's personal experience helped him contact more directly the consequences of alternative actions. Letting social interactions unfold at their own pace, as when watching a whole movie rather than skipping scenes, gives the client an opportunity to experience the satisfaction associated with listening to others.

Another way of ensuring that a metaphor is grounded in clients' culture and match the right functions is to use their own metaphorical language. We saw in Chapter 5 that often, clients spontaneously use metaphors to describe their experience, especially when this experience is difficult to describe. Therapists should pay great attention to these spontaneous metaphors since, by definition, they are guaranteed to belong to the client's culture and to functionally match the target. Sometimes, even a single word is an opportunity to unfold a whole story that powerfully resonates in the client's mind. Observe this process in the following exchange:

CLIENT: I can't stand how people look at me. It makes me feel self-conscious and very nervous. I just want to hide.

The client uses a metaphor to describe her response to social situations.

THERAPIST: As in a hide-and-seek game?

The therapist expands the client's own metaphor of hiding.

CLIENT: Yeah. Well, like in a hide-and-seek game where I really don't want to be found.

The client tracks her response further, using the expanded metaphor.

THERAPIST: How do you hide?

The therapist keeps using the metaphor to evoke further tracking.

CLIENT: I avoid conversations. I pretend I have something else to do. I leave. Or when I can't leave, I look away. I let other people talk to avoid being involved in the conversation.

THERAPIST: Does it feel like people are looking for you? Do they try to find where you're hiding?

The therapist continues to evoke tracking inside the metaphor.

CLIENT: Yes. It's like I'm behind a curtain, like a little kid who thinks she can't be seen, but in fact we can see her feet. It's cute when it's a kid. For me, it's kind of pathetic. I can never really find a safe place to hide.

The client notices the consequences of her actions by using the metaphor.

THERAPIST: Like a hide-and-seek game you can never win?

CLIENT: Exactly.

THERAPIST: How fun would it be to play hide and seek if you are never found?

The therapist draws the client's attention to unobserved consequences by using the metaphor again.

CLIENT: Hmm. I guess that would be boring. I never thought about it that way. I guess I'm playing a kind of fun hide-and-seek game in a way. I just never saw it as an enjoyable situation!

The client begins to open herself to other functions linked to social situations.

An Example

Let's go through an example and analyze the process of building a meta-phor based on these key principles:

The metaphor needs to target the appropriate function.
The dominant feature of the vehicle needs to fit the clinical target.
The missing events or functions in the target need to be dominant in the vehicle.
The metaphor needs to fit the client's background.

Imagine a client suffering with depression who is unable to express any interest in potential sources of satisfaction. She seems to have no motiva-tion for any activities and only decided to see a therapist when her partner said he would leave her if she didn't do anything to get better. When you ask her how she spends her time, she answers that all day long, she lies on the couch of her veranda, sleeping or mindlessly looking at the backyard. Together, you decide to aim for an improvement of the frequency and the variety of her activities.

As we saw in Chapter 7, the hardest part of this situation is finding appropriate means of motivation toward lasting sources of reinforcement when there aren't currently any obvious reinforcers in the client's life. One possible approach is to encourage activities even if they don't provide imme-diate satisfaction, assuming that they will become reinforcing again with time. This strategy requires that you evoke augmenting of reinforcement through symbolic processes, which motivate the client to engage in these activities, despite a lack of interest for them at the moment.

In order to build a metaphor that will encourage the client to engage in activities in which she has no interest in at the moment, it is useful to first identify the functional sequence included in her existing relational network. Right now, new activities don't bring satisfaction to her, but if she engages in them they may eventually be satisfying. In other words, there is a relation of condition between a behavior that is not satisfy-ing in the short term, as well as a long-term positive consequence. Thus, the metaphor will need to include a vehicle with this specific functional sequence.

We want there to be a deep, almost sensory connection between the dominant features of the vehicle and the target. In the example of the depressed client, the behaviors likely to bring satisfaction in the long term are topographically active (e.g., going out, working, seeing friends), and the client will experience them as effortful. Thus, a vehicle that was based on passive or easy behaviors would be undesirable even if they had the right sequence of a behavior that is not satisfying in the short term but that has a long-term positive consequence. It would thus be a bad idea to compare what the client can do to, say, not spending money now to be able to buy something expensive later. It would match the clinical situation functionally, but the dominant feature of the vehicle would not fit the target.

It is also important that a sense of enjoyment to come be dominant in the vehicle. If we want to be able to picture a day when life is meaningful again, the vehicle must have a rich, powerful, positive quality in the future it portends.

Finally, we need a metaphor that fits the client's experience. Unfortunately, the client's current experience is very limited since she spends her whole day on the couch sleeping or looking at the backyard. We faced a very similar situation with one of our clients, and the solution to this conundrum was found in the person's backyard—something that she saw herself. We asked her what she saw in the backyard during her long days on the couch. She started to describe how squirrels ran around the trees to find nuts. The exchange that followed became a metaphor for how she might move through her depression:

THERAPIST: What do they do with the nuts? Do they eat them?

CLIENT: No, they gather them and hide them somewhere.

THERAPIST: How come? Are they not supposed to eat them?

CLIENT: Well, yes, but they keep this food for the winter.

THERAPIST: So right now, there is no point to their work?

CLIENT: Well, no, but in the long term, it makes a big difference. They will eat the nuts later when it is too cold outside and there isn't any more food.

THERAPIST: So they do something that requires effort and is not satisfying right now because it will have some benefit later?

CLIENT: Yes, exactly.

There are many ways to use clients' experiences in a metaphor, and the more you know about their cultural and individual background, the easier it will be to find situations that match the therapeutic target. Following the steps we have described in this example will help you find what you are looking for. Fortunately, language itself is amazingly flexible: there is always something you can use.

Creating Metaphors by Working Backwards Experientially

There is always something to use because language is arbitrarily applicable. The number of possibilities for any situation is literally beyond calculation.

An experiential process can be helpful for the therapist to create powerful metaphors based on the flexibility of language. Once this process is habitual it is one you can deploy in the background even during sessions, because done skillfully it takes only a few moments and it parallels useful clinical empathy. Initially it is best to go through this process between sessions when planning possible directions for intervention.

Any child who loves to solve mazes will tell you that they are easier to solve if you do this simple thing: work from the end to the beginning. If we apply this idea to the development of metaphors, a good psychological inroad to finding the right vehicle is to dive into the form and function of clinical problems in an experiential way. This makes sense since the dominant feature and function of the vehicle will need to fit the target problem. So, start with the problems themselves. Try to feel them from the inside out. What sensations or thoughts are present inside this problem; does it feel active or passive; what functions dominate? Don't overthink it—allow your own judgment or analytic thinking to be loosened and seek instead an experiential connection with the struggle your client is having.

Then as you begin to feel this problem from the inside out, keep an experiential approach as you move on to the next therapeutic step. We want a vehicle in which the missing events or functions are dominant, and to find that connection we need to experience those events or functions in a visceral way. What would it feel like to take that therapeutic step? What sensations or thoughts are present; does it feel active or passive; what is driving action inside this new place?

Finally, remembering your client and everything you know about him or her, and staying in touch with your case formulation, what does this experiential contact with the problem and the therapeutic goal remind you of? What situation or event or object could integrate all of this? Here you need to loosen your thinking even more. Allow your attention to wander to films, stories, images, or symbols; to faces, colors, paintings, or snapshots; to memories, plays, actions, or exercises. You are deliberately loosening your style of thinking, as if allowing your own "unconscious" to speak to you. You want all avenues of information to be open.

Possible metaphors will begin to pop up inside this combination of experiential contact with the problem, the goal, and the client. These features will remind you of things you have seen, heard about, or thought about that contain all of these elements. The "associations" may be a bit loose, but they will not be random. There will be a connection.

To see how this process might work, suppose you have a client who is a workaholic. He spends a great deal of effort under the conviction that he is providing for his family, but he is driven, unhappy, and stressed. He has come into therapy in part because his spouse is threatening divorce on the grounds that he is unable to provide her with emotional support. But you have not yet worked out the specific therapeutic goal.

Your analysis of the situation so far is that the client had a critical upbringing in which being playful was criticized and only achievement was rewarded. A former military officer, he was successful as a soldier but has never dealt with the traumas he brought back with him from war. He loves his wife and daughter, but he fears he has nothing to give them other than money. He says he has always felt like a fraud, like he is just going through the motions: "I am afraid to look at myself—I'm afraid of what I might find."

As you delve into the problem behavior experientially—what it is like to be him at his worst—in your imagination you feel a heaviness and a narrowing of vision. It is as if you are carrying a burden. There is a rhythm to it—it is filled with urgency. You have a sense you can't see anything; you can't hear anything. You sense fear and urgency, as if slowing down is a threat and something bad will happen if you do. It's claustrophobic and encapsulated. It's hard work, but known and safe. It feels very, very old.

As you delve into what might be an improvement in the client's life, it feels like opening your eyes and sitting down. You yearn for the client to have a sense of openness, of self-kindness, of giving and receiving support, of play. The word that comes to you as you delve into what could be created clinically is "love," and as you sense that goal, you are surprised when you notice you are beginning to tear up.

Inside the problem, the goal, and the client, metaphors begin to pop up. One that emerges is this:

> "It sometimes feels in here almost as though your life has become an endless military march. Your head is down, and the rhythm of trudging feet is all that can be heard. You just need to keep marching until it stops. You are carrying this heavy sack on your back, which is supposedly provisions for people you care about such as your family—but while you're in this posture, they could be standing right to the side of the road and you might trudge by without even noticing them. And what is in that sack? Is it really provisions? Or is that heavy, old sack full of other things—things like unexamined moments, fear, trauma, pain, and self-criticism?"

If the client sees a connection between his experience and these metaphorical descriptions, you might conclude that

> "One of the things our work together might look at is this question: how long is this march going to go on? Is it really in your interests to keep marching carrying this heavy burden, or is now the time to put that burden down? Once it is off your shoulders, maybe we can find a place to sit. Maybe you can bring your head and eyes up and see who is around you. Maybe there is something to do with that sack full of your history that is kinder, gentler, and more loving."

HOW TO DELIVER A METAPHOR

Once you have chosen or built a metaphor based on the principles we presented in the previous section, you are halfway through the process of using it in therapy. The second critical part of this process is actually delivering the metaphor.

Here we have to be more speculative because the research work is sparse. From a theoretical point of view, however, there are new possible styles to explore.

In some of our examples so far, metaphors were presented in summary format, but in general a more experiential approach may work better, as it enables the client to see the concrete features of the vehicle more clearly. There are styles of presentation that take advantage of an effective metaphor as we have defined one in the previous section.

Taking the Client through the Story as a Role Play

Metaphors provide concrete situations that can be examined in the therapy room and provide new perspectives on behaviors. Whether the problematic behavior is primarily controlled by inappropriate rules or by short-term or variable contingencies, the client will need to recognize more favorable consequences in order to change her behavior. The way the metaphor is presented can make a difference in this regard. A metaphor is like a story, and telling it as a story makes the elements of the vehicle more vivid and easier to observe.

Imagine a therapist explicitly pointing out long-term consequences by saying, "When squirrels gather nuts, the benefits are long term rather than immediate. It requires effort now, but it brings satisfaction later." In this example, the therapist is using a rule that describes the long-term consequences.

There is nothing fundamentally wrong with that explicit approach because it still aims to get clients in touch with useful features in their experience. But by delivering the metaphor this way, the therapist directly provides a rule instead of giving clients an opportunity to observe their experience first. If clients are encouraged to see their own experience through the eyes of the therapist, social compliance can become central, and this can lead to problematic insensitivity (following the rule even when it is not effective).

You can diminish the risk of social compliance driving the client by presenting the metaphor as a quasi-role play, so that the client can track what is happening in the sequence directly, with less explicit intervention from the therapist. For example, in the metaphor of watching a movie that we used earlier, the therapist could lead the conversation in this way (some of these changes are subtle—you may need to look at the previous version on page 269 to see the differences):

THERAPIST: Let's imagine you are watching a suspenseful movie right now. Where do you watch movies generally?

The therapist invites the client to imagine being in the situation described by the vehicle and to contact concrete features of this situation.

CLIENT: In my living room. I have a big screen and a home theater. I make popcorn, and I lay on the couch.

THERAPIST: So you are comfortably sitting on your couch and enjoying your movie. At one moment, the hero of the movie is injured in a battle and falls in a hole. You don't know if he is dead or alive. What are you thinking right now?

The therapist begins to tell the story as if it was happening in the therapy room.

CLIENT: I am excited. I want to know what is going to happen.

THERAPIST: And what do you do?

CLIENT: I keep watching, I can't wait to know if the hero is still alive.

THERAPIST: Do you feel like skipping the next scene and going directly to the point where you will know what happened to the hero?

The therapist asks questions about the client's feelings and actions to involve him personally in the story.

CLIENT: Well, yes, in a way, but I never do that. It would ruin the movie.

Often it is even possible to act out the metaphor so that the client can have an even easier time seeing the concrete features of the situation. The principle is the same as in other metaphors, but here, the client doesn't have to imagine the situation—he can experience it directly.

Using the Present Tense

Since the situation in the metaphor is not actually present in the therapy room, clinicians often spontaneously tell the story using the conditional tense. For example, the therapist says, "Imagine that you stepped in the quicksand. . . . What would you do?"; or "Imagine that you were watching a movie and that the hero was injured and fell in a hole, what would you think?" This kind of presentation requires the client to make a supplemental step of derivation, and because of that, it can create more distance from the experience being observed.

This distance can be reduced by using the present tense. In this case the therapist would say something like, "Imagine that you are walking in the desert and that suddenly, you step in the quicksand. . . . What do you do now?"; or "Imagine that you are watching a movie right now and that the hero is wounded and falls in a hole. What are you thinking now?" Note that the therapist not only uses the present tense, but also grounds the story in the present (e.g., "now," "right now"), almost as if the metaphor is a kind of virtual reality experience. Part of the goal is to make the concrete features of the situation salient. Often, the client won't immediately imitate this form, but he can be gently brought back to the present where experiential observations are likely to be most powerful.

Here is a version of the same conversation we have been exploring that demonstrates how the therapist can help the client stick with the present tense (again, the differences are subtle, so you will likely have to compare these versions to see what has been changed):

THERAPIST: Imagine that you are watching a movie, comfortably sitting on your couch. Suddenly, the hero is injured in a battle and falls in a hole. What are your thoughts at that moment?

CLIENT: I would wonder what happened to the hero . . . if he is dead or not.

THERAPIST: Do you feel eager to know what just happened?

The therapist sticks with the present tense, without correcting the client.

CLIENT: Yes.

THERAPIST: Do you want to skip the next scenes to go directly to the conclusion?

CLIENT: No, that would ruin the movie.

THERAPIST: And yet, right now you really want to know what is going to happen.

CLIENT: Yes, I want to know, but I prefer to wait and let the movie develop.

The client is now using the present tense too.

THERAPIST: Why so?

CLIENT: Because I will enjoy the movie more if I let the story build.

Developing Direct Observation Using Experiential Cues

Noticing concrete aspects of the situation in the vehicle can be enhanced by drawing the clients' attention directly toward their own psychological reactions, such as emotions, sensations, and thoughts. This is similar to other techniques we present in this book for assessing psychological problems, improving functional contextual awareness, and delivering experiential exercises, where the therapist regularly evokes the client's observation, description, and tracking. As we ask the client about his current emotions and thoughts, it becomes more likely that he will stay in the present.

Here is an example of metaphor delivered with multiple experiential cues. The therapist uses a metaphor comparing the difficulty of not reacting to obsessive thoughts with the difficulty of playing football in an away game among a shouting crowd of opponent supporters.

THERAPIST: So, you hear the opponent supporters shouting at you as you come inside the stadium. What do they say?

The therapist evokes observation and description of the situation.

CLIENT: They say that we are going to lose.

THERAPIST: What does that feel like?

The therapist evokes observation and description of psychological experiences.

CLIENT: It's annoying, but that's the game. When we play against other in-state teams, it's worse.

THERAPIST: Imagine that you are on the field right now, playing against one of these teams, and you hear the supporters shouting. Try to picture that in your mind as if you were there right now. Can you hear them?

The therapist evokes observation of experiences.

CLIENT: Yes.

THERAPIST: What are they saying?

The therapist evokes description of experiences.

CLIENT: All kinds of insults toward us. They say that they are going to crush our team.

THERAPIST: How does that feel right now, as you hear them shout?

The therapist evokes observation and description of psychological experiences.

CLIENT: Really annoying.

THERAPIST: What kinds of sensations do you feel?

The therapist orients the client more specifically to sensations.

CLIENT: I don't know . . . I am tense.

THERAPIST: I see that you are frowning. Is it because you feel annoyed and tense as you hear them?

The therapist evokes tracking.

CLIENT: Yeah . . . Just thinking of it makes me a bit angry, I guess.

THERAPIST: And what do you feel like doing as you hear these supporters insulting you?

The therapist evokes further tracking.

CLIENT: Honestly? I feel like punching them!

THERAPIST: What does that feel like, inside of you?

The therapist evokes observation and description of sensations.

CLIENT: Punching them?

THERAPIST: Yes. What sensations come in your body when you feel like punching them?

CLIENT: Hmm . . . I clench my jaw. I feel the tension in my fists.

THERAPIST: And what do you do now?

The therapist evokes tracking.

CLIENT: Well, nothing. I'm not going to hurt anybody. They are stupid, but it's just a game.

Mixing Vocabulary from Vehicle and Target, and Limiting Explicit Comparisons

Clinicians often wonder while delivering a metaphor whether they should "explain" it to their clients or let them figure out what it means on their own. For example, a therapist may say, "The tension you feel when you hear insults from the opponent's supporters, it is like when you have urges to respond to your obsessions. It is hard, but it is possible to choose not to respond to them." The problem with explaining the equivalence between the vehicle and the target is that it may oversimplify the richness of the connection, turning an experiential process into a simple rule. If the client has not formulated this rule himself, it could be mistimed, or overstated; it could become a social goad, increasing the risk of problematic insensitivity due to pliance. RFT concepts do not specifically prohibit the therapist from stating a moral or a connection, since well-timed therapist statements will likely be useful. In general, however, it is safer to err on the side of letting the client see and verbally formulate the connections, so as to strengthen observation, description, and tracking skills. That being said, providing no guidance at all may not be workable in clinical practice because clients can become confused and frustrated.

A middle ground is to gradually mix the vehicle and the target as the client goes through the metaphor and processes it afterward. For example, the therapist might intentionally begin to use the vocabulary from the vehicle to talk about the target. This way, the relation of equivalence shared by the two situations is made more salient without directly explaining the metaphor. This also presents the advantage of bringing more concrete features from the vehicle to the target, which should help undermine the influence exerted by ineffective rules. With time, clients frequently begin to talk about their personal difficulties using terms from the metaphor. As this happens, it becomes easier to assess whether the metaphor is having a positive clinical impact since the client needs to generalize the metaphor to apply it with sophistication. For example, a client might say, "I heard the crowd shouting a lot this week. It was really hard not to punch them in the face. Still I kept my focus on the game." The detailed clinical vignette presented at the end of this chapter will show how to implement this technique.

Evoking the Extraction of Effective Rules

The point of using a metaphor is not just to tell a story, but to promote behavior change through changes in relations and functions. The ultimate goal is to replace a currently ineffective behavior with another behavior that brings more lasting satisfaction to the client. As in any experiential therapeutic technique, the choice of using a metaphor is made to favor the client's autonomy in the long term. If the client can observe her own experience and extract new tracks herself during the presentation of a metaphor, she will learn a sequence of behaviors that can be reproduced more readily outside the therapy room.

Helping the client extract useful verbal formulations based on a metaphor requires most of the techniques you have previously learned. In particular, the therapist can usefully ask questions that evoke the client's observation, description, and tracking such as, "What do you do in this situation?"; "What happens next?"; "What is the consequence of doing that in the short term?"; "What about the consequence in the long term?" Gentle guidance can help the client formulate rules that define new behaviors and their consequences in specific contexts. In the following alternative examples, observe the different degrees of involvement of the therapist in this process. In the first case, the therapist describes what she observes and tracks, to finally extract rules, while in the second case, she only evokes the client's observation, description, and tracking to help him extract new effective rules himself. These exchanges immediately follow the presentation of the quicksand metaphor.

Example 1: The Therapist Formulates Observations and Rules

THERAPIST: And when you start sinking into your anxiety, what do you do?

CLIENT: I do everything I can to relax, to not feel stressed.

THERAPIST: Like distracting yourself, trying to think of something else, right?

The therapist formulates an observation.

CLIENT: Yes.

THERAPIST: And what happens is that you feel even more anxious in the end . . .

The therapist formulates an observation.

CLIENT: Yeah . . . I guess it's like in the quicksand. I sink even more.

THERAPIST: Maybe the problem comes from avoiding your anxiety, then. What do you think?

The therapist formulates her own rule.

CLIENT: You think it makes things worse?

THERAPIST: If I listen to your experience, it seems like it makes things worse because you spend all your energy trying to feel less stressed and you are even more stressed in the end. Maybe a better strategy would be not trying to avoid your anxiety. What do you think?

The therapist formulates a rule and suggests an alternative response.

CLIENT: If I avoid my anxiety, it will make it worse. I understand. It is not easy to think that way. But I see what you mean. . . . It's like the quicksand.

Example 2: The Therapist Evokes Observation, Description, and Tracking

THERAPIST: And when you start sinking into your anxiety, what do you do?

The therapist evokes tracking.

CLIENT: I do everything I can to relax, to not feel stressed.

THERAPIST: Like what, for example?

The therapist evokes observation and description of behavior.

CLIENT: Like I said, I try to distract myself and think of something else.

THERAPIST: And what happens next?

The therapist evokes tracking.

CLIENT: I feel a little better.

THERAPIST: Do you mean that you feel better at first?

The therapist evokes tracking.

CLIENT: Yes.

THERAPIST: And then?

The therapist evokes tracking.

CLIENT: It comes back quickly.

THERAPIST: How is it when it comes back? Is it just as hard as it was before you tried to relax? Is it less hard? Harder?

The therapist evokes more precise tracking.

CLIENT: I don't know. . . . It is harder in a way because it is frustrating to feel the anxiety coming back again and again after it went away for a bit. It makes me feel like it will never go away.

THERAPIST: Are you saying that after it comes back, you feel frustrated in addition to feeling stressed?

The therapist evokes more precise tracking.

CLIENT: Yeah . . . It's even worse in the end.

THERAPIST: What else can you do then?

The therapist evokes tracking of alternative response.

CLIENT: I guess it would be better if I didn't try so hard to avoid feeling stressed.

THERAPIST: Why not? You said that you don't like feeling stressed.

The therapist orients the client to previous observation in order to improve tracking.

CLIENT: Yeah, but it makes things worse in the end.

THERAPIST: You are saying that struggling with your anxiety makes you sink even more?

The therapist reformulates the client's own observation.

CLIENT: Yes, it is like the quicksand in the end.

Note that both examples come to the same conclusion—that is, the formulation of a rule specifying the counterproductive consequences of avoiding anxiety. However, in the second example, the therapist never gave answers, but rather used comments and questions that helped the client observe his own experience and to formulate a new rule himself. Generally, this process takes more time since the answers come from the client, but the progress is more certain. In the first approach, sometimes clients will appear to understand but will later forget or deny what was understood. Focus efforts on helping clients observe their experience and draw their own conclusions about what works for them often is more sure-footed in the long run.

It is important to stay open to a variety of answers—the clinician needs to maintain an attitude of genuine interest and guided by the client. It is possible that the client doesn't experience any counterproductive effects from avoiding anxiety and that the metaphor doesn't actually match his difficulties. However, this apparent failure may be productive because it provides an opportunity to refine the assessment of the client's problems in a functional sense and may lead to revising the plan of intervention. Unless the client's capacity to observe is severely altered, the key clinical compass is his own experience.

USING FROZEN METAPHORS

We have emphasized in this chapter how you can use RFT to select, craft, and deliver metaphors, but we would be remiss if we did not relate these same ideas to the use of frozen metaphors in therapy. The vast majority of key ideas in psychotherapy are frozen metaphors (i.e., metaphors we use so often that we forget they are metaphors, such as when saying "I'm *inclined* to think that . . . "). Words do not entirely lose their metaphorical connotations, however, even when they transition into normal literal terms with a specific denotation. Because of the deep structure of language, even frozen metaphors carry some of their original meaning.

This realization allows clinicians to deliberately use word choices to tap into metaphorical information. Suppose a clinician has a lot of evidence that a client's problematic anger and aggression stems back to childhood issues of abandonment. The clinical goal might be to encourage more self-kindness that would allow the pain of feeling helpless and uncared for to be felt and attended to, much as one might care for a child in pain, but without striking out at others in order to escape the sense of vulnerability that results.

Many uses of language could convey this caring attitude toward oneself. Consider, for example, clinical requests to slow down and feel pain as if it is important and worth attention. Compare these two questions: "What if you stop and feel it?" versus "What if you take the time to *embrace* it and *hold* it?" The two questions are nearly the same, but the second uses terms that encourage self-care and treating oneself as if one is important. Even more directly, the second question uses terms that connote what a child might reasonably yearn for: being held or embraced when she is hurt.

If the client's experience of abandonment happened even earlier in childhood, this same question might be reworded again: "What if we look that feeling in the eyes and just kind of cradle it?" If the clinician wants to begin to suggest self-compassion as an alternative to defensive anger and attack, the question can be altered to pull for this comparison, but without having to state it explicitly: "What if you take the time to *embrace* it? Don't *grab* it or *clench* it *tight*. Don't *fight* it. Just see if you can gently *bring it close*."

The deliberate use of frozen metaphors generally flies completely under the radar screen of clients, but such metaphors can be powerfully evocative because word connotations matter. A person with a deep early childhood abandonment issue may tear up at the request to "cradle" an emotion and never realize that the vulnerability she feels comes from the deliberate use of a phrase that is almost the same as one would use to describe holding a very young child: "I looked the baby in the eyes and cradled it."

Once the clinician sees how to use frozen metaphors to probe a problem area or to advance a clinical agenda, their potential application is vast—almost every clinical statement provides an opportunity for their use. It can take some research and exploration (e.g., with websites such as thesaurus.com) to identify good alternatives but clinical themes are common enough across clients that as you initially work out how to use specific frozen metaphors with a given clinical situation between sessions, you will be able to gradually expand it into moment-by-moment language choices.

CLINICAL EXAMPLE

The following clinical vignettes present two approaches to delivering the same metaphor to a client suffering from fear of public speaking. In the first version, the metaphor is told in a didactic way, that is, with an explicit explanation of the equivalence between the vehicle and the target. In addition, the therapist goes through the story without involving the client in a role play, without using experiential cues, and without mixing the vocabulary of the two networks. Finally, he formulates the rule instead of letting the client extract it from his own experience. In the second version, you will see how integrating RFT principles can modify this technique with the goal of increasing the likelihood of impact.

Didactic Version

THERAPIST: Have you ever been on a roller coaster?

This simple question ensures that being on a roller coaster is part of the client's cultural experience.

CLIENT: Yes.

THERAPIST: Do you like riding roller coasters?

This is another simple question to ensure that being on a roller coaster will have useful functions to transfer to the target, which in this case, is the compatibility between experiencing difficult emotions and satisfaction at the same time.

CLIENT: Yes, it's fun. Scary, but fun.

THERAPIST: Have you noticed that your emotions go up and down like the roller coaster itself?

The therapist explicitly states the functions included in the vehicle.

CLIENT: Yes, There are moments when everybody screams.

THERAPIST: Like when you reach a very high point and it is about to go down again very fast?

CLIENT: Yes, that's pretty scary.

THERAPIST: But that is what makes it fun too, right?

The therapist explicitly states the equivalence between emotions of fear and satisfaction in the vehicle.

CLIENT: Yes.

THERAPIST: Have you noticed that emotions go up and down in life in general too? Like when you have to speak in public, it is like reaching the highest point of the roller coaster in a way . . .

The therapist explicitly formulates the equivalence between the vehicle and the target.

CLIENT: Yes, for me, that's definitely as scary as that . . .

THERAPIST: But what is interesting is that there are situations where we choose to be afraid because it is fun. Like going on a roller coaster or watching a scary movie. Could you imagine thinking of the fear you feel in public speaking the same way as you think of this kind of emotion?

The therapist again states the equivalence between the vehicle and the target. The transformation of function of the emotion of fear was explicitly suggested.

CLIENT: You mean, thinking of speaking in public like a roller coaster?

THERAPIST: Maybe not just speaking in public but life in general, actually. If you consider the different emotions you experience in your life to be normal variations, as parts of your life that make it interesting, you may be less bothered by your fear when you are about to speak.

The therapist formulates a rule specifying the advantageous consequence of seeing fear of public speaking the same way as fear in a roller coaster.

CLIENT: I have never thought about that, but it is true that there are fears that don't bother me or even ones that I like.

THERAPIST: If you see your fear of speaking in public and your emotions in general as ups and downs on a roller coaster, you may actually feel like choosing to live these emotions. They might be scary sometimes, but they are part of your life. Parts of what makes it interesting too.

Again, the therapist explicitly formulates the rule that may help the client change his behavior.

Experiential Version

THERAPIST: Have you ever been on a roller coaster?

This simple question ensures that being on a roller coaster is part of the client's cultural experience.

CLIENT: Yes.

THERAPIST: Do you like riding roller coasters?

This is another simple question to ensure that being on a roller coaster will have useful functions to transfer to the target, which in this case, is the compatibility between experiencing difficult emotions and satisfaction at the same time.

CLIENT: Yes, it's fun. Scary, but fun.

THERAPIST: Would it be okay if we did a little exercise like we do here sometimes?

CLIENT: Yes.

THERAPIST: Okay. I would like you to imagine that you are on a roller coaster right now. Can you picture that in your mind?

The therapist presents the metaphor as a role play by asking the client to imagine being on the roller coaster right now and by using a series of questions evoking the observation of concrete features of this situation.

CLIENT: Yes.

THERAPIST: Tell me what you notice around you.

The therapist evokes observation and description.

CLIENT: I am sitting in a kind of cabin. There are people behind me. I can see the rails in front of me.

THERAPIST: Has it started yet?

CLIENT: No. We are waiting for everybody to get in.

THERAPIST: Okay. Let's start it now. How do you feel?

The therapist evokes observation and description of feelings.

CLIENT: Excited.

THERAPIST: Yeah? What is it like? What sensations do you feel in your body?

The therapist evokes further observation and description of sensations.

CLIENT: Hmm . . . My heart is racing. I smile but I'm nervous . . . I hear people screaming. It makes it even more stressful.

THERAPIST: Do you have other sensations?

The therapist evokes further observation and description of sensations.

CLIENT: My hands are pretty sweaty.

THERAPIST: How do you like the ride so far?

The therapist evokes observation and description.

CLIENT: It is mixed. It is scary but fun at the same time.

THERAPIST: You are about to reach one of the highest points of the roller coaster now. It is moving very, very slowly. . . . Can you feel it?

CLIENT: Yeah . . . It is very stressful . . .

THERAPIST: What is it like in your body?

The therapist evokes observation and description of sensations.

CLIENT: Very tense. I can feel my heart pounding in my chest.

THERAPIST: Yeah? Are you having fun?

The therapist evokes observation and description.

CLIENT: (*laughing*) Yeah . . .

THERAPIST: Does that make you want to leave the roller coaster?

The therapist evokes tracking.

CLIENT: I feel like it because it's scary, but I don't really want to.

THERAPIST: Let's pause the roller coaster for a minute. I would like to ask you some questions again about your fear of speaking in public. Is that okay?

The therapist evokes the client's observation of the target without explicitly mentioning the analogy with the vehicle.

CLIENT: Yes.

THERAPIST: Could you tell me again what it feels like when you are on the highest point of a meeting, when you know you are going to have to talk in front of your colleagues?

The therapist evokes observation and description of psychological experiences in public speaking, in order to make the equivalence with the roller coaster more salient. Notice how the therapist uses the vocabulary of the roller coaster while talking about public speaking (the "highest point").

CLIENT: I feel very stressed, scared.

THERAPIST: How about the sensations in your body?

The therapist evokes observation and description of sensations.

CLIENT: I sweat, my heart races . . . I feel very shaky.

THERAPIST: And suddenly, the roller coaster goes down very fast. You have to talk now. How do you feel?

The therapist evokes observation and description while mixing again the vocabulary of the vehicle and the target.

CLIENT: It's even scarier.

THERAPIST: Do you hear screaming in your head?

CLIENT: (*smiling*) Yeah, something like that.

Often, clients start smiling or expressing their understanding when they perceive the equivalence between the vehicle and the target.

THERAPIST: What do you do then?

The therapist evokes tracking of the sequence included in the target.

CLIENT: I find a way to avoid speaking. When I can, I leave the room before.

THERAPIST: You leave the roller coaster because it gets too scary?

The therapist mixes the vocabulary of the two networks again so as to increase their functional equivalence.

CLIENT: (*smiling*) Yeah, that roller coaster, I don't stay on it.

THERAPIST: Does that make you feel better?

The therapist evokes tracking.

CLIENT: Not really. It is less scary now but . . .

THERAPIST: But . . .

CLIENT: I don't get to express my opinions in our meetings.

THERAPIST: Is that important for you, to express your opinions?

The functional equivalence between the roller coaster and public speaking implies that both situations can trigger difficult emotions and provide satisfaction at the same time. Therefore, the therapist evokes augmenting to connect public speaking with a meaningful source of satisfaction.

CLIENT: Of course, it's what makes that job interesting or else there is no point.

THERAPIST: Is it what makes your job fun?

CLIENT: Yes, but it's scary.

THERAPIST: Are you saying that the same thing that scares you is fun too?

The therapist reformulates the paradox of having emotions of fear and satisfaction at the same time. Whereas the client expresses this paradox as an opposition, the therapist reformulates it with a relation of coordination.

CLIENT: Yeah . . . I guess it is like the roller coaster. It's scary and fun.

THERAPIST: Would that be fun to be on a roller coaster if it was not scary?

The therapist helps the client see the connection between fear and satisfaction experienced on a roller coaster in order to indirectly transform the function of fear in public speaking. Next time he will have to speak in public, he may approach his fear as connected to the satisfaction this situation also provides.

CLIENT: Probably not.

THERAPIST: How do you feel about staying on the roller coaster next time you have to speak in public? Could that be fun?

The therapist evokes the client's tracking by asking him to explore the consequences of public speaking again but this time, with closer attention to the satisfaction it can provide.

CLIENT: (*smiling*) I can try.

THERAPIST: And see what happens . . .

The therapist again underlines the importance of tracking conse-quences in his experience to limit the possibility that the client will only engage in public speaking through pliance.

 **CHAPTER SUMMARY**

In this chapter, you learned how to choose, build, and deliver a metaphor to develop experiential skills in your clients. Here are the main principles to remember:

- Choosing or building a therapeutic metaphor requires taking into account the relevant clinical function and the client's background to ensure that the metaphor refers to an experience the client can relate to.

- Choosing or building a therapeutic metaphor requires that the dominant feature of the vehicle fits the clinical focus and the missing events or functions that you want to establish in the target are dominant in the vehicle. This is more effective if the dominant features are concrete and direct rather than abstract.

- Metaphors can be generated by the clinician by exploring the form and function of the problem and therapeutic goal experientially while main-taining context with relevant client details, allowing relevant vehicles to emerge spontaneously.

- A therapeutic metaphor will likely have more impact if delivered experi-entially. The main possibilities to explore are:
  - Presenting the metaphor as a role play.
  - Using the present tense.
  - Using experiential cues.
  - Mixing the vocabulary of the vehicle and the target while avoiding premature direct comparisons.
  - Helping the client extract rules rather than directly formulating them.
- Frozen metaphors can also be used deliberately in session, guided by RFT principles.

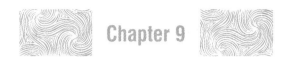

Chapter 9

Training Experiential Skills
through Formal Practice

All of the techniques we have presented in Chapters 4–8 are those you can directly integrate into natural exchanges, that is, without necessarily disrupting the course of a spontaneous discussion between you and the client. In this chapter, you will learn how to apply RFT principles to the use of formal experiential techniques that often require the substitution of specific exercises or instructions for natural exchanges. Formal practices or exercises in psychotherapy are also dependent on language processes. RFT provides principles to help you choose, build, and deliver such techniques with maximum effectiveness.

OVERVIEW

The Goal

Although significant changes can happen as a result of natural verbal interactions in therapy, it is often difficult for clients to consolidate these skills without more formal and regular practice. We can compare these distinctive forms of training to the way a coach shapes the skills of an athlete. For example, a tennis coach could hit the ball in specific directions in order to help a student refine his placement on the court, even while playing a casual game together. In contrast, he could set an exercise that requires the student to run very fast in specific directions to catch balls sent by a machine. In the former case, the student might not even realize that he is working on certain skills since his attention is all on the game. In the latter case, it probably feels more like working, but it is a great opportunity to improve more specific skills in a targeted way.

Students and beginning therapists often gravitate toward formal methods because they seem easier to learn and to deliver than informal ones. That is especially true of methods that can be written down as formal scripts or as tightly organized series of steps. In fact, almost the opposite is true if we focus on a therapist's competence and not merely adherence to a protocol. Indeed, it can be quite difficult to deliver formal techniques in a way that is well timed and that preserves the fluidity of the therapeutic relationship and the commitment and motivation of clients. As we will see, RFT provides useful guidance for how to do so.

At the highest level of abstraction, all successful forms of psychotherapy target awareness and change. Since clients persist in behaviors that are not effective and fail to adopt behaviors that would be effective, we need to help them notice the contextual variables that influence their actions and adopt more flexible and progressive strategies. Formal practice is extremely useful to raising a client's awareness; to changing behavioral patterns that are difficult to observe or to make more flexible, especially when they have become well practiced and habitual; and to instigating and retaining new actions. An old habit doesn't change in one day, and new skills often require practice before showing desired results (consider learning to play the violin). By setting a formal context, providing specific instructions or verbal guidance, and encouraging direct practice, we can help clients learn skills and change features of the context so that effective changes will transfer to the natural situations of their everyday life.

The scripts of formal exercises are generally easy to understand, but their deeper purpose or how they can be delivered to ensure effective impact without disrupting the therapeutic relationship is often not specified. Without these needed elements, formal techniques can feel awkward and arbitrary, and create a barrier between the therapist and her client. As we will see in this chapter, RFT principles can help avoid these dangers.

Why This Is Important, from an RFT Point of View

From an RFT perspective, formal and nonformal experiential techniques are not fundamentally different, since both include symbolic and non-symbolic learning processes that are used to establish behavior through alteration of the context. What makes formal practice special is the use of instructions and specific steps in a defined setting or period, steps that are being systematically followed in order to obtain the intended effect. How therapists deliver these instructions or the steps of a protocol is subject to more variability. Understanding how RFT principles operate at the core of formal experiential practice can thus help you make better functional moves when choosing, building, and delivering these techniques.

From an RFT point of view, it is essential that the practice fits the therapeutic goal, establishes an exemplar of the action or functional process, and is done in such a way that clients can replicate changes in their natural environments. Formal practice can undermine problematic actions and expand desired actions in new domains by creating contexts in therapy that are both functionally effective and overlap with the natural environment. If these exercises are cast in ways that fit the moment, they can enhance rather than interfere with the therapeutic relationship.

Formal practice often includes methods designed to draw the attention of the client to specific events or their characteristics. For example, asking a client to observe where in his body he feels anxious increases the influence of an intrinsic characteristic of this emotion, whereas asking him about the implications of his anxiety will amplify its symbolic functions. Instructions can also lead the client to expand a relational network so that new relations begin to influence his behavior in useful ways. For example, having a person practice a social skill while imagining doing it as a favorite actor (a method sometimes used in social skills training) alters the functions of specific actions by verbally imputing certain characteristics and comparisons. Formal practice of skills may include instructions to help establish their form, or may be based more on direct therapist feedback in order to select effective actions. Some practices may do both—for example, asking the client to breathe in a way that expands her abdomen both describes a form and gives a metric she can use in the future to examine breathing patterns—again, making transition to the natural environment more likely. Exposure exercises may deliberately organize how the stimulus is contacted, and direct attention toward features of the situation may be used to enhance response flexibility. Thus, formal practice involves symbolic events both as an input and as an output; it focuses on both the form of action and contextual control over action; it can alter the role of both antecedents and consequences.

How These Methods Touch on Various Clinical Traditions

Formal exercises have been used in different psychotherapeutic approaches for as long as there has been a field of psychotherapy. Classic skills development techniques (e.g., training social skills through practice and feedback) or formal exposure and problem-solving exercises are widely used to activate and strengthen behavior change. There has also been a concern over explicit skills methods for just as long a period, especially by humanistic, existential, or psychodynamic therapists concerned that explicit methods might overwhelm the therapeutic relationship. Some of those concerns seem to be weakening as experiential techniques have gained even greater attention more recently. For example, numerous mindfulness techniques (e.g., meditation) have been deployed in modern treatment packages applied to a variety of psychological difficulties in an effort to improve awareness and cognitive flexibility (Hayes et al., 2011). Nevertheless, we feel that both sides of this dialogue have a good point: experiential skills training can be useful, but it can also be done in ways that undermine the therapeutic relationship. The present volume has attempted to get beyond that polarized dialogue by digging down into the essence of these issues in a functional sense, so that practitioners can see the principles that underlie therapeutic methods more generally.

This chapter focuses on such methods as attentional training, mindfulness training, skills training, and formal exposure exercises. But beyond the cognitive-behavioral tradition, methods such as skills training, psychodrama, role therapy, and communication training, can all be included under the umbrella we intend to raise here. By getting clear on their functions and core purposes, we believe our main points will be relevant to virtually any skills training situation in psychotherapy.

How to Do It

In this section we will describe methods in a way that makes the underlying goals of formal experiential practice more evident, covering the areas of attention training, experimenting, expanding flexibility and contextual control, and establishing or altering symbolic relations.

Attention Training

Although attention is a relatively loose concept, for the purpose of this book we can approach it simply as the action of orienting toward events. These events can be external (as when listening to a piece of music) or internal (as when noticing a physical sensation). In behavioral terms, attention is a matter of stimulus control; what we attend to is what we are in interaction with. Attentional training is thus the process of learning how to broaden or narrow stimulus control voluntarily. With language especially, it becomes possible to disassemble complex stimulus situations readily into features and components, and to attend on purpose to particular features rather than others. Thus, attention training tends to improve the client's flexible sensitivity to the context, which is one of the main goals of our functional contextual approach to psychotherapy (see Chapter 3).

The opportunity for attentional training occurs informally during many moments of therapy—such as when the therapist asks his client to think of a good memory so as to augment contact with meaningful sources of reinforcement (see Chapter 7) or to focus on a painful memory in order to teach the client how to gain flexibility in contact with difficult experiences (see Chapter 5). All that is required to add attentional training to these moments is to help the client notice that attention is shifting and to note that this same shift is possible in other contexts.

Every experiential exercise that alters stimulus control contains the opportunity for attentional training in the same way. Since formal practices can be structured beforehand, it is worth thinking about the attentional training that can go on inside methods that are superficially for another purpose (e.g., exposure; skills training). On reflection, formal experiential practice often contains deliberate training of attention. Exercises may specify what to attend to, when, or for how long—these types of methods may augment or diminish certain forms of contextual control. For example, during exposure exercises a client might be asked to notice her body or to focus on her purpose for being in contact with difficult events (e.g., remembering she came to the mall to buy something for her child, not just to deal with anxiety).

The specific focus can be important. Learning to notice the interest of others, for example, can establish a consequence of action that can then aid in learning and shaping socially effective skills (Azrin & Hayes, 1984). In addition to the specific focus, however, *any* adjustment of attention in an experiential exercise is helping to disrupt existing attentional habits. If attentional targets vary to some degree within an exercise, or across exercises, then what is being trained in addition to attention toward these targets is the voluntary regulation of attention per se. Once this is seen, it is easy to add attentional training as a deliberate feature of experiential exercises. For example, suppose that during exposure exercises the client is asked to notice her bodily responses. The therapist might deliberately narrow or broaden attentional control by asking the client to notice just one specific bodily sensation (say how her stomach feels), stay with it for a period, and then shifting to another sensation (e.g., noticing her breath). This can be extended to shifting attention to another dimension (e.g., noticing thoughts; or watching people walk by) or expanding attention to two events at once. If events emerge spontaneously that capture attention involuntarily (e.g., "I'm starting to feel very anxious!") the methods in Chapter 5 can be used to break this large complex of events into smaller features that can be attended to one at a time, thus training more voluntary attentional control. Such attentional training can create more behavioral or emotional flexibility by establishing more skill in being able to choose what events capture attention: to narrow stimulus control when that is helpful and to broaden stimulus control when that is helpful.

Some experiential methods are mostly focused on attentional training. An example of such experiential practice is meditation. Focused forms of meditation narrow attention to a spot on the wall, or a mantra. Open forms of meditation ask the person to note without involvement the continuous flow of sensory and symbolic processes in the now.

Consider the practice of "following the breath." Attention quickly wanders, but when noticed the person is directed to gently bring attention back to the breath. In effect, that is a training trial of focusing, noticing loss of focus, and redirection of attention. The cycle continues endlessly—that is "the practice." With practice, the loss of attention may go down (said another way, the ability to narrow stimulus control voluntarily may go up), but equally important the ability to *notice* the loss of attention and then to redirect it may go up.

Training attention is useful to alter the client's sensitivity to different sources of influence. For example, a client with symptoms of posttraumatic stress disorder might have difficulties enjoying a pleasant activity because he is absorbed in memories of the trauma. In other words, his behavior is mainly influenced by a symbolic source of influence. Being able to redirect attention from difficult thoughts can help the client orient toward other events relevant to current activities and thus improve flexible sensitivity to the context and psychological effectiveness. But disengagement and redirection are not synonyms for suppression and distraction. As we saw in Chapter 2, trying not to think of something often leads to thinking about it even more, due to the derivation effects of language. Instead, the client is encouraged to expand his attention and observe alternative sources of influence so that effective actions appear more available. For example, noticing purpose and meaning may help the client stay engaged in an activity instead of quitting it to escape painful memories.

The ability to direct attention can also undermine ineffective rules such as, "If only it hadn't happened, then I would be happy," by reorienting one to other sources of influence than the rule (e.g., direct contingencies). It can increase flexible self skills (see Chapter 6), as the person is better able to notice internal and external events regardless of their valence as they unfold continuously.

Formal experiential methods can also direct the client's attention in useful directions by *altering* the impact of contextual events. In certain cases, the instructions lead the client first to build new relations in her symbolic networks and then to observe her reactions. For example, the client may be invited to derive deictic relations or to augment reinforcement and notice how it changes her perception of a given situation, which is useful to train self-awareness and meaning or motivation skills. Writing a letter to oneself is an example of an exercise that activates these types of derivations (Hayes, Strosahl, et al., 2012) The client may be led to imagine being 20 years older and to write a letter to her current self in order to express appreciation for the things that she is doing right now and that will have a positive impact in the future. The client thus needs to change perspective by imagining being at another time and to contact distant positive consequences (augmenting). As a result, the client notices which of her current actions are connected to these positive consequences and may decide to change her priorities.

Other techniques alter the impact of contextual events by reducing their symbolic functions. For example, a symbolic antecedent triggering painful emotions (e.g., a word related to a traumatic episode) can lose its function if the client is more in touch with its intrinsic characteristics (e.g., the sound that the word makes when it is spoken, or the shape of the letters when it is written). Noticing these distinctive characteristics helps the client broaden his range of possible responses to this event. In a classic exercise used in acceptance and commitment therapy, a client is asked to reduce difficult or entangling thoughts or self-judgments to a single word and then to repeat that word out loud very quickly. This can lead him to be much more in touch with the sound of the word than with its meaning, which will likely reduce both the distress it produces and its believability (Masuda et al., 2009). Part of that effect is likely attentional, and seen that way, it is easier to imagine how these skills might generalize. A person thinking self-critical thoughts might be able to focus only on their sound, or cadence, or what letters make up the words in these thoughts. This will reduce the transformation of stimulus functions produced by normal functional contextual cues. Increased awareness of different possible properties of symbolic events and increased ability to attend to various properties at will can be used to limit the influence of symbolic stimuli currently controlling the client's problematic behavior: attention itself can help regulate the transformation of stimulus functions.

Experimenting

Another type of process activated by formal experiential techniques and exercises consists of experimenting with different behavioral approaches to deal with a problematic situation or rise to new challenges. Sometimes, experimenting is used merely to help establish new skills, such as in communication training in couples work or social skills training with children. This is a simple case of response acquisition or response deployment under symbolic control. The use of motivational features of language, contingency tracking, and contextual control features—the subjects we have already covered in other chapters—are relevant to such tasks.

At other times, experimenting is done to notice discordance with existing rules or to establish rules that better match experience (i.e., promoting functional coherence; see Chapter 3). Thus, the therapist usually encourages the client to track the consequences of her actions, and it is quite common for these observations to be the focus of clinical work as the therapist helps the client extract rules that match the behavioral sequence as closely as possible (this approach is similar to functional contextual awareness and functional sense making skills presented in Chapter 5 through informal exchanges).

As an example of an exercise focused on rule discordance, consider the classic thought suppression exercise created by the late Dan Wegner.

Initially, participants are to avoid thinking of a white bear for the next 5 minutes and to note every occurrence of this thought during this period of time. Next, participants are told they can think of whatever they want while still noting the occurrences of a white bear in their thoughts. You can do this with a client. This experiment generally provides the client with an opportunity to observe that thought suppression is counterproductive: even if suppression works for a while, it rebounds. Noticing this relationship allows the client to develop a rule based on the experience of the conse-quences of suppressive actions, rather than a rule over extending strategies that are accurate elsewhere (e.g., trying to eliminate thoughts works differ-ently than trying to eliminate dirt on the floor).

Some classic methods employed in cognitive-behavioral therapy con-tain these same processes. For example, early in cognitive-behavioral ther-apy it is common to ask the person to engage in "behavioral experiments" while recording the results. A depressed person who says "I can't do any-thing" might eventually agree to test this thought by, say, trying to make breakfast for the family. The disconfirming evidence has been argued to help undermine the believability of the original thought and to reformulate beliefs. For example, Bennett-Levy et al. (2004) say that behavioral experi-ments in cognitive therapy "are primarily a means of checking the validity of thoughts, perceptions, and beliefs, and/or constructing new operating principles and beliefs" (p. 11). It is not yet known if behavioral experiments actually work this way (Longmore & Worrell, 2007), but it seems possible from an RFT point of view. RFT adds an emphasis on not allowing these processes to be linked to attempts to subtract or avoid symbolic functions. Indeed, the impact of cognitive reappraisal on psychological health is medi-ated by psychological flexibility (Kashdan et al., 2006), which suggests that what is key is the ability to think new thoughts based on experience, not the elimination of old ones as such.

Many exercises seem to fit this same pattern of experiences alter-ing thoughts based on rule discordance, including the use of paradoxical instructions, the use of exposure exercises designed to disconfirm cata-strophic thinking patterns, or the deliberate creation of cognitive desyn-chronies. An example of the later is to instruct a person to think "I can't pick up this pen" while doing so, in order to reduce the impact of automatic thoughts (cf. McMullen et al., 2008).

Expanding Flexibility and Contextual Influence

Experiential exercises can be used to create greater response flexibility or to alter sources of influence over responding. This kind of "expansion" goal frequently appears in what is perhaps the most common form of experien-tial exercise: exposure. Most people seem to believe that exposure refers to contact with emotionally distressing events in order to extinguish or habituate to emotional reactions. This traditional analysis is now known to be largely incorrect (Craske, Kircanski, Zelikowsky, Mystkowski, & Baker, 2008). An alternative way to view exposure is that it is organized contact with previously repertoire-narrowing events for the purpose of creating greater response flexibility (Hayes, Strosahl, et al., 2012).

This expansion agenda can be promoted by the use of the methods discussed in Chapter 5 (in the section on increasing response flexibility), helping the person during exposure to note details of their experience (bodily sensations, emotions, memories, thoughts, and so on) and to engage in new, more flexible forms of responding such as exploring sensations, watching emotions with curiosity, and engaging in additional behaviors (e.g., a person with panic disorder might watch people in a mall and guess what people do for a living).

Another form of expansion is learning to note antecedent or consequential events. For example, experiential processes such as communication training, training in perspective taking, or compassion-focused training may help sensitize people to the social consequences of their actions on others, which can then help shape more effective action over time. This is likely to be especially effective if the new antecedents or consequences are available in the natural environment.

Such an expansion process can be built into experiential exercises of all sorts once its role is appreciated. Take, for example, exposure exercises. If they are not being done to eliminate anxiety, but instead to create response flexibility, it is worth thinking about how contextual influence can be expanded to produce and maintain these more flexible patterns. Suppose an exposure exercise for a person with panic disorder involves going to the mall. It may be less important to take regular ratings of anxiety, hoping for spontaneous reductions, than it would be to measure response flexibility. Did the person buy a new and much wanted piece of clothing at the end of the exercise? Did she pick out a toy for a daughter's birthday, or did she have a nice cup of coffee? All forms of experiential work can in principle help construct effective actions linked to natural outcomes of importance, but the therapist will have to think in constructional and expansion terms to see how language can be used to orient the client toward those key features.

Establishing or Altering Symbolic Relations

Another process often involved in experiential exercises consists of establishing or altering the way a client relates experiences symbolically. At the most basic level, exercises aim to temporarily block the occurrence of a particular symbolic relation. For example, as in the exercise we mentioned earlier, a client might be invited to repeat a word very fast for 30 seconds until the relation of coordination between the sounds of the spoken word and the event it refers to is undermined. What the therapist hopes is that the client will eventually be able to relate to the word, or to words in general, in a different way (i.e., words will be seen as mere symbols, not the actual events they refer to). Another example is to invite a client to reformulate statements opposing feelings to actions with frames of coordination instead, in order to help alleviate barriers (e.g., from "I want to build a relationship *but* I am anxious" to "I want to build a relationship *and* I am anxious"). An exercise focusing on building a flexible sense of self might use hierarchical and deictic framing to help the client think of himself as the container and observer of his experiences rather than as the experiences themselves (i.e., from an equivalence between the self and the experiences to a conceptualization in terms of inclusion and perspective). For example, the therapist might invite the client to imagine himself at different ages and notice that beyond the changes that occur across time and space, there is a part of him that is stable, observes, and contains all experiences (Hayes, Strosahl, et al., 2012).

Both altering and establishing symbolic relations can also consist of building frames of coordination between the client's situation or difficulty, and concrete experiences that are easier to observe in the here and now of a therapy session. These kinds of connections also allow new learning experiences that occur in therapy to generalize to the natural environment. Note that these exercises are often in their essence therapeutic metaphors (see Chapter 8). Suppose, for example, that a therapist asks a client to bring her hand as close to her face as her thoughts are to her consciousness. This establishes a relation of equivalence between the distance that separates the client head and hand, which is an intrinsic characteristic easy to observe, and the symbolic, less salient distance that separates the client from her thoughts. By doing so, the client becomes more able to notice the distinction between what she thinks and who is thinking it.

Numerous formal techniques use this same principle. They draw parallels between the client's experiences and concrete objects that are easier to observe. For example, an exercise called "physicalizing" (Hayes, Strosahl, et al., 2012) consists of asking the client to imagine the color, the shape, or the movement of a sensation or thought. In another exercise, the therapist may ask the client to take a body posture that represents how she reacts to how she feels at her worst, and to adopt another body posture to express how she is at her best. The close versus open posture that the client will likely show can then be used to model the less tangible psychological posture of being emotionally closed or open.

Although the typology of processes activated by formal techniques that we presented in this section is not meant to be exhaustive, and these processes are often combined in a single technique, it provides a basis for understanding how most experiential exercises work. With these principles in mind, therapists can target more precisely the skills that their clients need most to improve as they choose, build, and deliver formal techniques. We will show how to do that in practice in the remaining sections of this chapter.

FORMAL EXPERIENTIAL TECHNIQUES IN PRACTICE

Choosing Formal Experiential Techniques

In this section, we will we examine the principles that guide the selection of experiential techniques by considering three different clinical cases. In each case, we will need to consider how to choose experiential exercises in ways that foster greater attentional control, experimentation to establish new actions or undermine undesirable rule control, expansion of flexibility or contextual control, new symbolic relations to establish more effective conceptualization of psychological experiences, and linking all of this to the natural environment.

In each of the following examples, we will start with a short presentation of a client, then build a brief case conceptualization and examine how to pick an exercise that fits the specific needs of this client.

Case 1

This first case involves a 43-year-old woman who comes to therapy because she devotes a considerable amount of time to obsessive rituals, which dramatically impacts her quality of life. When she wakes up, she immediately starts thinking about terrible things that might happen to her family. Because these thoughts make her feel very anxious, every day she engages in a number of behaviors aiming to ensure that everybody in her house will be safe all day. For example, she checks the electrical system, tests fire alarms, throws away any food item that was not bought the same day, calls her children and her husband repeatedly on the phone to be reassured they are safe, and spends hours on the Internet exploring websites about domestic safety. These behaviors have become a routine that takes more than half of her day. Her quality time with her family has shrunk to nearly nothing, and her relationship with her husband and her older children is strained. Although she acknowledges that she can't keep living this way, she also says that she must protect her family and doesn't see how to resolve this dilemma.

Although this presentation is short, we can make some hypotheses about the problems experienced by the client. First, it seems that her main problematic behavior is to escape and avoid her anxiety related to the harm and possible loss of those she loves. If all the things she does to ensure her family's safety were effective and didn't impair her well-being, escaping and avoiding might not be considered problematic. However, in this case, the negative impact of her rituals is quite obvious. We don't know exactly what effective behaviors are lacking, but we can imagine that the time she spends on rituals prevents her from engaging in other activities that are more satisfying in the long term (e.g., working, leisure, time with family, etc.), and there is some indication that paradoxically the very cost she fears most (harm to family) is happening via her actions, suggesting a lack of ability to engage in actions that contribute to deeper and more loving relationships.

Given the nature of this behavioral issue, we can logically hypothesize that the client is particularly sensitive to the short-term decrease of anxiety that follows her rituals. The thought "I must protect my family" doesn't clearly specify the behavior at play and its natural consequences, which increases the risk of pliance (the rule is followed regardless of the natural consequences). Further hypotheses could be formulated, but for the purpose of our demonstration, let's limit our case conceptualization to these few elements and see how we can choose an appropriate formal experiential technique.

Since the client seems to escape and avoid thoughts and emotions, the therapist could choose a technique that aims to train her ability to stay in contact with these psychological experiences (i.e., training response flexibility), and become more sensitive to new sources of influence, such as the long-term consequence of staying in touch with the emotion (i.e., attentional training). A meditation or exposure exercise could be useful because it would encourage the client to observe these experiences without attempting to change them.

However, the client probably already feels that she is constantly "in touch" with these experiences (which is why we generally call these thoughts "obsessive"). Even though the client tries not to have them, they are always on her mind. This suggests that distinguishing between observing a thought and being stuck with this thought might be difficult for the client. For this reason, it would be useful to choose an exercise that contains verbal instructions likely to increase the perception of distance between the client and her thoughts (i.e., establishing new symbolic relations). For example, an exercise widely employed in treatment packages using meditation consists of imagining one's thoughts as leaves floating on a stream or as clouds passing in the sky (thus establishing analogical relations between the client's experiences and something more concrete to observe, and deictic relations between thoughts and the self). With her eyes closed, the client pictures the scenery, and each time a new thought comes, she puts it on the leaf or the cloud and lets it go. Through persistent practice, the client learns to notice and distance herself from the psychological experiences that influence her behaviors in a problematic way. If this skill could be brought into actual exposure, it might be especially effective. The exposure might not be just to thoughts of harm, but to emotional vulnerability. Thus, it might be useful to develop exposure situations (initially in imagination) involving positive emotional situations with her family that would be disrupted if the avoidance of fears of harm was brought into them (e.g., playing with her family while they are eating food items that are safe but might be a few days old) and then practicing her mindfulness and attentional skills during these episodes.

Another possibility is to target the client's tracking by inviting her to experiment with different strategies to deal with anxiety and notice their impact on her well-being. An exercise such as *the passengers in the bus* (Hayes, Strosahl, et al., 2012) can be useful in this regard. The therapist asks the client to imagine driving a bus in the direction of what matters to her and to approach her psychological experiences as if they were passengers trying to take control of the bus. If she does what the passengers say, she ends up in a different direction than where she was heading to (establishing analogical relations between the client and something concrete to observe, and conditional and hierarchical relations to track the consequences of actions in terms of values). This exercise would be particularly useful to deal with the influence exerted by the rule "I must protect my family." After a clarification of what she cares about in her life (see Chapter 7), the client concretely observes the impact of her reaction to the passengers, which helps her notice that following the rule this way is not effective. She can also experiment regarding what it is like not to get rid of the passengers and focus on driving instead, and she can observe if the consequence of this new response is more desirable.

Case 2

The second case involves a 28-year-old man who comes to therapy after an overdose of heroin and several weeks in a rehabilitation center. He reports strong urges and starts to consider using heroin again. Even though he is well aware of the negative consequences of relapsing, he explains that having constant thoughts about heroin makes it impossible to resist the temptation. In addition, he explains that before the overdose, his whole life was about the heroin culture. He had found his place in a group of users who became close friends, and for the first time in his life, he was feeling good about himself until the overdose and the hospitalization. He says that he has a hard time "being himself" now and he feels forced to conform to social norms instead.

If we build a brief case conceptualization with these few elements, we can first identify that the client is at risk of engaging in a behavior that brings some positive satisfaction, but at the expense of other important areas of his life (adaptive peak). Some of the positive consequences being sought are harmful—addictive drugs—whereas in other areas the reinforcers are fine (having friends; feeling good about yourself) but the means to those ends are unworkable. At this point, he has not relapsed yet, but he is becoming increasingly sensitive to several misleading sources of influence. For example, the client mentions urges (thoughts and sensations) that work as antecedents indicating that he would feel better if he used heroin again. He seems to believe the rule that "constant thoughts about heroin make it impossible to resist using," even though he is not actively following it at this point. Although he has done hard things to quit using, he has cast them as a matter of pliance (being forced to conform) rather than as a means to accomplishing ends of importance to himself (sources of meaning). He is tempted to rebel against social conformity, but without being clear about what he actually wants in his life, this rebellion is likely to be self-destructive. The actual costs of his former drug use are foggy. He has a perception of himself that doesn't distinguish between psychological experiences and perspective taking on these experiences (see Chapter 6). Changes in experiences that resulted from quitting heroin are perceived as threats to the self, and the temptation is strong to use again in order to restore that sense. However, his sources of motivation are vague ("being himself") and are unlikely to promote effective behavior other than the same drug use that caused his problems in the first place.

On the one hand, urges and resistance against rules encouraging pliance ("counterpliance" is still a form of pliance) are beginning to have a strong impact, and it would be helpful to alter the client's sensitivity to this source of influence in order to limit the risk of using heroin again. On the other hand, motivation to change is weak, and the client is vague both about the costs of using and the benefits of quitting. Finally, alternative actions to achieve positive consequences (e.g., having friends; having an independent life) are weak.

Sensitivity to unhelpful symbolic influence can be undermined by increasing the impact of intrinsic sources of influence or other sources of symbolic influence (see Chapter 5). If we chose the first option, the therapist could use a technique that makes the formal, intrinsic characteristics of urges and rules more salient. For example, the client might be invited to write down the thought in a language that the client doesn't speak in order to help him see the distinction between the form and the function of a word or a sentence (alteration of symbolic relations). Although it seems impossible not to act upon the thought when it is written in its original form, it doesn't trigger any particular reaction when it is written in a language that the client doesn't understand. This exercise increases the awareness that a thought and the event it refers to are two different things and that the client has the option of not responding to his urges and rules since they are not *intrinsically* controlling his behavior. Other techniques that target distancing or "defusion" skills could be used in the same way, such as saying the thought very slowly, or writing each word of the thought both forward and backwards. These methods would hopefully select different functions of the thoughts and thus undermine their influence on the decision to use drug again.

The client's strong attachment to his concept of himself could be addressed with perspective-taking techniques that convey a sense of continuity beyond temporary definitions and evaluations about the self (see Chapter 6). For example, in a meditation-like exercise we mentioned earlier, the client is led to remember different moments of his life while adopting his own point of view in these different moments in the most vivid way (Hayes, Strosahl, et al., 2012). The client could thus imagine being a 5-year-old boy again, then an adolescent, and finally the person he was a month earlier. At each step, the therapist invites the client to notice his physical appearance and the way the world is arranged around him. At the end of the exercise, the therapist helps the client see that despite the multiple changes of his body and psychological experiences, there is a continuous sense of awareness that ties these together. "Being himself" is thus not based just on content—there is a sense of coherence that is outside rigid evaluations and definitions about himself (e.g., "I am a heroin user").

It would also be possible to encourage the client to establish or strengthen symbolic relations connecting his effective behaviors (abstinence in this case) to sources of meaning, by entering into a detailed description of his drug use and its costs and benefits, much as is done in Motivational Interviewing (see Chapter 7). As reinforcers such as having friends come up, the client could be asked to explore that territory experientially such as with the sweet spot exercise described in the next case, or the "finding meaning in others' actions" exercise we will describe in the section after that.

Case 3

The last case involves a 72-year-old woman who comes to therapy describing herself as depressed since she retired 6 years earlier. Although she used to devote most of her time to work, which she enjoyed very much, she has never been able to find any pleasure in other activities. She doesn't have much family and has progressively lost contact with her friends. She has been thinking a lot about suicide lately, but she doesn't want to kill herself because she doesn't want people to think that she is weak. However, since she doesn't see any good reason to live anymore, she is not sure that she will be able to "stay alive" much longer, which is the reason she decided to see a therapist.

In this situation, we can hypothesize that this client's main problem is a lack of effective actions connected to sources of meaning. The client seems to have a certain ability to engage in actions (as her decision to start therapy suggests), but she is unable to find a meaningful life direction. Possibly, she was not able to identify new actions to replace her work after she retired. It may be that the overarching goals and qualities of action she was pursuing while working were not clearly defined. As long as she could work, this may not have been a problem, but once this specific action became unavailable, she couldn't find a way to rebuild a satisfying life. It is also possible that she knew what mattered to her but was not able to broaden the range of actions serving the same sources of meaning because she had mainly focused on work for a very long time. As years passed, the variety and the frequency of her activities kept decreasing, leaving her with no reason to stay alive. Interestingly, she found motivation to seek help in the necessity to avoid a psychological experience (the shame of being seen as weak). Although going to therapy is probably the best thing she could do to avoid committing suicide and improve her well-being, this source of motivation is another indication that her behaviors are not often in contact with *positive* reinforcers.

A more detailed functional assessment may suggest different intervention paths, but based on this brief case conceptualization, it seems appropriate to work on meaning as a primary target. The client had always been very active before her retirement, and she doesn't seem to persist in particularly ineffective behaviors at the moment. Her main difficulty seems to be that she doesn't know what to do to find the kind of satisfaction she used to have in her life when she worked. In such a situation, formal exercises aiming to clarify and choose overarching goals and qualities of action can be very useful. For example, the *sweet spot* exercise we mentioned earlier (Wilson & Dufrene, 2009) consists of leading the client through a kind of meditation in which the client brings her attention to a moment of her life when she felt in harmony with what mattered to her (establishing deictic relations to connect to a past episode of her life and hierarchical relations to connect to a source of meaning). This memory could be that of a great achievement (e.g., finishing a very important work project) or a simpler, even casual moment in everyday life (e.g., going to the movies with a friend). As the client is remembering this episode of her life, the therapist encourages her to notice every feeling and sensation that comes up (i.e., attention training). After this phase, they can both explore what sources of meaning were connected to this special moment (e.g., sharing cultural interests with friends). The advantage of a formal exercise like this is in particular that it avoids excessive verbal analysis in the first phase of simple observation. If the client's life directions were not clearly identified when she used to work, talking about what was meaningful to her might be difficult and feel abstract. Giving her an opportunity to simply pause and observe her feelings and sensations can help get to the core of what used to matter, and maybe still matters in her life, in a way that is more vivid and essential.

Building Formal Experiential Techniques

Given the number of formal exercises available in treatment manuals, you could easily find several techniques perfectly adapted to the difficulties of each of your clients and never have to build a technique yourself. In addition, certain exercises are so effective that it would be a shame not to use them again and again. Yet, many therapists find that they can better deliver an exercise if they took part in its development; or they find more satisfaction in their work by creating their own techniques. After all, the giant toolbox of formal techniques that is now at our disposal exists only because thousands of clinicians decided to build their own techniques and to share them, thus contributing to the richness of our therapeutic interventions.

In this section, we will provide three examples of formal techniques we have built with the help of RFT principles. For each exercise, we will begin by clarifying our therapeutic purpose and then show step by step how using RFT guided the creation process. In a sense, we are "thinking out loud" in this section so that you can see *how* we created the exercises.

Given our own interests, these exercises are broadly related to acceptance, mindfulness, and values-based therapy, but our purposes in describing them here is more general. We think the same basic thinking processes would apply to a similar exercise put to the purposes of an existential therapist, or an analytically oriented one, or a cognitive therapist, and so on. That is, your focus as a reader should be more on *how* we arrived at what we did rather than on what we did per se.

Finding Meaning in Others' Actions

This first technique was created to help clients who have difficulty with identifying or choosing what they care about in their lives. Even evoking past events in their lives doesn't seem to lead anywhere. They may be unable to recall a moment when they felt happy, or this past episode seems now so disconnected from their current lives that it is difficult to use it as a start for a discussion on overarching goals and qualities of action. It also happens that the gap between what the client cares about and what he currently does is so important and so painful to acknowledge, that he has learned to avoid this topic altogether. In this case, targeting avoidance could be a therapeutic solution. However, it is often hard to motivate clients to drop an avoidant behavior when there is little reason to do so. In other words, without meaning, it is hard to see why one would be willing to contact difficult psychological experiences.

As we discussed in Chapter 7, there are always at least a few seeds of meaning in one's life. Coming to therapy is already an action that proves the client cares about something. However, whatever that is may not yet be formulated as an overarching and inexhaustible source of positive satisfaction. This is where working on identifying the higher function of a range of actions can be useful. A client might not be able to identify what he cares about, but he may still be able to express preferences among different objects or actions. These preferences can constitute a seed for developing meaning. In some cases, as in depression, even expressing a preference is difficult. Clients seem to have lost their ability to make choices because everything seems to feel equally plain. In such cases, it is still possible to extract preferences, then higher functions, and finally, overarching goals and qualities of action. The exercise we built targets this very process.

First, we needed to set a context encouraging the client to make choices among a variety of options in order to extract higher functions across multiple exemplars. Since we wanted this exercise to be useful in particular with clients who have difficulties talking about what matters in their lives, we decided to use materials involving other people. This way, instead of immediately talking about the client's life, the exercise could begin with a discussion about topics that put less pressure on the client. This approach led us to pick a series of 20 people, such as famous persons or characters from movies, books, or popular stories who are likely to be known by persons of the age, gender, and ethnicity of the client. We then put their names and/or their pictures on cards that we could put in front of the client in two random piles for the exercise. The instructions were as follow:

> "Here are two piles of cards in front of you. They both contain names and pictures of people you probably know. They may be characters from movies or stories, or actual famous people. What I would like you to do is to take one card from each pile and put them in front of you face up. Then, I would like you to take a moment to see if you know the person/character on these two cards and tell me which of these two characters' personality you prefer. There is no good or right answer, and sometimes you may find that it is hard to choose because perhaps you like or dislike both personalities equally as much. This is okay. In this case, I will ask you to try to make a choice, even if it doesn't seem to make a big difference."

Once the client has made the first choice between two cards, the therapist continues: "Okay, is this somebody you actually like?" If the client says yes, the therapist continues: "Can you tell me what you like about this person/character's personality?" If the client says no or doesn't express a strong opinion about the person/character on the card, the therapist continues this way instead: "Okay, could you try to tell me what made you choose this one instead of the other one? Is there something about his/her personality that you prefer in comparison to the other one?"

By doing so, the therapist encourages the client to identify qualities of action he may like. If the client makes a choice by default (e.g., "I chose this one because he is not as arrogant as the other one"), it is still possible to move on to the next step because a flaw can always be turned into a quality through opposition framing (see Chapter 7). For example, a client who rejects an arrogant person might care about humility as a quality of action.

Note that using the term "personality" helps to avoid choices based on physical appearance or on things that the person on the card possesses. Imagine, for example, a client who picks the picture of Frodo (from *The Lord of the Rings*) rather than the picture of Tony Stark (from *Iron Man*). He may then say that he likes both but prefers Frodo because he is more humble. If he had made the reverse choice, maybe he would say that he prefers Tony Stark because he is sharper and funnier. Obviously, there are infinite ways to justify one's choice, and the point is not to find a good reason but to find a characteristic linked to the person or character on the card that the client appreciates. This could be that they are nicer, more independent, more respectful of others, and so on. Once one or several personality traits have been identified, the therapist asks, "What kind of things does this person/character do that makes him/her _____ [complete with the personality trait]?" This way, the client's attention is directed toward actions rather than evaluations about the self (see Chapters 6 and 7). Then, the therapist asks, "Is this something that you care about in general?" in order to help the client establish this quality of action as an overarching reinforcer. Whether the client expresses a clear attraction to this quality of action or feels uncertain, the therapist can then ask, "Is there a moment in your life when you did something with _____ [complete with the quality of action]?" and follow up by asking him to describe feelings associated with this episode. If the client can't recall a moment when he expressed this quality of action, the therapist can ask him, "Is it something you would like to do in your life? Can you think of a moment when you had the opportunity to do something like that?"

This exercise can also be repeated by asking the client to choose the person who stands for something he prefers in terms of life purpose (e.g., Tony Stark stands for justice in the world; Frodo stands for the freedom of his people). This alternative approach can help identify overarching goals that the client may use as sources of meaning for himself by seeming to begin with questions that are external.

Black and Red Marks on Our Lifelines

This next exercise was built to help clients develop their observation, description, and tracking skills, and their capacity to make choices functionally coherent (see Chapter 5). More specifically, we wanted to help the client experiment and notice the consequences of attempting to suppress painful psychological experiences. As we saw in Chapter 2, suppressing thoughts, emotions, and sensations rarely works well in the long term due to the derivation processes of language. Not only do we end up having these painful experiences even more, but we also give up on important areas of our lives. One important phase of treatment is thus to help the client assess the effectiveness of her behavior and notice when it is not working or even counterproductive. However, noticing psychological experiences and responses to these experiences is not that easy. In fact, for many people, it is a very abstract thing to do because they are not used to thinking this way about what happens "in their heads." For this reason, it is useful to materialize these experiences by putting them in relations of equivalence with concrete things that the client can easily observe with one or several of her senses. This is what we did for the current exercise.

First, the therapist asks the client to represent her life as a timeline[1] on a sheet of paper. Then, in a meditation-like exercise, the client is invited to think of any episodes in her life that caused psychological pain and to put a red mark on the timeline for each episode. As she forms the red mark, the therapist encourages her to notice any psychological reaction such as thoughts (e.g., "I hate that it happened"), feelings (e.g., "I feel sad"), sensations (e.g., "I feel sick"), or urges (e.g., "I want to erase this red mark"). Then, the client is asked to think of all the things that she did to remove the pain and to put a black mark on the timeline for each of these attempts. Generally, there are quickly more black marks than red marks because for one painful episode, there are thousands of opportunities to think about this episode again, which often lead to attempts to escape and avoid these thoughts. In the last phase of the exercise, the therapist encourages the client to notice that the red marks have not disappeared and that black marks are all over the place on her timeline. By using these very salient cues, the client thus becomes more able to assess the effectiveness of her behavior. It is possible to go even further and encourage the client to notice what consequences the black marks have had in her life (e.g., breaking up with a boyfriend to avoid discomfort in an intimate relationship). Once formalized into a script with specific instructions, the exercise is presented this way:

> "Imagine a timeline that goes from your birth to this moment and draw this line on this sheet of paper. (*pause*) Notice that on this timeline, there are moments of happiness and also moments of pain. (*pause*) Now, with the red marker, put a mark on the timeline each time pain occurred in your life. Maybe there was disappointment, loss, rejection, fear, betrayal? Slowly, move along the line and put a red mark for each painful moment.
>
> "As you think about the pain you experienced in your life, you may notice reactions right here and right now—maybe the urge to

---

[1] This exercise shares some similarities with an exercise also built with RFT principles by Dahl, Plumb, Stewart, and Lundgren (2009).

erase or cross out these moments of pain. Think about all the things you have tried to escape or avoid this pain in your life. All the attempts to hide or forget, all the means you used to get rid of this pain and the risk of finding it again in your life.

"Now, take the black marker and put a black mark everywhere you struggled with this pain on your timeline. These black marks may be short, representing moments or days you spent struggling. Or they may cover long periods of time you spent trying to get rid of painful experiences.

"Now take a bit of distance to observe your whole timeline. Observe the link between the red marks, representing each moment of pain you had in your life, and the black marks representing all your attempts to escape or avoid your pain. (*pause*) What is the result of this battle? Have the black marks erased the red marks? Take a moment to observe the red marks and the black marks. (*pause*) How do you feel right now? What sensations, thoughts, emotions show up as you look at your timeline now?

"And as you observe the red marks, maybe still present before, during, and after the black marks, and the black marks covering days, weeks, and years of your life, ask yourself: What if your experience was right? No matter how much you try, you will never get rid of your pain. As long as you will be there, your life will be marked with red.

"But the timeline doesn't stop here. It continues to the unknown. We can't tell where this line will go and when the next red mark will occur. And you are here and now, with a black marker. What would your life look like if you quit this fight and embrace the complexity of life, sometimes marked with red, but not covered by black marks? What would fill these moments that were so far hidden by black marks?"

The Hierarchy of Self

This last exercise was built to train and distinguish the awareness of experience from taking perspective on this awareness. More specifically, we intended to help clients notice the impermanence of psychological experiences, while the "I/here/now" quality of consciousness, approached as a context for all these experiences, remains stable. As we saw in Chapter 6, conceptualized as a context, the self corresponds to the top of a hierarchical network that includes psychological experiences at its base. Although we don't need to teach technical RFT concepts to clients, it is possible to integrate some of these elements into concrete exercises. The representation of the self and the psychological experiences as a hierarchical network is a good example because it allows the client to visualize the variety of his experiences and the stability of the self at the same time. For this exercise, we thus decided to draw a kind of hierarchical network with "I" at the top, three verbs at the second level (am, do, feel), and empty columns below each verb (see Figure 9.1). The verbs were meant to encourage the client to identify different psychological experiences according to the ways he defines and evaluates his self ("am"), concrete actions he takes ("do"), and things he feels ("feel").

In order to help the client notice the variety and the impermanence of psychological experiences situated at the base of the hierarchical network, we decided to build a series of questions involving a variety of situations and leading to different definitions, evaluations, actions, or feelings. For example, one question was, "If you lost your job tomorrow, what would you be? What would you do? What would you feel?" Other questions could also refer to actual moments in the client's life, such as, "The day your son was born, what were you? What did you do? What did you feel?"

The exercise is proposed to the client using the following instructions:

"Here is a representation of you and the things you can be, the things you can do, and the things you can feel. I am going to ask you a series of questions about different moments and situations you have lived or may live in your life. In each case, I would like you to add everything you can think of that fits in each of the three columns of your experiences. For example, I could ask the question 'If it were this morning when you woke up, what would you be? What would you do? What would you feel?' You can fill the 'am' column with things that define you just in the moment, but also with things that already defined you

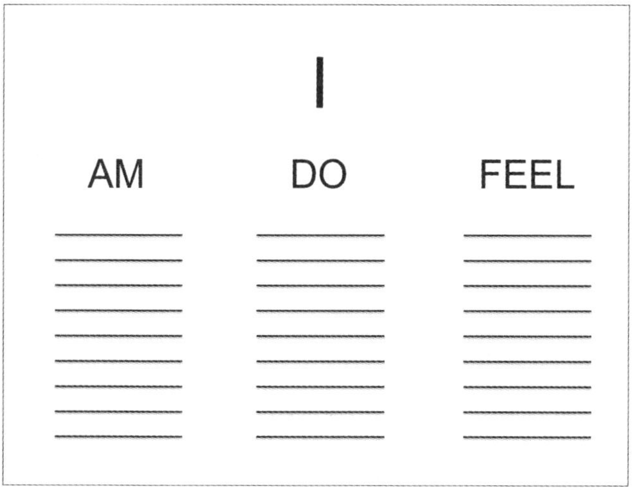

FIGURE 9.1

before and will still define you after. For example, if I answered this question, I could say, 'I am tired,' but also 'I am a therapist' or 'I am 33.' It is the same thing with the two other columns. For example, I could say, 'I get up' and 'I do therapy.' One thing happens just at this moment, and the other is more like a thing I do over a longer period of time. In the 'feel' column, I could say, 'I feel happy' or 'I feel scared,' which could be linked only to this particular moment or a more continuous feeling. Okay, let's give it a try and start with a first question if you like."

For each question, the client is encouraged to come up with at least several experiences for each column. As the client fills the columns, the therapist leads him to notice experiences that don't correspond to the new situation and to cross them out (e.g., if the client loses his job, he may want to cross out "happy"). If a subsequent situation leads to having this experience again, the client writes it in the column again. To make sure that most experiences can be crossed out at some point (in particular those the client tends to feel excessively attached to), it is important to use questions that are more likely to lead to a change of experience. For example, if the client tends to define himself as "a loser" because he can't find a job, the therapist could ask, "If you were hired for your dream job, what would you be? What would you do? What would you feel?"

Once a dozen or more questions have been asked (ideally until each experience has been crossed out at least once), the client can observe the variety of experiences reported in each column. On the one hand, certain evaluations and definitions have disappeared, and sometimes reappeared; certain actions were not possible to do anymore; and some feelings passed, came back, and passed again. On the other hand, one element has remained regardless of the situations and the experiences lived at the base of the hierarchy: the "I." Following this observation, the therapist can engage in a discussion using principles presented in Chapter 6 to develop a flexible sense of self.

How We Arrived at These Exercises

In each of these "thinking out loud" examples, we have started with an issue, dismantled it, and then created exercises that model the issue as understood from an RFT perspective. In the first exercise, we trained attention toward sources of meaning and created a context that encourages the establishment of hierarchical relations between actions and qualities of actions. We used an easy context first (displacing the target of awareness from the self to other people or characters through deictic framing) and then redirected attention to a more challenging one (the client's own qualities of actions).

In the timeline exercise, we externalized two functional classes of action: feeling pain and struggling with the feeling of pain. Those two classes combine in most people so tightly that they do not notice that struggle is a second type of action. Pain and struggle with pain seem like one thing, not two. But playing this out in a physical metaphor, we can see their independence and entanglement. Experimenting strategies inside the metaphor also helps gain awareness of the consequences of avoiding pain.

In the hierarchy of self exercises, we play out metaphorically the symbolic processes we think are key to distinguishing a continuously available sense of self as perspective taking from the continuously changing experiences of our lives. These processes are difficult to observe, and this is why, as for the previous exercise, we used a visual representation. Using a variety of relations that alternately establish and remove functions attached to the self directs the client's attention toward what is stable across these changing experiences.

Delivering Formal Experiential Techniques

Introducing an Exercise and Delivering Instructions

Introducing and delivering an experiential exercise is not as easy as it may seem. Even when the instructions are relatively simple and specific, there are still important gray areas in the way a therapist can best interact with her client. First, using an exercise often constitutes a disruption of the natural exchange, which a client can perceive as awkward or irrelevant. Then, the experiential nature of these techniques requires a delicate balance between explaining the purpose of doing an exercise and letting the client observe his experience and draw conclusions by himself. Of course, your social skills and your clinical experience alone can guide you in this process. Nonetheless, it is useful to identify a few principles ensuring that your formal techniques will be well received and understood, and will actually serve the function you are targeting.

As we mentioned in the introduction of this chapter, we can compare formal experiential practice to an athlete's workout. It is not an end in and of itself, but rather a way of training skills and bringing awareness to areas that are difficult to observe in natural settings. We believe that it is a fine way to present this aspect of therapy to clients, which aids in avoiding two opposing pitfalls: first, the risk that the exercise may be perceived as silly and irrelevant; and second, the risk that it is seen as magic or esoteric.

There is no reason to wrap techniques based on scientific principles in mystery. Even when techniques come directly from religious and spiritual traditions, they are integrated in a psychological treatment only because they are effective and because we can make sense of their effect, at least at a conceptual level. Thus, in the spirit of building a sense of experience, effectiveness, and autonomy, we generally try to present formal experiential practice with as much transparency as possible.

The difficulty, however, is to explain without explaining too much. Although a lot of exercises that aim to train a skill probably benefit from specific explanations beforehand, experiential exercises are different because their purpose is often to train the client's capacity to observe and draw conclusions by herself. For this reason, when introducing these types of exercises, it is better not to tell the client what she will experience but rather to encourage her to observe. Once a pattern of "let's try it and see" is established in therapy, even a few successes will embolden both the therapist and the client to explore even more. At their best, therapists using RFT principles are experts in observation, not in the client's experience. Conversely, the client is an expert in her own experience but is often not yet a good, or not an effective, observer. Therapy can help her improve in this domain, and formal experiential practice can be presented with this principle in mind. Here is an indicative example of how we do this:

> "As you know, in the kind of therapy I do, the point is to help you find out what works and what doesn't work for you in order to improve your well-being. In the course of our sessions together, I will sometimes propose that you do some exercises. At times, we will practice together during our sessions, and I will also give you some 'homework' if you are willing to practice between our sessions. You can see this as working out to improve a specific skill that you will then be able to use in your life. So, in many cases, exercises or experiments will be an opportunity to train your skills, in particular your capacity to notice what works and what doesn't work, and to then make choices that you think are best for you.
>
> "Finding a solution is not an easy thing to do, and once you have found it, the work is often not completely finished because even if you decided to change something that you are currently doing, it might take a while before what you learned has become a new habit. So you will probably find it useful to practice with exercises. Now, in the end, you are the only one who can tell if it is useful. Some exercises might be more useful than others. Some might make more sense than others, or you will just have a preference for some exercises and this is absolutely fine.
>
> "Another thing is that some of these exercises can be kind of surprising sometimes. This is because they mean to help you take a new perspective on things that happen and things that you do in your life. So, sometimes you will wonder what this is all about. You may even think that it is strange, or funny. This is actually part of what might be interesting to observe. And in any case, we will always have a

discussion about your experience doing these exercises so that you can tell me if this is helpful or not."

And here is an example of how we introduce a specific exercise (a meditation exercise in this case):

> "So, maybe you remember I told you that we would do some exercises together? I would like to propose that you do one now. Would that be okay?
>
> "In this exercise, the goal is quite simple in a way because all you have to do is to observe everything that comes to your mind during a few minutes. There are lots of things that can come to our minds even in a few minutes. We may think of different things, we may have feelings or sensations, notice emotions. . . . If you close your eyes, you may even picture a number of images in your head, and hear sounds, perhaps smell things. So, what I would like you to do, if you are ok to try this, is to just observe all these things. In the meantime, since it is the first time you do this exercise, I will guide you with a few instructions to help you stay on track. Are you willing to try this?"

Depending on the specific context in which this exercise is delivered, the instruction could also orient the client to certain aspects of his experience. For example, if the client acts upon physical sensations in ways that are problematic, the therapist could encourage him to notice urges to do so.

Shaping Observation, Description, and Tracking

During and after an exercise, the experiential process can be facilitated using the same principles presented in Chapter 5. Since one of the main goals of this practice is to develop the client's ability to assess the effectiveness of her behaviors and which elements of the context influence these behaviors, the therapist encourages her to notice what happens during the exercise with precision and to formulate rules that match her experience as closely as possible. As in the course of informal exchanges, the therapist avoids giving answers to the client. If it seems the client is not taking specific elements sufficiently into account, the therapist can draw the client's attention in the direction of these elements by asking more questions. Observe this approach in the following exchange:

THERAPIST: So, what was this exercise like?

The therapist evokes observation and description.

CLIENT: It was difficult, really.

THERAPIST: Yeah? What was difficult?

The therapist evokes further observation and description.

CLIENT: It was hard to keep observing what was going on in my mind because I kept being distracted.

THERAPIST: This is interesting. You noticed that you were distracted. What kind of things distracted you?

The therapist underlines the client's progress and evokes further observation and description.

CLIENT: Well, many different things. At first, I noticed that I was thinking of being here, doing the exercise with you. Then, I started thinking of my children because I need to pick them up after our session. And then, I was completely distracted. I started thinking of making dinner, helping the kids do their homework, all kinds of things. At this point, I was not really doing the exercise anymore I think

THERAPIST: What you are saying is really interesting, I think, because as you are telling me about your experience during the exercise, you are still noticing your experience. Even when you say that you were distracted, this is part of your experience. Did you see that?

The therapist shares her own observation to help the client track his behavior.

CLIENT: I think I see what you mean, but it felt like I was not really there, like I couldn't do the exercise right.

THERAPIST (*playfully*): Here is another observation! You felt like you were not really there, and you thought you couldn't do the exercise right. Do you see?

The therapist shares her own observation to help the client track his behavior.

CLIENT: I see. So I can observe everything?

THERAPIST: Exactly. In this exercise, this is all that matters. Can I ask you more about what you noticed?

CLIENT: Sure.

THERAPIST: When you started thinking that you were not able to do the exercise right, did you notice any feelings as well?

The therapist evokes observation and description of feelings.

CLIENT: Frustrated, a bit stupid I guess.

THERAPIST: Okay, so first you think you are not doing it right, and then another thought pops up "This is frustrating," "I am stupid," something like that?

The therapist reformulates the observation made by the client to help him notice this sequence.

CLIENT: Yeah, pretty much.

In this exchange, you can see that it is possible for the therapist to follow up on anything the client reports because the goal of the exercise is to observe all experiences. In fact, even if the client was completely distracted, or even if he fell asleep during the exercise, this would still be something to observe! Progressively, as the client repeats this kind of exercise and the therapist helps him notice each of his observations, his skills develop and lead to better awareness of what happens in his life.

In order to assess the effectiveness of a behavior with an experiential exercise, the therapist asks the client about what happened after a given action. For example, if the client said that after thinking that he was stupid, he tried to think of something else, the therapist could ask him if the thought went away. As we saw in Chapter 5, the point is not to demonstrate to the client that his behavior is not effective, but to help him judge this by himself. However, because he may not pay attention to important elements of the situation (e.g., short-term versus long-term consequences, variable consequences), the therapist helps him notice everything that may be relevant to draw a useful conclusion.

Sometimes the client may find satisfaction in an exercise because it seems to reinforce the impression that problematic behaviors are effective. For example, it often happens that clients use meditation exercises as relaxation techniques. Although there is nothing wrong with relaxing oneself, this could become a problem if it adds to the set of experiential avoidance strategies that have not worked so far. Because it is new, it may work for a while, but there is a good chance that these effects will wear off soon, especially if the goal pursued is the elimination of a psychological experience. In such a case, usually it is best to stay open to the client's experience and ask the client to do the same. Theory can provide guides about what is likely to work, but the client's experience is the ultimate arbiter. Taking an open stance will reinforce observation skills, so that the effectiveness of the method can be noted—a skill that can transfer to the natural environment.

Shaping Effective Change

Although increasing awareness is an important goal of formal experiential practice, it is not the only skill that can be shaped with these techniques.

The observation of what works and what doesn't work must lead to new effective behaviors if we want to bring more satisfaction in the client's life. Note that observing often constitutes in and of itself a new effective behavior, as when the client connects an action to an overarching goal or quality of action. However, many other behaviors imply not only observing but also changing a response to the sources of influence. For example, a client who usually escapes painful emotions and, as a result, disengages from meaningful activities may learn with a formal exercise to assess the effectiveness of his strategy *and* to do something different instead. The latter skill is often even more difficult to learn and maintain because it enters in conflict with powerful sources of influence, such as painful sensations, or rules that the client has been following for a long time.

To help clients gain flexibility in contact with misleading sources of influence and adopt more useful strategies during formal exercises, it is possible to use the principles of shaping presented in Chapter 5. Specifically, the therapist can help strengthen effective behaviors by reinforcing progress and connecting behaviors to natural consequences. He can also weaken problematic behaviors (through delivering and orienting to undesirable consequences, blocking, and extinction), and connect the therapy room to the client's life outside (through functional and symbolic generalization).

As in the course of informal exchanges, strengthening effective behaviors in formal practice needs to respect the client's own progression. Although it may be tempting to tell the client that his new behavior is appropriate in order to reinforce it more quickly, done crudely this would interfere with the general purpose of experiential practice, which is to teach the client to assess effectiveness and make choices on his own. This does not mean the therapist is there to simply give instructions and listen. At each step, the therapist can encourage the client to track the consequence of his action. Observe this approach in the following exchange:

THERAPIST: What did you notice, as you were staying in contact with this painful sensation?

The therapist evokes observation and description.

CLIENT: I noticed that it was hard.

THERAPIST: Can you tell me more about what was hard?

The therapist evokes further description.

CLIENT: I wanted the sensation to go away. *I* wanted to go away. So, staying in contact with it was unpleasant.

THERAPIST: I can understand that. It seems illogical to stay in contact with something painful, right?

The therapist normalizes urges to escape.

CLIENT: Yeah.

THERAPIST: Usually, what do you do when you have this sensation?

The therapist evokes tracking of the usual response.

CLIENT: I try to make it go away.

THERAPIST: And you did the opposite this time . . .

The therapist evokes tracking of the response in the exercise.

CLIENT: Yeah.

THERAPIST: What else did you notice, besides the pain?

The therapist evokes tracking of additional consequences.

CLIENT: It was a strange feeling not to do anything.

THERAPIST: You mean, as opposed to trying to make the pain go away?

CLIENT: Yeah. I hated feeling this sensation, but there was something a bit relieving about not needing to get rid of it. I still wanted to, believe me. But there was less . . . effort.

THERAPIST: Is it something you appreciate?

The therapist evokes the assessment of response effectiveness.

CLIENT: Yeah, I think so. I mean, it is different, not something I am used to doing. So, it is hard to know what I think about this right now. I guess it is an interesting approach.

THERAPIST: Would that make a difference in your life if you didn't have to make any effort to get rid of the sensation?

The therapist evokes further assessment of the response's effectiveness to expand toward broader contexts.

CLIENT: It would not be as exhausting. It would be painful though. But I would not need to do anything about it. I have been trying and trying, you know. If I didn't have to try, I guess my hands would be free.

Similarly, weakening problematic behaviors during formal practice follows the principles of delivering undesirable consequences, blocking, and extinguishing, as seen in Chapter 5. For example, if a client is tempted to disengage from a meditation exercise because the psychological experiences she is contacting are painful, the therapist can gently encourage her to stick with the task. To avoid putting the client in a situation where she might feel trapped, the therapist acknowledges the difficulty of the exercise, for example, using perspective taking (see Chapter 10) and always makes sure that the client feels free to quit. Observe this approach in the following exchange.

CLIENT: The meditation exercises I did at home made me even more aware of my obsessions, so I stopped doing them.

The client escapes difficult psychological experiences, in a similar way to rituals helping her to get rid of obsessive thoughts temporarily.

THERAPIST: I know you don't like noticing these obsessive thoughts, so I can understand it must not have been a pleasant experience.

The therapist normalizes the client's difficult experience.

CLIENT: Yeah, not at all.

THERAPIST: You know, these exercises are not meant to make you suffer. I hope you know that.

CLIENT: Yeah, I know. It is just that it is really difficult for me.

THERAPIST: Yeah, I understand. I would like to make sure you understand the point of these exercises. What do you think is the purpose?

CLIENT: It's like practicing skills?

THERAPIST: Yeah, exactly. Training our ability to observe our experience, so we can better see what works and what doesn't work.

In these last exchanges, the therapist clarifies the function of the exercise to help the client track with more precision.

CLIENT: I understand. I feel like observing doesn't work for me though.

THERAPIST: (*smiling with kindness*) Which is an observation too! Would you agree with that?

The therapist shares an observation to help the client track her behavior.

CLIENT: Ah! Yeah, I guess so.

THERAPIST: There is nothing wrong with not liking these exercises. In fact, I agree with you. If what you observe is unpleasant, it is understandable that you would not want to continue.

The therapist normalizes difficult experiences linked to the exercise.

I do want you to feel free to do these exercises or not.

The therapist makes sure the client feels free to quit.

However, I also know that practicing a new skill is often difficult and takes time. A little bit like people who decide to go to the gym, you know. At first, they will probably find it painful. If they persist though, they will start to see some results.

The therapist again clarifies the function of the exercise.

CLIENT: I see what you mean. It is like a phase?

THERAPIST: Maybe, yeah. You know, it is possible that painful thoughts will always be unpleasant to observe. But if you can notice what responses to these thoughts work best, you may find meditation useful in the end.

The therapist underlines the distinction between the function of the exercise (observing, describing, and tracking) and the psychological experiences that may be involved in the exercise (e.g., obsessive thoughts).

CLIENT: Right now, I feel like meditation is not working.

THERAPIST: I hear that. I think you have two possible options then. If you think you have enough information to know that it is not helpful, then maybe you can choose not to use it. The other option is to continue at least for a while and observe a bit more. I am open to both options because in the end, what I want is to help you find out what works best for you. I will always push you a little, gently, just to make sure that you are considering all your options carefully. But I will support your choice.

At the end of this exchange, the client still feels like meditation was not helping, and the therapist respects this observation because it is an opportunity to reinforce her tracking skills. Even though there is a risk that quitting meditation is part of the avoidance strategies, the therapist prefers giving the client the opportunity to draw conclusions by herself. Other formal exercises and informal exchanges will be used to decrease avoidance through different means, and meditation may actually be suggested again if the client is open to giving it another chance.

The last main principle of shaping effective change is to connect what is happening in the therapy room with what the client lives outside, using functional and symbolic generalization. This is a key aspect of formal practice because improvements that occur during the exercises need to spread to situations where new effective behaviors can make a difference. For the therapist, the difficulty is to help the client notice the similarity between the exercise and his own situation, while letting him draw conclusions by himself, based on his own observations. This is a process that was discussed in the previous chapter on the use of metaphors, since drawing parallels between two situations is at the core of this technique. The main principle is to go back and forth between the two situations without explicitly formulating contextual cues that may turn the similarity between both situations into a simplistic and potentially rigid rule. By helping the client observe both behavioral sequences in detail and mixing the vocabulary from the two situations, functional and symbolic generalization is made more likely as the client progressively extracts rules that can be followed in life outside therapy. We will demonstrate this approach in the vignette that closes the chapter.

CLINICAL EXAMPLE

The following vignette involves a 21-year-old woman with a history of trauma and currently presenting with generalized anxiety. The exchange begins immediately at the end of the "black marks on your life" exercise (presented earlier in this chapter) and focuses mostly on the functional and symbolic generalization of what happened during the exercise to the client's life.

THERAPIST: How are you doing?

The therapist evokes observation and description.

CLIENT: I feel kind of crushed.

THERAPIST: Are you upset by what happened during this exercise?

The therapist evokes tracking.

CLIENT: Yeah.

THERAPIST: What is difficult right now?

The therapist evokes observation and description.

CLIENT: Feeling like I have been spending so much effort trying to make my life work and it was all a waste of time in the end.

THERAPIST: As you were looking at the black marks, you felt like you had wasted time in your life?

The therapist mixes elements from the exercise and the client's life to establish coordination between the two situations and facilitate tracking.

CLIENT: Yeah.

THERAPIST: (*gently*) Can you tell me more about these black marks?

The therapist evokes further observation and description, still using the vocabulary from the exercise.

CLIENT: I am constantly thinking about terrible things that could happen. I feel like I am constantly running, hyperactive, trying to make sure that nothing bad happens again.

THERAPIST: It feels like you are filling your life with the black marker?

The therapist reformulates the client's description with vocabulary from the exercise.

CLIENT: Yeah . . .

THERAPIST: What about the red marks? Are they still there?

The therapist evokes observation and description using the exercise's vocabulary.

CLIENT: Always there. That's the big problem. I keep covering my life with black marks, and all I can see is the red marks.

THERAPIST: And this is what makes you feel crushed, right? Feeling like you keep trying and . . .

CLIENT: And I waste my time in the end.

THERAPIST: How frustrating! I am with you, you know. Red marks are painful. Why wouldn't you want to make them go away?

The therapist normalizes painful experience and urge to escape.

CLIENT: This is what I have always wanted.

THERAPIST: (*gently*) So, what do you think you can do? What does this exercise tell you?

The therapist evokes the assessment of response's effectiveness and extraction of new functional rules.

CLIENT: That I need to stop running, I guess. It seems like a relief in a way, but what am I going to do? I can't just let bad things happen again.

THERAPIST: You know that what we are trying to do here is to look at what can help you. And what can help is what works, right? So far, you have been using your black marker because this is what makes more sense, and I am pretty sure I would have done the same thing as you did. We all first try to do what makes sense to us.

The therapist normalizes urges to escape through perspective taking (deictic framing).

But maybe another thing we need to take into account is if the black marks allow you to remove and prevent the red marks from happening in your life. What do you think?

Here, since the client is a little stuck, the therapist adopts a style slightly more didactic but only to clarify the purpose of their work together (in particular, looking for and adopting strategies that work).

CLIENT: I agree that I need to do something that works better. But I don't know what to do.

THERAPIST: You talked about the waste of time that the black marks have caused in your life. What could you do if you were not putting black marks on your timeline? If you dropped the black marker, what would you fill your life with?

The therapist uses distinction framing to evoke tracking of alternative response and consequence.

CLIENT: I don't know. I have been doing this for all my life.

THERAPIST: What if we explored that together? What if filling your life with something other than black marks, with something that would bring satisfaction in your life, was our objective here?

The client's avoidant behaviors have taken her away from sources of meaningful satisfaction, to the point where she has difficulties identifying what she cares about besides not suffering. Thus, the therapist sets the context for working on overarching goals and qualities of action in future sessions.

CLIENT: Yes, I think I would like that.

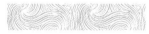 **CHAPTER SUMMARY**

In this chapter, you learned to choose, build, and deliver formal techniques allowing your clients to improve their experiential skills. Here are the main principles to remember:

- Formal experiential techniques are used in therapy to increase awareness, establish new actions, and change existing actions. Although there are a great variety of techniques (attentional training, mindfulness training, skills training, formal exposure exercises, and so on), the processes they activate can be categorized into four main areas:
  - Attention training.
  - Experimenting.

- ○ Expanding flexibility and contextual control.
- ○ Establishing or altering symbolic relations.
- Choosing formal experiential techniques requires:
  - ○ Building a case conceptualization.
  - ○ Choosing a technique that can alter the context of psychological experiences and transform their functions in ways that fit the client's needs.
- Building formal experiential techniques requires:
  - ○ Identifying the function you want to target and the ways the context can be altered to create behavior change.
  - ○ Building your own tools based on the processes activated by formal techniques (attention training, experimenting, expanding flexibility and contextual control, establishing or altering symbolic relations).
- Delivering formal experiential techniques requires:
  - ○ Providing instructions with a balance between explaining the general purpose of experiential practice and letting the client observe his experience on his own and draw conclusions by himself.
  - ○ Shaping effective change by:
    - ▪ Reinforcing progress and connecting effective behaviors to natural consequences.
    - ▪ Weakening problematic behaviors.
    - ▪ Connecting the experiences lived in therapy to the client's life through functional and symbolic generalization.

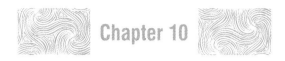

Chapter 10

Empowering
the Therapeutic Relationship

In this chapter, we will explore how to apply RFT principles to the therapeutic relationship. Each interaction that the therapist uses with her client
to help him change his behavior constitutes an element of the relationship.
Thus, all the techniques we covered in the previous chapters pertain to
the therapeutic relationship. However, there are certain key principles that
deserve specific attention if we want to set a powerful context to deliver
clinical interventions. We believe RFT can provide some useful guidance
to do that. First, we will explore how the principles applied to our clients
can be useful to therapists themselves. Then, we will see how to establish
a stance that fits your own style while remaining linked to useful RFT
principles.

APPLYING RFT PRINCIPLES TO THE THERAPIST

There is no fundamental barrier between the therapist and his clients in
terms of psychological functioning. People suffering from psychological
difficulties may not be functioning effectively in their lives, but in most
cases the processes that led to this impairment are also involved in the lives
of those not in psychological treatment. Everybody, including therapists,
can be victims of the downsides of symbolic and nonsymbolic learning
processes: problematic behaviors can be maintained despite obvious detrimental consequences, and effective behaviors can be blocked, despite their
benefit in the long term. The techniques that worked to help clients be

more in touch with their experiences and engage in more effective behaviors apply to therapists as well.

Awareness, Sense Making, and Flexibility

Exactly like their clients, therapists can get stuck in the attempt to maintain coherence in language in ways that are not useful. A typical trap is to look for the Truth with a capital T (essential coherence—see Chapter 3), while neglecting to assess for effectiveness and to maintain relational flexibility. This trap leads us all to adopt behaviors that seem right because they are in line with "True" thoughts, but nevertheless are not effective in bringing lasting satisfaction. For therapists, getting stuck in nonfunctional coherence can appear in the form of excessive attachment to their clinical model, to the hypotheses they formulate about their clients, or to the traditions in which they were trained. Thinking from the perspective of a specific model is useful, of course, because it helps us organize the information we gather in therapy sessions, and provides guidance for the next therapeutic moves. That is part of why clinical science matters. However, doing what is coherent *within* a model and doing what works can sometimes be at odds: we may faithfully deliver a treatment and yet observe client deterioration, not improvements. If therapists are more concerned about being true to their model than about doing what is effective, they end up in another version of the same trap that language sets for their clients. This is another reason why clinical science matters—it can provide principles that guide therapists in knowing when and how to adapt treatment when it is effective to do so. A pragmatic and broadly flexible stance seems to be demanded of clinicians in precisely the same way that life itself demands it of our clients.

In Chapter 5 we described how we might improve the contextual sensitivity of clients. These same methods apply to clinical work itself. Tracking with precision the behavioral sequences happening in the room and their consequences short and longer term can help differentiate between clinical moves that help clients make progress and those that don't, even if they felt like it was the "right thing to do" in the moment. Being able to do that requires paying attention to sequences in therapy (and using the scientific literature to help in that cause), but it also requires that we hold models lightly enough that their costs and benefits can be appreciated over time.

Narrow language processes can also get in the way of effective clinical work when difficult emotions, thoughts, or sensations are triggered by the experiences that clients have or report in session. For example, hearing a client talk about a traumatic event can be extremely stressful for a therapist, even following him after the session and into his personal life. The derivational power of language can lead the therapist to suffer a kind of second-order trauma if that pain is mishandled. Trying to escape a painful story or image newly added to the therapist's relational network is as doomed to failure in the long run as is that same move made by clients.

Mishandling difficult experiences is particularly likely if the emotions, thoughts, or sensations have resonance with the clinician's history—as concerns over "countertransference" have long underlined. It is thus useful to approach difficult psychological experiences of the therapist in much the same way one might approach the experience of clients: as normal reactions to events in our lives. A clinician trying hard not to feel distressed by what her clients tell her may end up avoiding certain topics or disconnecting herself from the conversation, even unconsciously, to limit access to the emotions. And if bringing up these topics would be useful for the client's progress, prioritizing avoidance of the therapist's psychological experiences can become a serious problem for the therapeutic work.

Functional coherence can be regained by connecting with the importance of instigating, modeling, and supporting greater openness in clients. When a clinician experiences difficult reactions in therapy, it need not be so much a problem as an opportunity to do just that. Consider the following exchange, in which the therapist does this very directly:

THERAPIST: It is extremely hard to hear that. Part of me just wants to run and hide as I hear it—it is that painful.

CLIENT: That is the world I live in all the time. In fact, I think that's what I've been doing: running and hiding.

THERAPIST: Then let's not either of us do that in here. Even if we don't quite know what to do. And I don't want you to rescue me. Instead, let's walk into this together, even if it is hard territory for us both.

Of course, identifying and engaging in effective action can be difficult when psychological experiences are particularly strong. Issues such as attraction, anger, and fear can be hard to manage. This is particularly true when judgments are involved, either those of the client or of the therapist. It can be helpful for therapists to apply the techniques described in Chapter 5, such as changing or diminishing the function of the symbolic sources of influence to gain response flexibility. For example, suppose a practitioner has the thought, "I'm failing as a therapist—I don't know what to say." The therapist can notice the intrinsic characteristics of these symbolic constructions, undermine some of its symbolic functions (i.e., backing out of the idea that you have to know what to say to be effective), or alter the likelihood of them producing disruptive functions, and quickly return to the work at hand. For example, the clinician might mentally restate "I'm failing—I don't know what to say" in his voice as a school-aged child and then redirect his attention toward the client. This technique alters the impact of a thought by the use of functional cues—we would naturally listen with compassion to a child who yearns to be effective and fears he is not, and this thought probably occurred many times before this moment in this session with this client. Sometimes it can work to use that very content as a reflection of the processes the client is experiencing too:

> THERAPIST: My mind tells me I'd better quickly come up with answers or I'll fail you as a therapist. But this is a hard area. It may not be a matter of a simple "answer." Is the urge to find a quick answer there for you as well?
>
> CLIENT: My mind practically screams it at me. "If you don't find an answer soon, your life will be a failure."
>
> THERAPIST: Wow. In me that urge to "figure it out or else" is pretty old. I can find voices like that inside me even as a young child. How old is that thought in your case?
>
> CLIENT: I can't remember a time when I didn't feel different; odd; confused. It's old. Very, very old.

Flexible Sense of Self

Like their clients, therapists can rigidly identify with a limited number of psychological experiences and form a conceptualization of themselves that narrows the range of their actions in therapy. Typical problems caused by a strong attachment to this kind of "self" include the tendency to only make therapeutic moves that fit one's identity as a _____ therapist. That blank can be filled with therapeutic approaches such as behavioral, psychodynamic, humanistic, and cognitive. It can be filled with traits such as calm, knowledgeable, kind, even-tempered. It can be filled with positive or negative judgments such as wonderful, world class, lousy, incompetent.

The presence of terms to fill in blanks of that kind is not uncommon and not abnormal. If any of these terms are embraced in a rigid way, however, they can lead to ineffective therapeutic moves (e.g., referring a client to another therapist despite having the competency to treat him, terminating too early, not terminating when appropriate, and so on). Even seemingly objective definitions such as "I am a man," "I am white," or "I have a history of trauma" can get in the way of therapeutic interactions with a client if they seem to be incompatible with providing care in this situation. For example, a therapist may think that being a white man prevents him from relating to what a black female client is going through, when, in fact, careful attention and listening may open up a new space that is healing.

Conversely, a therapist may think that having had a history of trauma and still being bothered by it prevents her from helping clients who have similar difficulties, when the issue may be more how that history is handled. We are not arguing that these self-descriptions are to be ignored or that they should not enter into decisions about how to help clients, whether a referral would be useful, and so on. Our point is that we need to be open to what works best when dealing with our own issues and to keep the focus on what is good for clients, not just what is comfortable and habitual within our own symbolic networks.

Another form this takes is an unbalanced sense of agency that can lead the therapist to feel excessively responsible or hopeless in her work. On the one hand, the therapist might think that everything that happens to her clients is under her control, and therefore beat herself up when progress is not being made or when the situation deteriorates. On the other hand, she might feel like nothing she is doing will ever improve the client's condition. As we addressed in Chapter 6, neither of these two extreme positions captures the interactive nature of the relationship between people and their environment. For therapists, it is necessary to find balance in their sense of agency since they can indeed alter a number of variables to help clients change, and, at the same time, they don't have access to the whole range of relevant variables.

As with clients, a useful alternative approach is to consider flexible dimensions that, together, promote stability, variability, and balanced responsibility. Practicing awareness skills fosters the recognition that psychological experiences are varied and often transient. Noticing the perspective-taking activity inherent in consciousness itself helps create stability in an aspect of self that remains stable across times and situations. Expanding the hierarchical network in which self is a container of all psychological experiences allows a functional coherence to emerge even with experiences that are seemingly contradictory. Finally, noticing the impact that contextual variables have on one's behaviors and, in turn, the impact that behaviors can have on contextual variables allows clinicians to foster a balanced sense of responsibility that prevents the excesses of hopelessness or therapeutic narcissism.

Meaning and Motivation

Like their clients, therapists can suffer from a lack of awareness of what matters to them in their clinical work. Even when they have a clear idea of the general directions they want to take, they might still have difficulties identifying actions consistent with these directions. And when specific actions are identified, difficulty with motivation to actually engage in these actions may remain. RFT principles can help foster meaning and sustainable motivation in therapeutic work, much as they did in Chapter 7 with clients.

What are your overarching goals as a therapist? What qualities of action do you want to infuse in the pursuit of these goals? It is safe to assume that most therapists want to help people improve their lives, and to do so ethically, but this may not constitute the most powerful source of motivation and satisfaction for all therapists at all times. A therapist may, for example, scrupulously comply with ethical rules, not because he experiences ethical rule compliance as meaningful per se, but because it serves a higher function for him (e.g., another quality of action such as "with professionalism"). This distinction is important because an action will be meaningful only if it is connected to its higher functions. Thus, if the therapist must take a painful decision in order to follow the ethical rules, he can still find satisfaction in his action if he relates it to professionalism. Conversely, acting ethically may be taken as a given and not as a source of satisfaction if it is not clearly connected in his mind to the quality of action he cares about.

In the same way that it is important for the client's motivation to be positive (moving toward), and not only negative (moving away), it is important that this is true for the therapist. In the rush of moment-to-moment clinical work, this kind of motivation can be lost. Knowing this fact can encourage therapists to think carefully before each session about the positive qualities of their own actions that they want to make manifest in their work.

To increase the chances that clinical work remains a meaningful experience, it is thus useful to have a personal vision of *what* you want to contribute to and of *how* you want to do it. You can then identify a variety of actions hierarchically connected to your overarching goals and qualities of action. This can prove especially useful when the therapist is feeling ambivalent about the best move to make in therapy. For example, a therapist may include in the range of actions she can take to improve her client's life the action of reporting to the police an imminent attempt to commit suicide, even if she thinks that it will harm their relationship.

This kind of situation, as well as all the difficult moves we have to make in the therapy room (e.g., exposure to painful emotions), requires the therapist to connect his action to overarching goals and qualities of action as he anticipates, executes, and remembers this action. Techniques presented in Chapter 7 to foster motivation with clients apply here in a similar manner, using augmenting processes that give actions their reinforcing qualities, independent of the current context.

Formal Experiential Practice

Therapy work in the end is a set of actions and skills, linked to a purpose. Mindfulness practice, exposure work, skills practice, and so on can all contribute to therapeutic ability. As we noted in the last chapter, these can be done in ways that promote attentional flexibility, create a spirit of experimentation that fosters practice and undermines unnecessary or discordant rules, expand repertoire flexibility and relevant contextual control, and extend across clients and setting via symbolic generalization. All of these are ways of strengthening skills that require regular practice to stay effective.

There is no clear dividing line between the therapy setting and clinicians' lives. It is not by accident that most clinical approaches based on mindfulness (e.g., dialectical behavior therapy, mindfulness-based cognitive therapy, acceptance and commitment therapy) strongly encourage therapists to regularly practice meditation exercises. The exercises made available to clients should be explored by therapists, too, when they target general processes. Exposure to fears of contamination for a client suffering from obsessive–compulsive disorder while fostering psychological openness and behavioral flexibility is not fundamentally different from guiding a session into territory where a therapist feels confused or incompetent while fostering psychological openness and behavioral flexibility. Thus, virtually everything in this volume applies to both clients and therapists, each in their own way.

It is not possible to determine a priori the amount and the type of formal practice that therapists need to remain effective in their work. As in working out, some people can gain muscles easily but are not very flexible, whereas it is the opposite for others. A different practice might be needed depending on what one wants to improve. The advice offered in this volume, however, has been less focused on the details of "what" and more on the details of "how" and "why." We see no dividing line between the work we do for clients and the work we do on ourselves.

BUILDING A FLEXIBLE THERAPEUTIC RELATIONSHIP

After looking at how therapists can apply RFT principles to themselves, we now turn to the techniques that allow them to establish a stance most compatible with the use of these principles in clinical interventions. The relationship is not defined solely by the targets of clinical change or by the stance of the therapist—it includes clinical transactions and interactions themselves.

Finding Trust in Effectiveness, Normalization, and Commonality

The therapeutic relationship is a kind of haven of trust and intimacy. Clients need to trust their therapists to be able to share what is going on in their lives, to share what they feel and care about, and to work together on a new approach to deal with their difficulties. RFT principles can be used in therapy to foster trust and intimacy in the therapeutic relationship. Trust means that the therapist is reliable and respects the rules of the therapeutic framework. Intimacy means that there is an ability to share values and vulnerabilities with a sense of understanding and empathy. Defined this way, trust and intimacy are a common basis of all effective psychotherapies.

In some approaches, the therapist must also appear credible as a source of information in the eyes of the client. This is true of the approach presented in this book, but to a notably lesser extent.

From an RFT perspective, too much emphasis on credibility can lead to excessive rule giving and rigid rule following, which can result in insensitivity to useful sources of influence that go beyond simple rules. This is an even greater risk if the therapist gives topographic rather than functional advice to the client.

It can be helpful to share scientific information with clients, but we need to be wary of the degree to which advice of this kind could lead to pliance instead of tracking. Even if the client contacts advantageous consequences with a new strategy that is described or directly recommended by the therapists, there is a risk he will keep doing it because he trusts his therapist, not because it works. And even if *that* is not true, he may be somewhat less likely to learn by observing his own experience and assessing the effectiveness of his actions. Thus, even accurate rules can at times have less long-term utility than trying to shape an ability to generate rules linked to one's own experience over the long term.

Rules directly given by therapists may be helpful when science has shown effects in the *very* long term that outstrip the ability of experience to be a reasonable guide (e.g., eating breakfast appears to have health benefits that may take decades to contact), when strategies have short- or medium-term effects different from long-term ones, or when a strategy works well but in the long run another would work even better. In more typical situations, however, in which consequences are detectable over a reasonable time span, shaping awareness and sense making in a more experiential fashion (see Chapter 5) should be enough for the person to generate accurate rules on their own. These details will have to be worked out by research, but as a default mode it is safer for therapists to present themselves more as experts in training observation skills than as experts in knowing what to do.

In the experiential approach presented in this book, when a client seems to engage in behaviors because she thinks that this is what she is "supposed to do," the therapist can reorient her to the natural consequences outside the rule. Each time the client wonders about the decisions she *should* make ("Do you think I should do *x*? Am I supposed to do *x*?"), the therapist can encourage her to assess the effectiveness of her options and to make her own choices. And each time the client seems to make progress, the therapist helps her notice it and avoids arbitrary praise in favor of orienting toward natural consequences that might sustain progress. These principles were included in many vignettes that you read in the previous chapters (see in particular the section on tracking, and reinforcing tracking over pliance in Chapter 5). Let's observe them again in the following exchange:

THERAPIST: So, did you go to your date as you had planned to?

CLIENT: Yes! I was nervous, you know, and it was hard. But I went because I didn't want to come today and tell you I failed.

THERAPIST: I can imagine that it was hard. I remember you said you were quite scared last week. And still, you went to your date. How did that make you feel to go there despite feeling nervous?

The client shows signs of pliance but the therapist chooses to ignore this part of her response to reorient her instead to the natural consequences of her action.

CLIENT: I was proud of myself.

THERAPIST: Yeah? You seem happy as you say that.

The therapist doesn't praise, but orients the client's attention to natural consequences.

CLIENT: Yes, I am happy because I was able to do something that seemed completely unfeasible to me not that long ago.

THERAPIST: It must feel really good, does it?

Here again, the therapist doesn't praise but evokes observation of natural consequences.

CLIENT: Yes!

THERAPIST: And beyond accomplishing something difficult, did going on your date bring other kinds of satisfaction?

The therapist encourages the client to explore the natural consequences further.

CLIENT: It was a really nice evening, yes.

THERAPIST: So, would you say that not listening so much to your anxiety was a good thing for you in the end?

The therapist encourages the client to assess the effectiveness of her action.

CLIENT: Yes. Absolutely.

The client's experiential skills can also be improved by the therapeutic relationship when the therapist models these skills in the course of a natural exchange. Disclosing your own personal experiences and engaging in effective actions that your client can witness provide an opportunity for him to learn from you in an experiential way—a way that is likely to be more flexible than learning based on simple linear rules, as might happen if you tell the client what to do. Expressing your own experiences, as well as the pain and the difficulties that they may bring also allows the client's painful emotions, sensations, and thoughts to be normalized. If the therapist can feel anxious, sad, or have difficult thoughts, then perhaps the client doesn't have to fight these experiences to live a satisfying life. Observe these techniques in the following exchange:

THERAPIST: Would you like to tell me more about what happened to you?

CLIENT: I would rather not talk about this. It was a horrible episode of my life and every time I think about it, I am very upset.

THERAPIST: Yeah, talking about painful experiences of our lives is often very upsetting. You know, asking you about it makes me feel upset too, actually. Even if it didn't happen to me, knowing that it happened to you makes me feel sad.

The therapist normalizes the client's feelings by disclosing her own psychological experiences.

CLIENT: Yeah. I can see in people's eyes that they are very upset when I talk about that part of my life. They try to reassure me, but I can tell that they prefer not hearing about it. I don't blame them. I would rather not either.

THERAPIST: We all have urges to avoid painful feelings. We both feel like we would rather not talk about this part of your life. Right before I asked you this question, I could already feel some tension in my stomach. And I started to think "Hmm, maybe I should not ask her about it. This is going to be painful." I have seen many clients who have been through very hard events in their lives. Every time it feels hard, and I have the same thoughts that maybe I shouldn't ask about it. And I still ask because I have seen my clients improve in the past when I do so.

The therapist discloses urges to avoid painful feelings. She then emphasizes the effectiveness of not responding to these urges and models response flexibility in contact with urges to avoid.

CLIENT: Maybe I'm just broken. Damaged goods. This is so hard for me.

THERAPIST: Ah, so it isn't just that it is emotionally hard. These memories pull you to categorize yourself and to judge yourself very harshly. And when that happens, what do you feel pulled to do?

The therapist notes and normalizes the spread from emotion to judgment, and asks the client to examine the consequences of that spread.

CLIENT: I feel like giving up.

THERAPIST: Me too. When I notice that, it is sometimes hard to sit with my clients. When they are in pain, my mind starts telling me that means I'm a lousy therapist. So we are kind of together here in a way. Maybe that can actually help us.

The therapist shares a parallel process and models how to use these experiences to foster greater effectiveness.

Another ingredient that promotes trust and intimacy in the therapeutic relationship is ensuring the client feels understood and seen. The therapist cannot consider himself an expert of the client's experience a priori; rather, what is important is to attend to what the client communicates about this experience and to reflect back what the therapist has understood in a way that shows good perspective-taking and empathy skills. This aspect of the therapeutic work is common to most clinical approaches, but it has been extensively formulated in dialectical behavioral therapy (Linehan, 1993; Koerner, 2011) as part of the set of *validation* skills, in nonviolent communication (Rosenberg, 2003), and in humanistic therapies. For the purpose of this current section, the main principle we will emphasize is to be attentive to the client's psychological experiences (expressed either explicitly through statement or implicitly, for example, through facial expressions, tone of voice, or posture) and to let the client know that these experiences are being noticed as matters of importance.

Clients and therapists form a social system. When therapists notice experiences, it helps the client to notice these experiences too. When the therapist treats these experiences with openness and curiosity, the client is more likely to frame them as natural reactions to current and past events that are worth attention. This therapeutic posture helps reduce the client's ineffective attempts to control and suppress these experiences, and helps him focus on more useful actions. Observe these techniques in the following exchange:

CLIENT: I don't know if I will be able to do that (*Does not look at the therapist, and rubs her hands against each other.*)

THERAPIST: You seem worried. Are you?

The therapist communicates to the client that he notices her emotion, but he also asks for confirmation to limit the risk of imposing his interpretation.

CLIENT: Yeah. I guess. It freaks me out a little bit. It's a big step.

THERAPIST: I can understand. It *is* a big step. Doing something for the first time is often scary.

The therapist normalizes the client's feeling by underlining the contextual variables responsible for this experience and by stating that what she is going through is common to other people.

Building a Flexible Sense of Other

As we saw in Chapter 6, identifying oneself with psychological experiences (e.g., I worry → I am a worrier) is responsible for a number of problems because self-concepts become entrapped in narrow definitions. A similar conceptualization process can happen in social interactions if one identifies others with their experiences (or an interpretation of these experiences). Just as we tend to define ourselves with a limited number of concepts that don't reflect the variety of our experiences, we often put labels on other people that capture only a small part of what they are, do, and feel. Although categorizing people according to certain characteristics or patterns of behaviors can have some utility, it also increases the risk of stigmatization. For example, if you meet a person for the first time and notice that she doesn't speak much, you may think that she is distant. In the future, you may think of her as a distant person and act around her according to this label (e.g., by being distant too), while she may have simply been tired the first time you met her. If you report your first impression to people who don't know her yet, they may also act around her according to this label, while they have actually never seen her as being distant. All the categories created by our language and transmitted in our cultures similarly contribute to narrowing our perception of other people and can even lead to prejudice if the labels we use demean others.

Because of its social nature, the therapeutic relationship is not spared by this process. Not only are therapists influenced by cultural categories like anybody else, but they are also often encouraged to sort their clients into categories of disorders or personalities, which increases the risk of seeing them through the lens of narrow labels. This could lead to a client "having" the attributes of a personality disorder label, before these were even observed in session. The cognitive efficiency of labels can easily overwhelm the context sensitivity of a therapist's observations, which reduces her ability to notice useful information that contradicts hypotheses and expectations. The stigmatization of people suffering from psychological difficulties is so pervasive in our cultures that even therapists' ability to foster a caring relationship can be impaired. This is one reason stigmatization of clients links to therapist burnout (e.g., Hayes et al., 2004).

Fortunately, RFT principles that help clients build a flexible sense of self can be used to foster a flexible "sense of other." First, noticing the client's flow of experiences helps to see him as an individual and fosters feeling and expressing empathy, as we saw earlier. Noticing the client's experiences can be achieved the same way we notice our own experiences, that is, by observing with precision, moment by moment or across different contexts. Because we don't have access to others' private experiences, it is also useful to adopt their points of view or to ask them how they feel and what they think. Observe this technique in the following exchange:

CLIENT: (*not expressing any emotion*) Things didn't go as I was expecting this week. I was supposed to go out on Friday night with my husband, but we had to cancel. And then, we had friends over for dinner on Saturday, but it was not as much fun as I thought it would be.

THERAPIST: This must be quite disappointing.

CLIENT: Yeah.

THERAPIST: If it happened to me, I would be sad. How about you?

The therapist adopts the point of view of the client and asks about her own observation.

CLIENT: (*frowning*) Hmm no, not sad.

THERAPIST: What just happened? I noticed that you frowned. Was there something I said that upset you?

The client denies feeling sad and seems to express another emotion immediately after the therapist's question. The therapist thus asks her again how she was feeling in that moment.

CLIENT: Yeah . . . I don't want to be sad. I don't like letting things hit on me. I just need to move on.

In this vignette, it is interesting to notice that the therapist's assumption was not directly confirmed by the client. It is possible that denying feeling sad is a way of avoiding this emotional experience. However, we don't all react the same way to similar events, and perhaps the client was not feeling sad in this moment. Thus, asking for confirmation and remaining open to the client's own observation even when they are surprising is important.

A second principle that can contribute to developing a flexible sense of other consists of noticing the client's perspective taking on her own psychological experiences. Although it is impossible to directly access this private activity, experiential exercises can help improve the sense of perspective taking in another. For example, in session it can be helpful not just to notice the client, but also to actively notice the client noticing you; or at a deeper level noticing that the client is noticing you noticing her (and so on). Perspective taking is mutual and reflective—that is part of how and why it was established in the first place. Being conscious of the consciousness of a client establishes a sense of interconnection that is uplifting. People want to be seen, and they want to be seen from the inside out. We cannot know all of the history of a client, but we see their awareness and its interconnection with our awareness. That is a powerful ground for addressing the content of therapy work.

This interconnected sense of perspective taking can then be integrated into a conceptualization of the other as a conscious context for difficult material, using hierarchical framing exactly as we did with the contextual sense of self in Chapter 6. From this view, both the therapist and the client are conceived as containers of their own psychological experiences, rather than put in equivalence with them. This approach helps open oneself to the variety of behaviors and feelings that the other experiences and, at the same time, fosters a sense of other as stable and continuous. At the level of the relationship, an interaction happening from a self and other as "conscious containers" increases the sense of commonality between the therapist and the client beyond specific definitions, behaviors, and feelings. The therapist can contribute to fostering such context in the therapy room by referring to the relationship with metaphorical phrases based on hierarchical framing. Observe this technique in the following exchange:

CLIENT: I don't know if you can understand. I think it is something you have to go through yourself to really know what it is like.

THERAPIST: I think you are right. I can never know what it is like for you to have these experiences. I can imagine what this would be like for me, but I can't be in your shoes. Even if had been through the same difficulties, I would still have my own experiences, which may not be exactly the same as yours.

The therapist talks about psychological experiences as things they have in order to undermine the identification with these experiences (hierarchical framing to build a contextual sense of self).

CLIENT: Yeah . . . This makes me feel disconnected from other people. Even from people I love. They just can't understand.

THERAPIST: When we look at these experiences from above (*drawing an imaginary circle right above the floor with her hand*), it feels like there are so many differences across people . . . the way they feel, what they do, their history. And this can make it hard to feel close to other people.

*The therapist uses gestures and metaphorical speech to establish
a hierarchical network that puts the relationship on top and their
experiences at the base.*

CLIENT: Yeah. I feel like there are walls around me.

THERAPIST: Yeah . . . If we look at each other through these experiences, it can be difficult to feel connected sometimes (*now drawing the circle at the level of their eyes*). But if we look at each
other at this level (*drawing the circle at a much lower level and
raising her head above to demonstrate how she looks at the client at a higher level*), all our experiences are there (*pointing the
circle much below their eyes*) and we are connected in another
way. What do you think?

*The therapist continues with hierarchical framing through gestures
and metaphorical speech to conceptualize the relationship as a context of their experiences.*

CLIENT: It would be nice to put all these things aside, for sure. I wish
I could erase them and be like everybody.

THERAPIST: Yeah, if all our differences were erased, we would be
exactly alike. And maybe there is a way to be here together,
without erasing anything. You and I, we could look at these
experiences from above (*pointing again the circle below their
eyes*). Maybe we can find this connection there.

*The therapist emphasizes that approaching their relationship as a con-
text of their experiences can improve the connection between them.*

A nonverbal process you can also use to amplify this point is to move
your chair so that you sit right next to the client, as a metaphor for shared
perspective. In this approach, the dialogue above could begin with disparate content being like objects on the floor, but after moving the chair to sit
next to the client, the focus could shift to the common commitment to look
at that content together, each sharing consciousness of it from a point of
view, much as two people sitting together are both looking out at the world.

Finally, considering the interactive relationship that we all share with
our past and current context can help the therapist see that the client is
neither fully responsible nor hopeless, no matter what he is going through
(see Chapter 6). This is particularly useful when treating clients who have
done reprehensible actions or are acting in ways that displease the therapist.
In this case, the therapist notices the impact of contextual variables, such
as the chain of events that led the client to behave as he did in the past and
to become the person he is now. The therapist can even adopt the point of
view of his client and realize that with the same history, he may have likely

ended up at the same place. Engaging in this process privately helps change the therapist's responses in the therapy room (e.g., expressing more care and empathy). It is even possible to communicate this process to the client as a way to reduce the risk that the client feels judged when sharing experiences he is ashamed of. Observe this technique in the following exchange:

CLIENT: I drank again last weekend and I passed out as usual. . . . You must think I am a big failure.

THERAPIST: You seem really disappointed.

CLIENT: Yeah. I don't know why I keep doing this. I say that I am going to change but I keep doing the same thing. You must think you are wasting your time with me.

THERAPIST: I think if I were in the same situation, I mean, having strong urges to drink, I would also have an extraordinarily hard time sticking with my commitment not to drink.

The therapist adopts the point of view of the client to emphasize the impact of contextual variables on the client's behavior.

CLIENT: You think so? When you say that you will do something, you do it. I can always rely on you. But me? I am the most unreliable person.

THERAPIST: I appreciate that you say I am reliable. And I guess I am lucky that I had a history that strengthened this in me. Strengthening that in the face of strong urges is a lot harder.

The therapist emphasizes the impact of contextual variables on his own behavior.

Emphasizing the interaction between the client and his historical and current context is also useful when the therapist finds himself doubting the capacity of his client to ever change, notably due to variables that seem impossible to overcome (e.g., a social environment that reinforces ineffective behaviors, or limited financial resources). In this case, the therapist's attention must be brought to the effective impact of the client's behaviors, even if it is still limited at this point. Here again, the therapist can privately engage in this process to change his responses in the therapy room, but also communicate it to the client. Observe this technique in the following exchange, which directly follows the previous vignette:

CLIENT: So, since I didn't have the same history as you had, I guess I will never be reliable.

THERAPIST: Well, your history is done and can't be changed, but what about what is going on in your life right now?

The therapist orients the client's observation to the variables that may be impacted by his behaviors.

CLIENT: Right now, I am not reliable.

THERAPIST: Okay. What could be changed so that you become reliable?

The therapist evokes tracking to identify behaviors that can have an impact.

CLIENT: I don't know. Every week I swear that I won't drink during the weekend, but I always end up drinking.

THERAPIST: What has worked in the past for you? Like, for example, what do you do to come here every week? You have never missed a session so far.

The therapist evokes tracking to help the client notice the impact of his current behavior.

CLIENT: I don't miss any session with you because I want things to change. I want my life to change.

THERAPIST: And for this to happen, you make the effort to come here every week, even though you said in the past that it was hard for you, right?

The therapist shares an observation to refine tracking.

CLIENT: Yeah.

THERAPIST: How is it working so far?

The therapist evokes further tracking, focusing on the impact of behaviors.

CLIENT: Well, I haven't changed much yet, but I have made some progress.

THERAPIST: So, this is an area where you made a commitment that you kept and that helped you make some progress?

The therapist reformulates to underline the effectiveness of the client's behavior.

CLIENT: Yeah.

THERAPIST: How about we try to figure out together how to do the same thing with drinking?

CLIENT: That would be good.

Fostering and Sustaining a Meaningful, Positive Relationship

In order to engage in the difficult process of therapy, both the therapist and the client need to clarify the purpose of their collaboration and to allow that purpose to infuse their interactions. In many clinical approaches, the main goals of therapy are laid out in the therapeutic contract established during the first session. These goals depend on each situation, but RFT principles can help guide the goals and qualities of action that are of most importance in the therapeutic relationship, and to make sure that clinical transactions manifest those very goals and qualities.

In Chapters 5–7, we organized clinical interventions according to three overarching goals: developing a sense of experience and effectiveness to activate behavior change; promoting a flexible sense of self to establish stability and variability; and fostering meaning and motivation to bring lasting satisfaction in clients' lives. Experience and effectiveness are served by a relationship based on awareness, curiosity, and pragmatism; flexibility is fostered by a relationship characterized by openness, acceptance, and compassion; and meaning and motivation are fostered by care, commitment, and perseverance linked to the deepest yearnings of others. By conducting interactions in the therapy room with this stance, the therapist encourages the client to join her on this path. This sense of travelling together increases the hope that obstacles that will show up on the way can be overcome.

One way to test the viability of these methods and goals is to think of times when you felt uplifted and empowered by your relationship with another person. Picture the person and what that relationship was like and see if it isn't the case that you felt as though the other person was aware of you, curious about your experiences, and deeply wanted things to work out for you. See if it isn't the case that you felt accepted for who you are rather than being judged, and that your feelings were noticed and mattered. Finally, see if what you cared about was given attention by the other person and you could do things together in ways that fostered what was important. If the answers fit with the structure we have outlined, then it is likely that they will be true for your clients as well.

The purpose of therapy can become unclear if the overarching goals and qualities of action of the relationship are not sufficiently stated, or if they are stated in a way that excessively emphasizes narrow purposes, social desirability, or avoidant motivation. In this case, therapist and client should look together for the higher function of the stated goal, ensure that it serves the client's life satisfaction beyond others' approval, and connect effective actions to positive motivation. Meanwhile, the therapeutic exchanges themselves need to manifest these qualities. Observe these techniques in the following exchange:

THERAPIST: I have been thinking about the work we are doing here and what we came to do together, and I was wondering if you thought we were heading in the good direction for you. What do you think?

CLIENT: Yeah, I think so. I mean, it is important that I go to therapy.

The purpose of therapy doesn't seem clear to either the client or the therapist.

THERAPIST: At the beginning of our work together, we agreed on certain directions that we wanted to follow together. I wonder if we still have them in mind. I feel a bit uncomfortable putting this on the table because I'm not sure I've been attentive enough to those goals, but our work here is too important for me to just pretend. I am asking you this because somehow I have had the feeling that maybe together we have drifted a bit away from these directions, and I would like to make sure that we stay on track in a way that is useful for you.

The therapist encourages the client to restate the purpose of their work and simultaneously holds himself accountable to that same standard, sharing his feelings and goals in the process.

CLIENT: Okay, I understand. I think that what we had decided was that I should no longer hide my feelings from my wife because my wife doesn't like that.

The goal is too narrow and specific (not connected to an overarching and inexhaustible source of reinforcement), and it is stated as an avoidant goal (negative reinforcement). In addition, the goal seems linked to an arbitrary social consequence for rule following per se, suggesting pliance rather than tracking.

THERAPIST: In the long run, what is the purpose of changing this? If this was entirely between you and the person in the mirror—like no one else could tell you that was the wrong answer—what is most important here as a purpose of our work?

The therapist reorients the client to the higher function and to the personal choice behind this specific goal.

CLIENT: To have a better relationship with my wife . . . and maybe not just with her but others as well.

THERAPIST: Okay. And what would be positive about that? What are the qualities of relationship you yearn for?

The therapist reformulates and orients the client to positive sources of reinforcement.

CLIENT: I want us to be more connected, more like we used to be at the beginning of our marriage. I want to learn how to be close.

THERAPIST: Okay, I get that. I see that yearning for closeness. If that is what you want, how do you think sharing feelings can improve your relationship with your wife?

The therapist encourages the client to consider the effectiveness of the behavior he wants to improve.

CLIENT: My wife always complains about me not saying anything about my feelings.

THERAPIST: And on your end? Would you notice any positive changes between you if you shared your feelings more with her?

The client still seems strongly connected to the sources of negative reinforcement (wife's complaints), so the therapist reorients him again to positive consequences and makes sure these were personally relevant.

CLIENT: I think that since I have started to do it more, things have gotten better between us, yeah. It think I've actually gotten better in being more open.

THERAPIST: I think I've seen that in here too. And how has it been for you to see these changes happen?

The therapist reinforces focus and orients the client to his own satisfaction to increase tracking over pliance.

CLIENT: I've felt closer to her. I have been happier in my life in general too. I think I'm learning how to be myself.

THERAPIST: So, would it make a positive difference in your life to keep working in this direction? Developing your skills at sharing your feelings with your wife in order to improve the connection between the two of you?

The therapist reformulates the purpose of their work together as an overarching goal bringing positive reinforcement. Asking "would it make a positive difference in your life?" was meant to help the client connect to the intrinsic consequences rather than to social approval.

CLIENT: Yes. I want to get better at sharing—letting my wife see who I am at a deeper level. I think it would be good for me to keep learning how to do that. I've noticed that I learn things about me when I'm more open and honest. And my relationship with my wife just seems softer and more caring. But I'm not always attuned to that.

The client augments and extends positive motivation, noticing more subtle and broader purposes inside the goal of therapy.

THERAPIST: Me neither, but I'm moved by what you are saying. This is worth our attention.

The therapist models openness and commits the therapeutic relationship to the client's extended and elaborated goals.

Another difficulty sometimes arises when therapist and client notice discrepancies between what they each care about. It is usually possible to find a common ground because the therapist cares first about helping the client choose her own directions and make effective steps on these paths. However, the client's directions or actions may be so different from the therapist's that there is a risk of disconnection in their relationship.

To prevent this disconnection from happening, the therapist can use two main approaches. First, if she can relate to the client's overarching goals and qualities of action but feels judgmental about the way the client turns them into actions, it can be useful for her to remember the hierarchical nature of these life directions. A variety of actions can serve the same overarching source of satisfaction. For example, the client and the therapist might share the same overarching goal of contributing to people's well-being in their community, and yet, have very different views about what to do to accomplish this. This might happen, for example, if a very liberal therapist realizes that her client is an extreme conservative. By focusing on the shared goal, judgmental thoughts that might distract the clinician can be more easily put to the side.

Sometimes, the overarching goals chosen by the client are quite different from those of the therapist. This difference could create difficulties in the relationship if it became a central focus. In this case, the therapist can benefit from noticing similarities in the ways they follow their respective goals. For example, a therapist could recognize in the client's persistence to always improve his athletic performances his own persistence to improve his knowledge about psychology. The quality of action is the same even if the overarching goal is different. Here again, recognizing what is common between them helps foster connections in the relationship. Observe how the therapist uses this technique in the following short exchange:

CLIENT: I know it is hard for other people to understand, but my faith is what is the most important in my life. I don't expect you to understand either. You are a scientist, and you probably think I am stupid to spend so much time reading religious books.

THERAPIST: There may be different things I care about in my life, that's true. But your dedication to your faith is something I can relate to. You seem to care about approaching your faith with depth and care.

The therapist identifies a quality of action.

CLIENT: Yes, with depth.

THERAPIST: Well, this is something I care about too. You said that I am a scientist. It is true, and I try to approach my science with depth and care. I spend a lot of time reading to learn more about psychology.

The therapist underlines the quality of action they have in common, although applied to different overarching goals.

CLIENT: Do you sometimes feel like nobody can understand what you care about?

THERAPIST: Sometimes, when I am completely absorbed in a topic, I feel like I am the only one caring about this very topic, yeah. And sometimes others do not understand me and why this is important.

The therapist underlines similar experiences associated with their common quality of action.

CLIENT: That is how it is for me. Some of my family thinks I've just gone overboard. But it matters to me.

Even when therapist and client find a clear and common ground in the purpose of their collaboration, they may still have difficulties actually engaging in effective actions together. Exactly as one person may lack motivation and satisfaction before, during, or after performing an action, two people can find themselves unable to make effective moves in the context of their relationship. For example, it is not rare that at the end of a session both the client and the therapist leave each other with the feeling that they have not accomplished anything significant. They felt connected and talked about different topics, but they didn't do what they had planned to, such as an exercise of exposure or skills training. As we saw earlier, this could be due to psychological experiences being perceived as barriers to action (e.g., difficult emotions leading to avoidance). It could also be caused by a lack of connection between the action and the higher purpose this action is supposed to serve. In this case, it often becomes necessary to state or restate together how the action will help make progress in the therapeutic work (see Chapter 7). Although the relationship as a whole is involved in this process, it is primarily the job of the therapist to notice this lack of motivation and to initiate the reconnection of their actions to the purpose of therapy. However, including the client in this effort is important to strengthen the collaborative dimension of their relationship. Observe this approach in the following exchange:

THERAPIST: I am noticing that we have been talking for about 15 minutes now, and I have very much enjoyed our conversation.

CLIENT: Me too!

THERAPIST: At the same time, I have the thought at the back of my head that we had planned to do an exposure exercise together today.

The therapist brings the client's attention to the effective action.

CLIENT: Yeah . . .

THERAPIST: (*smiling*) It seems like you are not so excited about doing that? Are you?

The therapist evokes the client's observation of her motivation.

CLIENT: No, not really . . .

THERAPIST: I think that I have the same feeling as you are having. For some reason, I find it more appealing to keep talking with you than doing this exercise. At the same time, I wonder if this is the most helpful for our work together here. What do you think?

The therapist shares her own lack of motivation and evokes tracking to assess the effectiveness of their current actions.

CLIENT: I think I'm dreading doing this exercise because I know it will be hard. And it is hard to see the point of doing something hard right now.

THERAPIST: Yeah, I see what you mean. We are having this nice conversation, and we wonder why we would do something that will likely be difficult, right?

CLIENT: Yeah . . .

THERAPIST: So, maybe we could look again together at why it might be useful to do this exercise?

The therapist evokes augmenting, which bridges the exercise to its purpose.

CLIENT: Okay.

THERAPIST: What do you think is the point?

The therapist continues to evoke augmenting.

CLIENT: Well, I know that if I keep avoiding the things that I am afraid of, there is no way I can get better.

The client engages in augmenting through negative reinforcement.

THERAPIST: Okay, and what kind of positive things do you expect from this exposure work? What is it even for?

The therapist evokes augmenting through positive reinforcement.

CLIENT: Being able to spend more time with my family and to be more successful in my work instead of doing my rituals all the time.

The client engages in augmenting through positive reinforcement but limited to specific goal.

THERAPIST: Okay. And even that—what is important for you inside time with your family or success at work?

The therapist evokes the exploration of a higher function.

CLIENT: I want this to change because I want to build a family where we share things together, and I want to be successful to give my family the things they need.

THERAPIST: I am here to help you make the changes that matter to you. That's what I'm up to. So, what do you think? Do we keep having this really nice conversation, or do we do the exercise?

The therapist lets the client make the choice of action in order to increase her motivation.

CLIENT: (*smiling*) I guess we should do the exercise.

THERAPIST: (*smiling*) Is this what you want?

The client shows possible signs of pliance ("we should"), so the therapist reorients her to what she wants to do.

CLIENT: Yeah. I am a bit scared, but I know this is what I actually want.

THERAPIST: (*smiling*) Let's go then?

CLIENT: Okay.

It is also possible to reconnect the action to its purpose while performing or debriefing an action. You can use the principles laid out in Chapter 7 in a similar way, but this time involving the whole relationship (client and therapist work together at clarifying and reaffirming their motivation).

Mindful Preparation for Sessions

Caring relationships require perspective taking, empathy, and enough openness not to withdraw when things are emotionally difficult (Vilardaga et al., 2012). The last of these three features clinicians need to work on over time, but the first two can be worked on regularly before psychotherapy sessions. Vilardaga and Hayes (2010) provide an example of how this might be done: taking the time in the minutes before a psychotherapy session to picture:

> Being the client on the way to session and sensing what the client might be hearing, seeing, and feeling.
>
> Connecting what the client might be thinking or feeling about the upcoming session and the problems the client faces.
>
> Noticing how historical these reactions are—how these themes of emotion and cognition have been with the client for many years.
>
> Catching that the client is viewing her own experiences from an "I/here/now" perspective, even if the client doesn't know that.
>
> Noticing emotions, thoughts, and judgments that you may have about the client or the client's presenting problem.
>
> Noticing how historical these reactions are too—how these themes of emotion and judgment show up inside you, related to many clients (and not just clients).
>
> Noticing your own sense of "I/here/nowness" and noticing the continuity between this sense and the same sense in your client.
>
> Remembering the values you bring to your work and connecting with what you hope to bring to the client in her journey. If all goes well, what would the client have taken from your time together, say, 5 years from now?

CLINICAL EXAMPLE

In the following vignette, you will see that the therapist uses several principles presented throughout this chapter. This exchange happens with a 33-year-old female with borderline personality disorder.

> CLIENT: I need to see you more often. You have to do something! Change your schedule . . . I don't know . . . You have to figure something out to help me!
>
> THERAPIST: I sense that you are worried about being on your own this week. Is this how you feel right now?

The therapist shares an observation about the client's experience and asks for confirmation to build mutual understanding.

> CLIENT: Yes, of course! I am terrified! You don't know what it's like for me. You are not alone all the time.
>
> THERAPIST: If I was alone all the time, I would certainly feel scared and probably sad too. Do you feel sad when you are alone?

The therapist uses deictic framing to build mutual understanding and normalize the client's experience.

CLIENT: Yes.

THERAPIST: I hear that you would like to see me more often. It is understandable that you worry about spending this week on your own and that you want to see me more. At the same time, what we agreed on is to have a phone check every other day now, you remember?

The therapist normalizes the client's experience and evokes tracking.

CLIENT: Yes, but I don't think I am ready for that. I need special care! I can't be on my own.

THERAPIST: You know, it is hard for me to know that you are alone. I feel sad to know that you are sad and worried. As I notice that I feel this way, I also have the urge to say "Okay, let's meet another time this week." And at the same time, I try to remember what we agreed about the purpose of our work together. Do you remember it?

The therapist self-discloses his own current experiences to normalize the client's experience, improve commonality, and model response flexibility. Then, he evokes augmenting to connect their work to its higher purpose.

CLIENT: I know . . . I need to be more independent. I need to deal with my problems.

The word "need" and the absence of consequence explicitly stated suggest possible pliance.

THERAPIST: Well, that is one way of saying it. Would that make a difference in your life if you could be more independent?

The therapist evokes exploration of intrinsic reinforcement associated with independence in order to undermine potential pliance.

CLIENT: Yeah. But it terrifies me to be on my own.

THERAPIST: Of course. It is something new for you. Most of us are scared of doing things for the first time. For you, it is being independent. For other people, it might be having a first child or starting a new job. And what is difficult is that we *want* to do these things. If we didn't care about them, they would not be difficult at all.

The therapist normalizes the client's experience again, but this time by emphasizing the role of contextual variables on her reaction.

Then, he targets the transformation of function of the difficult experience into a sign that a source of meaning is involved.

CLIENT: Yeah, it's true. I want to be independent even if it is scary. But I don't know if I am ready for that just now. Maybe we could wait a bit longer?

THERAPIST: I think that if we waited, we would both feel better in this moment.

The therapist shares an observation about the short-term effect of responding to their urges.

CLIENT: Yes!

THERAPIST: What I wonder is if the purpose of our work together is to feel better right now. What about learning to be more independent?

The therapist evokes the assessment of response effectiveness with regard to the client's overarching goal.

CLIENT: Maybe it is better to wait.

THERAPIST: What I promised you when we started this work together is that I would not tell you what you should do but that we would look together at what works and what doesn't work for improving your life.

The therapist restates the principle of effectiveness and experience that bonds their relationship.

CLIENT: Yeah.

THERAPIST: What have you noticed when you waited in order to feel better?

The therapist evokes tracking.

CLIENT: It makes things worse . . . I know.

THERAPIST: Yeah. And I know it is hard for you right now. It is hard for me too. Like I said, if I listen to what I feel just now, I want to say "Okay, let's schedule another meeting this week."

The therapist normalizes the client's experience by self-disclosing his own urges.

CLIENT: But you are not going to do it . . .

THERAPIST: Not if I want to help you become more independent.

The therapist models flexible response to urges and connects action to meaningful purpose in order to increase motivation.

What do you want to do? Are you willing to stick with our plan? Checking in on the phone until next week?

The therapist evokes choice of action.

CLIENT: Okay . . .

THERAPIST: Let's make this bold move together then. Let's work at improving your independence! Are you in?

The therapist again connects their work together to its meaningful purpose.

CLIENT: Okay.

THERAPIST: Wow. Bold. Scary. New.

CLIENT: Tell me about it. But I'm doing it.

 **CHAPTER SUMMARY**

In this chapter, you learned to apply RFT principles to yourself as a therapist and to the relationship with your clients. Here are the main principles to remember:

- As a therapist, you can experience difficulties caused by language processes the same way as your clients do. Since the processes are similar, the methods used to help clients can be applied to yourself too:

  ○ Problems linked to insensitivity, essential social or coherence, and narrowed repertoires of actions can be addressed through functional contextual awareness, functional sense making, and increase of response flexibility.

  ○ Problems linked to the therapist's self-concept can be addressed through the four principles of the flexible self (awareness of experiences, awareness of perspective taking, coherence grounded in context, and responsibility grounded in interaction of person–context).

  ○ Problems linked to meaning and motivation can be addressed through identifying and building overarching goals and qualities of action associated with clinical work, and broad patterns of actions connected to these meaningful directions in a hierarchical network. Motivation to make the most effective therapeutic moves can be built and sustained through augmenting, which bridges these actions to their higher purpose (using positive and intrinsic reinforcement).

  ○ Formal experiential practice can help strengthen therapeutic skills, and many of the exercises used with clients can be applied to the therapists themselves.

- Problems experienced at an individual level can also concern the relationship. RFT principles are applied in this case by involving both the client and the therapist:
  - Finding trust in effectiveness, normalization, and commonality.
    - Trust in the relationship can be established through the common agenda of identifying and improving effective actions.
    - Mutual understanding can be communicated through perspective taking and acknowledging psychological experiences.
    - Psychological experiences can be normalized through perspective taking and self-disclosure.
    - Response flexibility can be modeled through appropriate and well-timed self-disclosure.
  - Building a flexible "sense of other."
    - Noticing the client's flow of experiences improves the therapist's empathy and awareness of the various experiences lived by the client.
    - Noticing the client's perspective taking allows the therapist to perceive stability in the client, across and beyond psychological experiences, and to relate to the client in a way that is more interconnected.
    - Seeing the client as a container of content allows the therapist to integrate variability and stability in the way the client is conceptualized.
    - Seeing the interactive relationship between the client and the context allows the therapist to consider the client's responsibility with balance.
  - Fostering and sustaining a meaningful positive relationship.
  - The purpose of the therapeutic relationship involves overarching goals and qualities of action that are intrinsically and positively reinforcing.
  - Identifying overarching goals and qualities of action shared by the therapist and the client increases connectedness and alleviates judgments.
  - Client and therapist's motivation to perform therapeutic moves together can be sustained by restating the connection between these actions and their purposes (in terms of positive and intrinsic sources of reinforcement).

Epilogue

The clinical conversation is a universal mechanism of action in all psychological interventions. Yet to date, there are no guides to the use of language in psychotherapy that are systematically linked to basic behavioral research programs in human language.

There is a reason for that. Basic researchers in human language and cognition have just not focused that much on where these abilities come from within the lifetimes of individuals, nor on how they can be regulated by context, nor on their pragmatic impact on behavior. Instead, language and cognition are argued to be products of mental processes or brain process; the structure of language is examined in great detail, but not its function. The robust and worthy intellectual traditions already focused on human language and cognition rarely tell clinicians what to do in psychotherapy work in any moment-to-moment sense. That is not really a criticism: they were not designed to do that.

The purpose of this book is to extend some of the implications of a functional contextual analysis of human language, relational frame theory, into the normal work of psychotherapy. Precisely because it is a functional contextual theory, it *is* designed from the beginning to be contextually focused and pragmatically useful. RFT argues that human language is a learned ability to build, understand, and respond to relations among events that go beyond the mere form of those events or our direct experience with them. It partitions this ability into simple elements: relating events mutually, combining them into networks, and changing functions. It appeals to contextual control over derivation and contextual control over functional transformation. And it views all of that as learned behavior, based on but stepping forward from ancient learning mechanisms.

At this point in the volume, we hope you will agree that this ability is a relatively simple set of evidence-based processes. Like a formula for a fractal, however, this simple set of processes extends endlessly. It extends across different events, different relations, different networks, different functions, and different clinical issues. Relational framing impacts on contingency learning and the emotional and behavioral effect of much older learning processes, such as respondent and operant learning. In the area of human behavior it changes . . . everything.

RFT has historically been tied to acceptance and commitment therapy, and there is no denying that they evolved together. We are excited to think of how our colleagues who are interested in ACT will apply, extend, and test the analysis in this volume. Nevertheless, we have bent over backwards to avoid writing this book as an ACT book. ACT is an evidence-based psychotherapy based on psychological inflexibility as a model of pathology processes, and psychological flexibility as a model of psychological growth processes. In this book we have touched on some of those ideas regularly. But we did not write this book to explain ACT, justify ACT, or promote ACT. We understand that some readers will focus on areas of apparent difference between ACT writings and the present volume, but in our view nothing in this book is ruled out by ACT, nor by any other evidence-based psychotherapy and the principles that drive them. This effort stands on its own, and it appears to comport with the broad evidence base in psychotherapy.

Ironically perhaps, in order to fulfill our promise of a book that is focused on general clinical methods, we had to orient the reader to ideas drawn from behavioral psychology and its umbrella of evolution science. We used these principles as a foundation to understand the broad range of ideas in clinical psychology, not as a fence between traditions. We have repeatedly appealed to ways of creating healthy psychological variation, to situate action in its context, to link it to selection criteria that are desired, and to practice action so that it is likely to be retained. In our view, these are simply ways of stating the conditions under which living systems evolve, whether we are talking about species, repertoires, or cultures. We have focused on broad issues of antecedents and consequences, and of function and long-run outcomes—wary of inducing behavior change that is superficially helpful but forced by compliance with the therapist or other short-term fixes, instead of promoting skills that can be generalized and retained better, leading to long-run improvement. We have addressed multiple response dimensions (overt behavior, thought, emotion, sensation) and multiple levels of analysis (the individual, the therapeutic relationship, cultural processes). All of these points are central to any endeavor in behavioral or applied evolution science.

We understand that it is not always easy for those who are not trained in these ways of thinking, but if these evolutionarily and behaviorally sound principles can be embraced enough for the basic points to be made (and the behavioral language barriers overcome), we feel that almost *any* approach to clinical work can use some or all of these principles to foster gains without sacrificing their core beliefs and orientation.

Efforts of a somewhat similar kind have been made in the history of psychology, such as Dollard and Miller's (1950) attempt to understand neurosis and psychotherapy using neo-behavioristic principles. With the benefit of hindsight, these efforts are often viewed merely as translations—of saying what is already known in fresh terminology. That is not our present purpose. With RFT we are focused only on how language is used in psychotherapy, and in that limited domain we are not merely reinterpreting what many clinical traditions do, we are attempting to provide them with a flexible, coherent, and pragmatic framework based on the implications of a small set of evidence-based principles. It is true that in broad terms much of what we end up recommending is not fundamentally new and exists to a degree in many depth-oriented clinical traditions, once the relevant terms are translated. But our primary contribution is to address old issues in a way that is linked to evidence-based principles about human language that have specific implications, so that interventions can be guided and changed. It is one thing to be concerned over issues of self—it is another to use deictic and hierarchical symbolic relations deliberately; it is one thing to see the value of metaphor in psychotherapy—it is another to know the language processes that make metaphors apt and experiential; and so on through the range of issues we have covered. In every broad area we addressed, we think the present analysis suggests new concrete steps that might be taken. We believe clinicians in these traditions will be able to assess the value added.

A concern we expect is that RFT sometimes states the obvious in complicated ways. We understand the concern: instead of saying, "The word 'apple' refers to actual apples," we say, "The sound 'apple' is in a frame of coordination with actual apples," and so on. Even at that level, RFT labs can show through experiments where things like "frames of coordination" actually come from, while "reference" is just a term. And it is in complex clinical areas that the value of technical concepts such as framing really is felt. Approaches of language that are grounded in common sense terminology, such as referential theories that emphasize clear concepts or logical reasoning are easier initially but have been notorious for their lack of precision and scope—and as a result, as they are scaled into the complex topics psychotherapists deal with, they either revert to increasingly common-sense terms or they become vague or even silent about important details. A fair measure of the value of an RFT approach is the ability to maintain precision and scope across the range of empirical topics relevant to human language. It should stand or fall on that basis, and seemingly simpler approaches need to do the same.

By viewing symbolic events in this bottom-up way, we can see the outlines of another kind of evidence-based clinical practice: one that is both empirically based at the level of principle and yet tied to the details of individual clients behaving in the moment. We are not arguing that these ideas are yet "evidence-based practice" in the sense meant by lists maintained by the American Psychological Association or by U.S. government agencies. This approach can be integrated with such methods easily however, and seems likely to empower their application. We encourage that exploration.

But there is another sense in which practice can be evidence based. Clinical work of the kind encouraged by the present volume is empirically based in the much same way as applying learning principles to individual needs has always been viewed as evidence based. If desired outcomes are measured and known processes of importance are used, empirical commitments of practitioners can readily be made manifest. Of course, doing formal outcome research on this approach would be important and useful, but a more proximal target is linking the advice in this volume to indications of variation and selective retention, context sensitivity, motivation, and the like. Those links do not need to wait until they appear in the distant future—practitioners can assess them *now*, with clients they are treating *now*. If practitioners see healthy processes move, that in itself is a worthwhile outcome.

This pragmatism was part of the original vision of behavior therapy and clinical behavior analysis. It struggled due to the rise of psychiatric nosology and treatment packages, on the one hand, and the failure of functional principles to climb the mountain of human language and cognition on the other hand. Psychiatric nosology and technologically based treatment packages are now staggering under their own weight, however, and it is obvious to many that asking practitioners to learn myriad packages for endless lists of topographically based syndromes and subsyndromes is neither viable nor progressive over the long run.

Direct contingency principles can do a great deal in guiding practitioners toward effective interventions, but what has been needed to make that original vision of evidence-based practice more realistic is a functionally and contextually robust approach to language and cognition. If RFT is the theory we think it is, it may be time to revisit the original vision and to begin to carve out a form of evidence-based practice that goes beyond packages and procedures to principles and people.

Quick Guide to Using RFT in Psychotherapy

In this quick guide, you will find a review of the skills targeting the core areas of clinical work, as presented in Chapters 4–7. Each section is illustrated by examples of typical phrases you might say to your client in this context. We encourage you to use this quick guide as a cheat sheet while practicing specific skills in role plays and supervisions, or before a session with a client.

In our experience, the best way to integrate new skills into your clinical repertoire is to pick one and practice it repeatedly until a satisfying level of mastery has been reached. For example, if your goal is to improve your ability to help clients observe and describe their experiences through perspective taking, you may want to rate your competency at baseline on a scale of 10, then practice perspective taking for this purpose in role plays or in actual sessions, and rate yourself each time, until you systematically reach a score of at least 8. Then, you can move on to another skill, using the same approach.

PSYCHOLOGICAL ASSESSMENT (CHAPTER 4)

Creating an Experiential Context for Assessment

Focus on the Client's Experience

- Encourage the client to make his or her own observation and description.
  - Ask questions that evoke observation and description (e.g., "How were you feeling in that moment?"; "How did you respond to this situation?"; "What do you feel like doing next?").
  - Offer reformulations that refine the client's observation and description (e.g., "So, you are saying that. . . . Is that right?").
  - Remain clearly open to the client's view while sharing your own

observations (e.g., "I'm seeing a lot of anxiety right now. Is that what you are experiencing?"; "I noticed you never talk about your wife, and I was wondering if it's a topic you would rather avoid. Is that the case?").

- Improve mutual understanding.
  - ○ Reflect back (e.g., "It seems what you are saying is. . . . Is that what you meant?"; "I would like to make sure I understand what you are saying. Can I reflect back what you just said?").
  - ○ Use perspective taking (e.g., "If I were in your shoes, I would feel quite anxious. Is that how you are feeling?"; "I would like to see this situation from your perspective. Can you help me picture what it's like for you?").

Connect the Therapeutic Process to the Client's Life

- Use coordination framing to draw attention to similar experiences (e.g., "Is what you are feeling now similar to what you experienced in the situation you described earlier?"; "I noticed you change the topic of our conversation a few times. Is that what you also do when you talk with your friends about your personal life?").
- Use analogical framing to draw attention to similar functions (e.g., "So, if you avoid looking at me, then you are less anxious about what I might think. Could it be that drinking alcohol has a similar effect on your anxiety about work?").
- Use perspective taking to bring different situations to the therapy room.
  - ○ Interpersonal deictic framing (e.g., "Imagine I am your partner and we are having a casual conversation. What would the tone of your voice be like now? Can you show me?").
  - ○ Spatial deictic framing (e.g., "Imagine you are alone in your apartment right now. How are you feeling now?").
  - ○ Temporal deictic framing (e.g., "Imagine you travel in time and you are 2 hours from now. What thoughts are in your mind now?").

Assessing Context Sensitivity

Assess Sensitivity to Antecedents

- Use temporal framing to identify what happens before a response (e.g., "What happened right before you began to feel this way?"; "What did you notice in your body before you left the room?"; "When do you tend to have these reactions?").
- Use spatial framing to identify situations (e.g., "Where do you have these kinds of urges?"; "In what places do you tend to feel this way?").
- Use conditional framing to identify triggers of a response (e.g., "What do you feel if someone criticizes you?"; "How do you respond to your wife if she says she loves you?").

Assess Sensitivity to Consequences

- Use temporal framing to identify what happens after a response (e.g., "And then, what happened?"; "What did you notice after you did that?").
- Use conditional framing to identify the consequences of a response (e.g., "What happens as a result of avoiding talking about painful memories?"; "What impact did canceling your date have?").
- Use distinction or comparison framing to identify changes resulting from actions (e.g., "What is different after you drink alcohol?"; "Do you feel more or less depressed after you watch television?").
- Use temporal framing to explore long-term and short-term consequences (e.g., "And then, what happened?"; "What about in the long term?").
- Use temporal framing to explore the variability of consequences (e.g., "How often does that happen as a result of doing that?"; "Would you say that what happens after you do this happens always, often, or from time to time?").
- Use spatial framing to explore consequences in different domains (e.g., "So, not trusting other people prevents you from being hurt at work. What about in your intimate relationships?"; "You are saying that doing these rituals decreases your anxiety when you are at home. What avbout when you are at work?").

Assessing Coherence

Assess Relational Fluency and Flexibility

- Assess coordination framing (e.g., "What else is happening in this moment?"; "Could these two things come together?"; "Do you see any similarity between what you are feeling here and what you are feeling when surrounded by strangers?").
- Assess distinction framing (e.g., "Do you notice any difference?"; "What is not there?"; "How do you know when you are not happy?").
- Assess opposition framing (e.g., "What is the opposite of being bored for you?"; "What could you do instead of leaving?").
- Assess comparison framing (e.g., "Are there moments where you are less confident?"; "Do you feel more or less anxious now?").
- Assess temporal and spatial framing (e.g., "Where do you feel this sensation?"; "When do you have these urges?").
- Assess conditional framing (e.g., "What would happen if you let her spend time with her friends?"; "What would you do if you had all the time in the world?").
- Assess deictic framing (e.g., "If you were me, how would you respond to this question?"; "If you were 10 years from now, what would your life look like?").

- Assess hierarchical framing (e.g., "Is there something bigger that includes this goal?"; "What part of yourself tells you that?").
- Assess analogical framing (e.g., "If this work were a journey, would you want to travel alone or with a fellow?"; "It seems you are at a crossroad. What direction do you want to take?"; "Is there a picture that might represent how you are feeling now?").

Assess Rules and Rule Following

- Explore rules.
  - Ask what the client is thinking before/during/after a behavior (e.g., "What did you have in mind as you were about to leave the room?"; "What are you thinking now?"; "What thoughts come to your mind as you reflect on what you did?").
  - Ask how the client explains or justifies a behavior (e.g., "Why did you want her to know how you were feeling?"; "Why did you decide to stay in bed instead of going to work?"; "I'm curious to know more about what led you to do that.").
- Explore rule following.
  - Pliance.
    - Use distinction/opposition framing to remove social influence (e.g., "If nobody cared about what you should do, would you still make this decision?").
    - Use coordination framing to make social influence noncontingent (e.g., "If your parents were happy no matter what you did with your life, would you still think you should go to college?").
    - Use perspective taking to explore contexts with lower social influence:
      - Interpersonal deictic framing (e.g., "If you were someone who didn't care about what people think, would you still believe this is the right thing to do?").
      - Spatial deictic framing (e.g., "If you were in a community where people don't ever judge what you do or believe, would you still want to do that?").
      - Temporal deictic framing (e.g., "Imagine you are 60 years from now. You are not a teenager who listens to his parents anymore, but the old grandfather who is listened to by his children. What do you feel is right now?").
  - Inapplicable tracking.
    - Use conditional framing to assess the feasibility of following the rule (e.g., "If this is right, then what should you do next?"; "And can you actually do that?"; "Have you tried to do that?").
    - Use interpersonal deictic framing to distinguish rules *others* can follow from rules *the client* can follow (e.g., "Is this something you should do or something other people should do?"; "So, if you were her, you would handle this situation differently? What do you want to do then?").

○ Inaccurate tracking.

  ▣ Use conditional framing to identify the consequences of following the rule (e.g., "And when you use this strategy, what do you experience as a consequence?"; "Does it work to follow this rule?").

  ▣ Use temporal framing to identify the consequences of following the rule over time (e.g., "So when you follow this strategy, it seems to work in the moment. What about in the long term?").

  ▣ Use temporal framing to explore variable consequences of following the rule (e.g., "Are there times when following this strategy doesn't work?").

  ▣ Use spatial framing to explore the consequences of following the rule across situations (e.g., "So, you experience that sharing your opinion with your colleagues is not appreciated. What about with your friends?").

  ▣ Use perspective taking to shift the context of rule following.

    ☐ Interpersonal deictic framing (e.g., "Would you advise your best friend to follow the same strategy?").

    ☐ Temporal deictic framing (e.g., "If you make decisions in your life upon this belief, do you think that in 10 years, you will look back and say you were right?").

○ Tracking leading to adaptive peaks.

  ▣ Use spatial and temporal framing to explore the cost of following the rule across situations and over time (e.g., "Are there areas of your life that suffer from living this way?"; "So, using drugs helps you perform better at work. What impact will it have on your health in the long run?").

  ▣ Use coordination framing to explore other sources of satisfaction neglected by following the rule (e.g., "Are there other things that might bring satisfaction in your life that you can't have or do because you are living your life this way?").

  ▣ Use comparison framing to explore greater sources of satisfaction neglected by following the rule (e.g., "Is it what you were dreaming of, or do you wish your life were more exciting?").

ACTIVATING AND SHAPING BEHAVIOR CHANGE (CHAPTER 5)

Increasing Functional Contextual Awareness

Shape Observation of Experiences

• Use nonverbal orienting.

  ○ Visual cues (e.g., Pointing to parts of the body, facial expressions).
  ○ Auditory cues (e.g., Pace, tone, and volume of voice; bell).
  ○ Tactile cues (e.g., Touching a part of the body).

- Use verbal orienting.
  - Spatial cues (e.g., "Notice what is going on here."; "Observe the sensations in your body."; "Focus on your breath."; "Picture your home and how you feel when you are there.").
  - Temporal cues (e.g., "Notice how you are feeling now."; "Can you remember how you were feeling then?"; "Observe what's going through your mind at this moment."; "Remember how you experienced feeling alone when you were young.").
- If the client gets stuck:
  - Use analogical framing to make observation more concrete (e.g., "Imagine you are listening to this sensation."; "Look at this thought like it's a painting.").
  - Use perspective taking to gain insight.
    - Interpersonal deictic framing (e.g., "Think of a time when your wife was sad, and observe what you can see on her face."; "Imagine you were one of the persons who saw you have one of these panic attacks.").
    - Spatial deictic framing (e.g., "Let's switch chairs in our minds, and observe what we can see from these different points of view.").
    - Temporal deictic framing (e.g., "Imagine you are 2 hours from now and you remember this moment.").

Shape Description of Experiences

- Encourage neutral description.
  - Use coordination framing to name experiences ("What do you feel?"; "What do you hear?"; "What were you thinking in that moment?"; "What is this sensation like?").
  - Use hierarchical framing to categorize and label experiences (e.g., "You're having an emotion . . ."; "What thoughts do you notice?"; "Is it a sensation of fatigue or excitement?").
- Encourage more precise description.
  - Use distinction framing to explore differences (e.g., "How is this sensation different from that one?"; "Any feelings we can rule out?").
  - Use comparison framing to explore differences along dimensions (e.g., "Is it more or less intense?"; "Is it closer to irritation or rage?"; "Do you feel this sensation more in your chest or in your throat?").
- If the client gets stuck:
  - Use analogical framing to make description more concrete (e.g., "If this emotion had a size, a shape, and a color, what would they be?"; "Imagine this feeling were a scene, how would you describe it?"; "Can you take a posture that represents this feeling?"; "Can you draw this emotion you are having?"; "What song would best say how you are feeling?").

○ Use perspective taking to gain insight.

  ※ Interpersonal deictic framing (e.g., "If your daughter were experiencing that, how might you help her describe it?"; "What do you think I might be noticing right now?"; "If you heard what you told him from someone you love, how would you be feeling?").

  ※ Temporal deictic framing (e.g., "When you leave my office and you remember these feelings you're having during our conversations, what words come to mind?").

  ※ Spatial deictic framing (e.g., "If you were sitting there looking at yourself now, what would you see?").

Shape Tracking of Functional Relationships among Experiences

• Encourage observation and description of contingency (antecedent → response → consequence).

  ○ Use temporal framing to identify correlations among experiences (e.g., "How do you feel right before you leave the room?"; "What happens when you look at her this way?"; "What did you notice after you decided to stay home?").

  ○ Use conditional framing to identify causal relationships (e.g., "What happens if you drink alcohol when you feel anxious?"; "What triggers this feeling?"; "What happens as a result of not talking?").

• Encourage more precise description.

  ○ Use distinction framing to explore differences (e.g., "What do you not experience after you call your friend for help?"; "What is different after you respond this way?").

  ○ Use comparison framing to explore differences along dimensions (e.g., "Did you feel more or less depressed after you canceled your meeting?").

  ○ Use temporal framing to draw out additional consequences (e.g., "And then what happens?"; "What about in the long term?").

  ○ Use spatial framing to explore various situations (e.g., "In social interactions at work, you feel scared and stay quiet. What about in social interactions outside of work?"; "In what situations are you more likely to respond to your fear by escaping?").

• If the client gets stuck:

  ○ Use analogical framing to make functional relationships easier to observe and describe.

    ※ Metaphors (e.g., "If feeling anxious were like stepping in quicksand, what would be your next move?"; "If you had filmed this moment with a camera, what would we see on this film?").

    ※ Gestures (e.g., Moving a hand from the left to the right while reformulating the contingency).

○ Use perspective taking to gain insight.

■ Interpersonal deictic framing (e.g., "If someone said that to you, how would you be feeling?"; "If I asked your wife, what would she say you do when you feel uncomfortable?").

■ Spatial deictic framing (e.g., "Imagine you were on the other side of the table during that meeting. What would you have seen happen? Try to describe the scene step by step.").

■ Temporal deictic framing (e.g., "Imagine you could travel in time. What would you like to have done differently in the past year?"; "What do you think your life will look like in 10 years if you were to make this decision?").

Making Functional Sense

Normalize Psychological Experiences

● Use coordination framing to turn disturbing or confusing psychological experiences into normal experiences of human life (e.g., "That's a normal reaction."; "Of course you feel sad!"; "Yes, it is hard.").

● Use conditional framing to link responses to historical and current context (e.g., "I can understand why you would think that based on the feedback you get at work."; "This response helped you avoid troubles when you were a child.").

● Use perspective taking to establish commonality (e.g., "I would feel that way too if I had been through these life experiences"; "Anyone who grew up around that much violence would be scared in that situation"; "If your best friend had lost her husband too, do you think she would be upset? Would that be understandable?").

Encourage the Assessment of Response Effectiveness

● Use conditional framing with consequences to assess the effectiveness of responses (e.g., "And when you do this, what impact does it have on . . . ?"; "Does that help?"; "What result did you get with this strategy so far?").

● Use comparative framing to assess the effectiveness of alternative options (e.g., "On the one hand, you can do [action A] and [consequence A] happens; on the other hand, you can do [action B] and [consequence B] happens. Which option works better for you?").

● Use hierarchical framing to connect responses to a higher purpose (e.g., "Is doing that a way of serving an important part of your life?"; "When you do that, do you feel connected to your values?").

Increasing Response Flexibility

Change the Context around the Source of Influence

- Alter the context with no additional framing (e.g., Word repetition, saying a thought out loud with another voice, with a different tone or pace).

- Use coordination framing to make psychological experiences compatible with meaningful actions (e.g., "You want to tell her you love her and you feel scared.").

- Use opposition framing to create a lighter context (e.g., Irreverence, humor: "What a great experience!"; "I see you are eager to do some exposure!"; "Who wouldn't want to feel so scared!").

- Use hierarchical framing to transform experience through labels and categories (e.g., "Interesting thought!"; "That's the kind of emotions we can feel in these situations.").

- Use analogical framing to import useful functions from other situations (e.g., Metaphors: "Try to imagine your thoughts as leaves on a stream."; "Let's surf on this emotional wave.").

- Use perspective taking to create distance (e.g., "If you heard what you said from somebody else, what would you think?"; "What will you think about this thought in 5 years?").

Change the Context around the Response

- Alter the context with no additional framing (e.g., Reflective listening, silences, changes of posture).

- Use coordination framing to evoke additional responses (e.g., "While you do [current response], can you also do [different response]?"; "And how does that make you feel, when you notice that you don't want to talk about . . . ?").

- Use distinction framing to evoke different responses (e.g., "What if we tried something different?").

- Use temporal/conditional framing to make the current source of influence a cue for a new response (e.g., "Every time [source of influence] appears, let's try to do something meaningful.").

- Use analogical framing to set a context for curiosity and playfulness (e.g., "Let's approach this as a game."; "Let's begin this journey together.").

Reinforcing Progress

Reinforce Step by Step[1]

- Use coordination framing to make positive qualities of action more salient (e.g., "That's great."; "Good for you!"; "That was a big step, don't you think?"; "It's nice to see you make progress.").

- Use distinction framing to differentiate effective responses from problematic responses (e.g., "I'm glad you tell me you are angry because I care about how you feel, but when you yell it is hard for me to listen to you."; "So, you were able to get up everyday. That's a great improvement, congratulations. Let's see if we can help you get out of your apartment a little bit next time. What do you think?"

- Use conditional and temporal framing to link action to desirable consequence (e.g., "So, it seems you felt closer to your partner as a result of listening to her. Is that right?"; "When you slow down, I understand you better.")

Reinforce Tracking over Pliance[2]

- Encourage the observation of benefits associated with new effective actions.
  - Use coordination framing to notice positive experiences (e.g., "What was that like to make this new step?"; "How does it feel to take the bus on your own now?").
  - Use conditional framing to notice desirable consequences (e.g., "What improvement did you notice as a result of going to sleep earlier?"; "What consequence did it have on your relationship when you decided to spend the holidays with your husband?"; "How is your health better as a result of quitting smoking?").
  - Use perspective taking to increase awareness of desirable consequences.
    - Interpersonal deictic framing (e.g., "What do you think that was like for your children to be hugged?"; "If you observed somebody else make this big effort, what would you like to tell them?").
    - Spatial deictic framing (e.g., "Imagine you had been there when your parents opened the card you sent them for Christmas. What do you think you would have seen?").
    - Temporal deictic framing (e.g., "If you look back in time since you've started to make these changes in your life, what improvement do you notice?").
- Encourage the checking of the correspondence between predicted and experienced contingency (antecedent → response → consequence).

---

[1] See also sections on performing and debriefing actions in "Fostering Meaning and Motivation."

[2] See also sections on "Observing, Describing, and Tracking."

○ Use analogical framing to compare expectations to actual experience (e.g., "Last week, you said you wanted to stick with your schedule to avoid procrastination. Did this plan work as you expected?"; "Last time, you decided you would go for a walk if you started to feel angry in order not to escalate arguments with your wife. Was that as helpful as you were hoping?").

○ Use perspective taking to assess the value of a rule, advice, or idea.

▪ Interpersonal deictic framing (e.g., "Would you give the same advice to your best friend in a similar situation, then?").

▪ Temporal deictic framing (e.g., "What would you say to the 'you' that thought it would be a good idea to start exercising again last month? You were right or you were wrong?").

Weakening Problematic Behaviors

Deliver and Orient to Undesirable Consequences

● Use coordination framing to make negative qualities of action more salient (e.g., "That might be problematic."; "I see how that could be hurtful.").

● Use conditional or temporal framing to link an action to an undesirable consequence (e.g., "When you withdraw, it becomes difficult for me to help you."; "Do you remember that your wife said you won't be able to see your daughter if you drink again? Would that be a problem for you?").

● Use perspective taking to increase awareness of undesirable consequences.

○ Interpersonal deictic framing (e.g., "How do you think you would feel if you were yelled at by your boss in front of your colleagues?").

○ Spatial deictic framing (e.g., "Imagine you had been at home when your wife received your harsh text on her phone. How do you think you would have seen her react?").

○ Temporal deictic framing (e.g., "Imagine that a year from now you are still avoiding seeing your parents. How do you think your relationship with them will be then?").

Block[3]

● Use coordination framing to maintain contact with relevant contexts ("What if we stuck with this topic for a moment?"; "I asked you a question earlier, and I think we got a bit off track. Do you mind if we come back to this question again?").

● Use distinction/opposition framing to redirect toward more useful contexts (e.g., "I suggest we don't try to solve this problem right now, and instead we slow down for a moment").

---

[3]See also the section on "Increasing Response Flexibility."

Extinguish

- Use nonverbal responses (e.g., Silence; no visual contact; facial expression that doesn't match the client's expectation).

- Use verbal responses (e.g., Changing the topic of conversation; responding while intentionally ignoring the client's problematic action).

BUILDING A FLEXIBLE SENSE OF SELF (CHAPTER 6)

Finding Variability in the Awareness of Experiences

Stabilize Perspective Taking

- Encourage the observation of self experiences in the here and now (e.g., "How do you feel now?"; "Do you feel like you are _____ [self-concept] with me right now?").

- Then, encourage the observation of changes and the variety of experiences.
  - Use distinction framing to draw attention to differences (e.g., "Is this the same or different now?"; "Do you notice changes or variations?").
  - Use comparison framing to explore differences along dimensions (e.g., "Are you feeling more tired now?"; "Are you in less pain at this moment?").

Shift Perspective Taking

- Encourage the observation of self experiences across a variety of contexts.
  - Use interpersonal deictic framing to explore different social contexts (e.g., "How do you feel when you are the leader of the group?"; "How do you feel when you are not in charge?"; "What are three typical adjectives that describe the way you are when your primary role is to be a father, a husband, a friend, a coworker?").
  - Use temporal deictic framing to explore different times (e.g., "How were you feeling this morning?"; "What do you think you will be experiencing in your body at the end of this long day of work?").
  - Use spatial deictic framing to explore different locations (e.g., "How do you feel when you are at home?"; "How do interact with others when you are around people you know?").

- Then, encourage the observation of changes and variety of experiences.
  - Use distinction framing to draw attention to differences (e.g., "Are you the same or different in these different situations? At these different moments?"; "Do you notice variations? Changes?").
  - Use comparison framing to explore differences along dimensions (e.g., "Do you feel more or less sad when you are in this different context?").

- Encourage observation of the same experience from different points of view.
  - Use interpersonal deictic framing to explore different social contexts (e.g., "If you were me and you heard what you are saying right now, what would you think/feel?").
  - Use temporal deictic framing to explore different times (e.g., "A year ago, what did you imagine you would be like today?"; "Tomorrow, remembering how you feel right now, what will you be thinking?").
  - Use spatial deictic framing to explore different locations (e.g., "Imagine you were sitting over there, watching yourself right here. What would you see?").
- Then, encourage observation of the transformed experience.
  - Use distinction framing to draw attention to differences (e.g., "When you look at this from another point of view, is this sensation the same or different?"; "Do you see yourself the same way or differently when you take these different points of view?").
  - Use comparison framing to explore differences along dimensions (e.g., "Do you feel more or less critical when you observe yourself from different moments?").

Finding Stability in Perspective Taking

Encourage the Observation of the Common Perspective-Taking Activity across Experiences

- Use coordination framing to draw attention to similarities (e.g., "What remains the same?"; "What doesn't change?"; "What is common across all these experiences?"; "Is there something you always do in these situations regardless of what you think and experience?").

Encourage the Observation of the Common Perspective-Taking Activity across Points of Views

- Use coordination framing to draw attention to similarities (e.g., "What is common across all these points of view?"; "Is there something you always do no matter where you stand?").

Finding Coherence in the Context

Emphasize the Hierarchical Dimension of the Self

- Use hierarchical framing between the self and the experience (e.g., "You were having the thought that you were stupid?"; "There is a part of you that doesn't feel comfortable here?"; "You're saying that one of the roles you have in your life is to be a mother.").
- Use analogical framing to make the hierarchical dimension of the self more concrete (e.g., "What if you were like the sky and your thoughts and sensations were like the weather?").

Emphasize the Distinction between the Self and the Experiences

- Use distinction framing between the self and the experiences (e.g., "If you can feel this sensation, then you are not this sensation, or at least not just this sensation, right? So, what is the part of you that is not this sensation?").

- Use coordination framing to redirect self-evaluations toward the experiences (e.g., "You said you were stupid. What did you do that you found stupid?"; "What kind of sensations do you feel when you are crushed?").

Finding Responsibility in the Interaction

Encourage the Observation of the Contextual Variables' Impact

- Use conditional framing to explore antecedents and history (e.g., "What do you think led you to act this way?"; "What happened just before?"; "What in your history might explain this reaction?").

- Use perspective taking to improve awareness of antecedents and history:

  ○ Interpersonal deictic framing (e.g., "If you were me, what would you think caused your behavior?"; "If your best friend reacted the same way, how would you explain it?").
  ○ Temporal deictic framing (e.g., "Remember when you were a kid and you had the same reaction in this kind of situation. What would you say was the cause of this reaction?").
  ○ Spatial deictic framing (e.g., "If you were in the audience listening to your own speech, what is the first thing you would think of that explains why your voice was shaking?").

Encourage Observation of the Behaviors' Impact

- Use conditional framing to explore action–consequence relationships (e.g., "What happens when you do _____?"; "How do you manage to do _____?"; "Is it hard? What do you do to make it anyway?").

- Use perspective taking to improve awareness of consequences.

  ○ Interpersonal deictic framing (e.g., "If your wife spoke to you the way you just spoke to her, how would you feel?").
  ○ Temporal deictic framing (e.g., "What do you think you will see a year from now, as you look back at what happened since you made this decision?").
  ○ Spatial deictic framing (e.g., "Imagine you are watching a movie that shows that whole day when you decided to get up and go to work. What consequences of getting up would you see in that movie?").

FOSTERING MEANING AND MOTIVATION (CHAPTER 7)

Building Life Meaning

Help Identify and Build Lasting Sources of Meaning (Qualities of Action and Overarching Goals)

- Explore sources of meaning.
  - ○ Encourage the derivation of lasting sources of meaning from specific actions and goals.
    - ▪ Use coordination framing to draw attention to similarities (e.g., "What do all of these actions/goals/interests have in common?").
    - ▪ Use distinction framing to draw attention to differences (e.g., "Why this goal and not another?").
    - ▪ Use comparative framing to explore differences along dimensions (e.g., "What about this action is more rewarding than that action?").
    - ▪ Use analogical framing to explore similar and different functions (e.g., "How is the purpose of this action similar/different from the function of this other action?").
    - ▪ Use conditional framing to identify function of actions and goals (e.g., "If you achieved that goal, how would your life be improved?").
    - ▪ Use hierarchical framing to identify higher purpose (e.g., "What is this action part of? What does it contribute to?").
  - ○ Encourage the reconnection with sources of meaning through perspective taking.
    - ▪ Use interpersonal deictic framing to explore different social contexts (e.g., "When you were holding your newborn baby, what did you wish for her?"; "If I asked your best friend what matters most to you, what would they say?"; "If you were [someone the client admires], how would your life be different?").
    - ▪ Use temporal deictic framing to explore different times (e.g., "When you were a kid, what did you imagine for yourself as an adult?"; "If you could time travel and visit yourself in 10 years, what would you want to see?"; "Take me back to a time in your life when you were most satisfied.").
  - ○ Encourage the creation of sources of meaning by exploring potential actions and goals.
    - ▪ Use conditional framing to encourage imagination (e.g., "What if anything were possible?"; "If you had a billion dollars to donate or invest, where would you put your money?").
    - ▪ Use conditional and comparative framing to encourage imagination through comparison (e.g., "If your life got bigger, what would you have room for?"; "If you had more time for yourself, what would you be doing?").

- Emphasize intrinsic reinforcement.
  - ○ Undermine pliance.
    - ▪ Use distinction/opposition framing to remove social influence (e.g., "If nobody knew you got this degree, would you still work toward getting it?"; "If no one was watching, what would you be doing?").
    - ▪ Use coordination framing to make social influence noncontingent (e.g., "If everybody loved you no matter what you chose, what would you want to do with your life?").
  - ○ Undermine the influence of external consequences and self-concepts.
    - ▪ Use distinction/opposition framing to remove outcomes (e.g., "If being nicer to your partner didn't make her want to spend more time with you, would you still want to be nice to her?").
    - ▪ Use coordination framing to make outcomes noncontingent (e.g., "If you could make a lot of money regardless of the job you did, what job would you choose?").
    - ▪ Use coordination framing to transform self-concepts into qualities of actions (e.g., "So, you would like to be a cool guy. How would you act as a cool guy?").
- Emphasize positive reinforcement.
  - ○ Use coordination framing to draw attention to added experiences (e.g., "What is positive about doing this action/reaching this goal?"; "Are there other things than relief that you experience when you do this action?"; "Are there things that are added to your experience?").
  - ○ Use opposition/distinction framing to remove sources of negative reinforcement (e.g., "In what ways would your life be better if that burden were removed?"; "What would you be doing if you were not bothered by this stuff?").
  - ○ Use analogical and opposition framing to import useful functions from other situations (e.g., "If pain was one side of a coin, what do you think you'd find if you flipped it over?").

Building Patterns of Meaningful Actions

- Encourage the connection between actions and the top of the hierarchy.
  - ○ Use hierarchical framing to derive parts from a whole (e.g., "What are the things you could do that would be part of living a life with [quality of action]?").
  - ○ Use conditional framing to identify steps toward broad qualities of action and overarching goals (e.g., "If you were being [quality of action], what would you be doing?"; "What is one action you could take now that would take you in the direction of that goal?").

○ Use perspective taking to increase awareness of potential actions.

■ Temporal deictic framing (e.g., "If you look back on your life a year from now, how will you know if you were living with compassion?").

■ Interpersonal deictic framing (e.g., "Who is the most patient person you know? What do they do that makes you admire their patience?").

● Help build variability at the base of the hierarchy.

○ Use coordination framing to discover a range of actions with a common higher function (e.g. "What other things could you do in the service of . . . ?"; "What else could you do that would still be part of . . . ?").

○ Use comparison framing to identify actions with various amplitudes (e.g., "Is there something you could do that takes 5 minutes rather than 1 day, and would still serve . . . ?"; "If you had less money, what could you do that serves the same purpose?").

○ Use distinction/opposition framing to discover alternative actions (e.g., "What would still be possible if you were sick and could not do . . . ?"; "How could you act with love toward your spouse even if you didn't feel loving?"; "If you were injured and couldn't go for a hike, what else could you do to connect with nature?").

Fostering Sustainable Motivation

Preparing Actions

● Help track and augment reinforcement.

○ Encourage the connection between future actions and sources of meaning.

■ Use hierarchical framing to connect a possible action to sources of meaning (e.g., "If you did that, what would it contribute to?"; "What would calling your mom be in the service of?"; "If that action were like adding a brick in the wall of a house you are building, what would this house be in your life?").

■ Use conditional framing to connect a possible action to a specific goal linked to an overarching goal (e.g., "If you do this action, will it be like taking a step closer to your goal? Which goal? Is this goal linked to something even bigger in your life?").

○ Encourage the connection between positive experiences and future actions.

■ Use coordination framing to draw attention to positive experiences (e.g., "What do you think it will be like to talk to your mom for the first time in 2 years?"; "What are some positive sensations you remember having the last time you spent some time with your husband?").

■ Use distinction/opposition framing to draw attention to differences (e.g., "What are some pleasant feelings you usually have when you share your feelings with your partner that you don't have when you keep them to yourself?").

- Use comparative framing to draw attention to differences along dimensions (e.g., "What do you hope to experience more at work if you change jobs?").
- Use analogical framing to import useful functions from other situations (e.g., "What picture or song might represent the way you feel when you hold your child in your arms?").
- Use deictic framing to explore different interpersonal, temporal, and spatial contexts (e.g., "What do you think your daughter will feel when you tell her you will be there for her soccer game?"; "What do you think you will feel at our next session if you come back telling me you have been to that job interview?").

- Exploring and overcoming barriers[4]

  ○ Encourage observation/description/tracking.
  ○ Encourage functional sense making.
  ○ Increase response flexibility by turning barriers into opportunities for action and into markers of progress (e.g., "What if the criticisms from your partner were an opportunity to enact compassion?"; "Perhaps your fear is a sign that you care about doing this?").

Performing Actions

- Help track and augment reinforcement.

  ○ Encourage the connection between current action and sources of meaning.
  - Use hierarchical framing to connect action to overarching goals and qualities of actions (e.g., "Can you tell me again why staying in contact with dirt without doing your ritual is important to you?").
  - Use conditional framing to connect action to goal steps linked to sources of meaning (e.g., "How is sharing your feelings with me now a step toward building intimacy with your wife?").

  ○ Encourage the connection between positive experiences and current actions.
  - Use coordination framing to draw attention to positive experiences (e.g., "What is it like to be doing something that matters to you right now?"; "What do you feel in your body?").
  - Use distinction/opposition framing to draw attention to differences (e.g., "What are some positive feelings you are having now that you didn't have a moment ago?").
  - Use comparative framing to draw attention to differences along

---

[4]See the section on similar skills in "Activating and Shaping Behavior Change."

dimensions (e.g., "Is there something you are feeling more than earlier?"; "Are the sensations you feel in your body more pleasant than before?").

- Use analogical framing to draw attention to useful functions from other situations (e.g., "If what you are feeling now were a picture or a song, what would that be?").

- Use deictic framing to explore different interpersonal, temporal, and spatial contexts (e.g., "In 2 hours from now, how do you think you will feel about having made this step?")

- Help overcome barriers.[5]

  ○ Encourage functional sense making.
  ○ Increase response flexibility by turning barriers into opportunities for action and into markers of progress (e.g., "What if this urge to argue were a signal to listen?"; "Only a person with a lot of [quality of action] would do [meaningful action] even though [barrier].").

Debriefing Actions

- Help track and augment reinforcement.

  ○ Encourage the connection between completed actions and sources of meaning.

    - Use hierarchical framing to connect actions to overarching goals and qualities of action (e.g., "What was calling for help instead of harming yourself in the service of?").

    - Use conditional framing to connect action to goal steps linked to sources of meaning (e.g., "What goal were you pursuing by doing this action? How is this goal connected to one of your values?").

  ○ Encourage the connection between positive experiences and completed action.

    - Use coordination framing to draw attention to positive experiences (e.g., "What was that like to tell your child you love him?"; "What sensations were you feeling when you were chatting with your friends?").

    - Use distinction/opposition framing to draw attention to differences (e.g., "What different experiences did you have while having this special moment for yourself?").

    - Use comparative framing to draw attention to differences along dimensions (e.g., "Was there any feeling or sensation that was more pleasant to have when you got up instead of staying in bed?").

---

[5]See the section on similar skills in "Activating and Shaping Behavior Change."

- Use analogical framing to import useful functions from other situations (e.g. "If the moment when you did that action were an episode of your favorite show, would it be a pleasant episode to watch?").
- Use deictic framing to explore different interpersonal, temporal, and spatial contexts (e.g., "If there was a picture of you while you were doing this action and we could look at it now, what facial expression would we see on your face?").

- Help overcome barriers.[6]
  - Encourage observation/description/tracking.
  - Encourage functional sense making.
  - Increase response flexibility by turning barriers into opportunities for action and into markers of progress (e.g., "You showed a lot of quality of action when you did [action] in the presence of [barrier]"; "That's like muscle soreness after lifting weights; a sign of gaining strength.").

---

[6]See the section on similar skills in "Activating and Shaping Behavior Change."

Practical Definitions of Terms Used in This Book

With this glossary we hope to get readers started by defining terms using relatively common-sense language. The definitions are meant to be practical in the context of this book, rather than the authoritative canon of RFT and contextual behavioral science concepts.

Adaptive peaks: Advantageous results of an adaptation that fails to provide a platform for beneficial future development. For example, parents might successfully punish a child when she has bad grades at school in order for her to have better results, but meanwhile, prevent her from developing a desire to learn that will last beyond school.

Analogical framing: Category of symbolic relational responses establishing the coordination or equivalence between two sets of relations. For example, in the sentence "Trying to deny your emotions is like trying to push a ball under water" there is a relation of equivalence between two conditional relationships ("if you deny your emotions, then they will come back" and "if you push a ball under the water, then it will come back").

Augmenting: Form of relational framing (i.e., language and cognition) leading to a new symbolic consequence, or to an alteration of the impact of an action's apparent consequence. The consequence can become more or less aversive, and more or less desirable. For example, telling oneself, "I will work late tonight so that I won't have to work this weekend and I will be able to relax" makes the consequence of working late more desirable. Connecting an action to a source of meaning is a form of augmenting (e.g., "I will spend the evening at home because it will contribute to building intimacy with my family").

Behavior: Anything a person does in response to the context—for example, eating when feeling hungry because doing so makes us less hungry. Behavior includes "mental actions" such as thinking, remembering, attending, feeling, perceiving, and sensing.

Coherence: A core property of language and cognition (i.e., relational framing) defined by the relative consistency of relational responses. Symbolic relations must be sufficiently consistent with each other within the same network to allow for mutual and combinatorial entailment to occur. For example, if the word "chair" is equivalent to an actual chair, and a cadeira is also equivalent to an actual chair (as it is in Brazil), then the word "cadeira" must be equivalent to the word "chair." Saying that the two words are not equivalent or that the actual chair is not a "chair" or a "cadeira" would be considered incoherent. Some degree of coherence is necessary in language because speakers and listeners must derive similar relations in order to understand each other (i.e., when the speaker says "chair" or "cadeira," the listener must be able to understand that these words mean an actual chair).

Combinatorial entailment: A core principle of relational framing according to which symbolic relations can be combined into networks. For example, if we learn that "silla" is the Spanish word for "chaise" in French, and that "chaise" is the equivalent of "chair" in English, then we can derive that "silla" means "chair." Combinatorial entailment can emerge from an infinite number of relations, as long as there are at least two established relations connecting at least three events.

Comparative framing: Category of symbolic relational responses establishing that an event is higher or lower than another or more events along a given dimension. For example, in the sentence, "The horse is bigger than the cat," "horse" and "cat" are in a relation of comparison according to their sizes.

Conditional framing: Category of symbolic relational responses establishing that an event conditions another or more events. For example, in the sentence, "If you open the window, it will be cooler in this room," opening the window and the temperature of the room are in a relation of condition.

Context: The historical and situational sources of influence on a person's behaviors, including biological, social, and cultural bases, development and learning history, and the person's current internal (cognitive and affective) and external environment. For example, a feeling of hunger that comes after several hours of not eating is a context likely to influence the behavior of eating.

Context sensitivity: The degree to which we notice and respond to the various elements of the context.

Contextual behavioral science: A modern holistic version of behavior analysis that is based on functional contextualism as a philosophy of science, relational frame theory as an approach to language and cognition, a reticulated development strategy rather than purely bottom up, and that views behavior analysis as part of modern evolution science.

Contextual cues: Elements of the context evoking relational responses or altering their features. Some cues can evoke a particular derived relation (called "Crel" for the "relational context" in RFT literature). For example, the cue "is" in the sentence, "The cat is black," evokes a relational response of coordination between cat and black. Other cues specify the functions relevant to transformation of stimulus functions (called "Cfunc" for the "functional context" in RFT literature)—for example, the cue "smell" in the sentence, "What does the flower smell like?"

Coordination framing: Category of symbolic relational responses establishing two or more events as coming together. This might be justified, for example, by their equivalence, similarity, or compatibility. For example, in the sentence, "The cat is black," "cat" and "black" are in a relation of coordination.

Deictic framing: Category of symbolic relational responses establishing that an event is in a relation of reference or perspective with another or more events. For example, in the sentence, "I am right here behind you; I can see you there," "I" and "you" are in a deictic relation (interpersonal perspective), as are "here" and "there" (spatial perspective).

Derivation: The production of a symbolic relation that has not been directly trained. For example, if we are told that "chaise" means "chair" and that "chaise" means "silla" (directly trained relations), we are able to derive that "silla" means "chair" (not directly trained relation).

Distinction framing: Category of symbolic relational responses establishing two or more events as different from each other. For example, in the sentence, "The cat is not black," "cat" and "black" are in a relation of distinction.

Essential coherence: A way of reaching coherence that is based on *intrinsic relations of equivalence* between symbolic relational networks and the claimed properties of events. Thus, in essential coherence, people consider that their concepts or ideas are coherent if they *intrinsically correspond to their experiences*. For example, a person who rejects gay marriage because "marriage *is defined* as the union between a man and a woman" is likely driven by essential coherence.

Experiential avoidance: Behavior aimed at reducing, removing, or escaping contact with unwanted feelings, emotions, or sensations. For example, a client drinks alcohol to reduce anxiety.

Experiential psychotherapy: Psychotherapy that emphasizes the use of techniques helping clients contact and observe their own experiences over the use of rules, didactics, and psycho-education.

Flexible sensitivity to the context: Capacity to notice various features of the context and to respond to what is most relevant. For example, a driver stopping at a crossroad even though the light is green because a child is standing in the middle of the road would show flexible sensitivity to the context.

Function: The function of a stimulus is its impact or effect on behavior. For example, a loud bell ringing may have the function of making one startle. The *symbolic* function of a stimulus can also be understood as the *meaning* of this stimulus due to relational framing. For example, the loud bell ringing could mean that class is over.

    The function of a behavior is the impact, or effect, it has on the context. For example, drinking alcohol can have the function of reducing anxiety.

Functional coherence: A way of reaching coherence that is primarily based on *relations of condition* between symbolic relational networks and the claimed properties of events. Thus, in functional coherence, people consider that their concepts or ideas are coherent if *their impact on experiences matches their goals*. For example, a person who uses a shoe's heel to hammer a nail is revealing functional coherence.

Functional contextualism: A pragmatic philosophy of science proposing that behavior (including the behavior of scientists) can only be understood in functional relation to its context, and setting out prediction and influence with precision, scope, and depth as its analytic goal.

Habituation: Decrease of a reflex response due to a prolonged or repeated exposure to the stimulus triggering this response (e.g., not startling anymore after hearing a loud noise several times).

Hierarchical framing: Category of symbolic relational responses establishing that an event is in a relation of hierarchy, inclusion, category, or attribution with another or more events. For example, in the sentence, "Cats belong to the family of felines," cats and felines are in a relation of hierarchy (category).

Inaccurate tracking: Following a rule in order to contact the consequences it specifies, while these consequences don't match actual experience. In this case, rule following is reinforced by other natural consequences not stated, or not clearly stated, by the rule. For example, a client drinks alcohol to improve his social life, and yet it actually hurts his relationships in the long term. The use of alcohol might be reinforced by the reduction in anxiety that immediately follows drinking. The difference between short-term and long-term consequences is not stated by the rule.

Inapplicable tracking: Attempting to follow a rule in order to contact the consequences it specifies when it is actually impossible to do so. In this case, rule following is reinforced by other natural consequences not stated, or not clearly stated, by the rule. For example, a client ruminates about a car accident she was involved in, wishing that she had not driven so fast and hoping for a different outcome (ruminating might be reinforced by a brief reduction of anxiety, but not by a change in what actually happened).

Intrinsic relations: Relations based on characteristics that are independent of the social context (e.g., a black cat and a black dog are in an intrinsic relation of similarity based on their color, which doesn't depend on social context). Some nonhuman animals are able to derive these types of relations.

Language and cognition: The learned behaviors of building and responding to symbolic relations among events. In RFT, these behaviors are synonyms of "relational framing."

Mutual entailment: A core principle of relational framing according to which a symbolic relation between two events must be bidirectional. This bidirectionality allows for the derivation of mutually entailed relations. For example, if we learn that "chaise" means "chair" in French, then we can derive that "chair" means "chaise" in English.

Operant learning: Learning under the influence of a history of actions in given situations being followed by given consequences (e.g., learning to avoid heights because doing so decreases fear).

Opposition framing: Category of symbolic relational responses establishing two or more events as opposed to each other, often along a dimension. For example, in the sentence, "I would like to go out but it is cold outside," going out and the temperature outside are in a relation of opposition; they are described as incompatible.

Pliance: Following a rule because there has been a history of others noting and rewarding the consistency between the action specified by the rule and the performed action. In pliance, social approval for following the rule per se is the primary source of reinforcement (e.g., stopping at a red light even when there is no other car around, *because that is what people are supposed to do*).

Relational frame theory: A contextual behavioral theory that approaches language and cognition as learned behaviors influenced by the context.

Relational framing: Building or deriving symbolic relations among events (i.e., language and cognition).

Relational learning: Learning under the influence of intrinsic or symbolic relations among events.

Respondent learning: Learning under the influence of pairing between stimuli (e.g., learning to fear cars after having had a car accident because car and pain have been associated).

Rule: Set of symbolic relations that specify conditional relationships between an action and its context (e.g., If you open the window, it will be cooler).

Social coherence: A way of reaching coherence that is based on relations of equivalence between symbolic relational networks and what is expected by the social community. Thus, in social coherence, people consider that their concepts or ideas are coherent if they *correspond to what is socially approved*. For example, a person who rejects gay marriage because "marriage between two persons of the same gender *is not the norm in our community*" is likely driven by social coherence.

Social learning: Learning under the influence of others' behavior (e.g., learning how to find the bathrooms in a restaurant by watching other customers open a door).

Symbolic generalization: Generalization of a stimulus function to another stimulus through the process of relational framing. For example, a child learns to fear ants because he is told that they are like spiders.

Symbolic relations: Relations not based solely on intrinsic characteristics of the events being related, but also on the context established by social convention and cues. For example, a physically smaller coin, like a dime, can be said to be larger in value than a physically bigger coin, like a nickel.

Tracking: (1) Following a rule because there has been a reinforcing history of contacting the consequences specified by this rule. For example, using the recipe of a delicious cake that actually allows you to make a delicious cake. (2) Observing and describing functional relationships among psychological events (e.g., noticing the consequence of a behavior; drawing out rules based on observation) that could then function as tracks in the first sense. For example, modifying a recipe after having used new ingredients that made the cake even more delicious.

Transfer of function: A stimulus function is considered transferred when its impact (i.e., effect, meaning) spreads to other stimuli. This can result from different contingency learning or relational learning processes. For example, the fear experienced while performing on stage may begin to appear when speaking to small groups or while being looked at by fellow bus passengers.

Transformation of function: A stimulus's function is considered transformed when its impact (i.e., effect, meaning) changes due to its involvement in relational framing. A tickling sensation that is experienced as pleasant while being teased by a friend can cause fear and disgust when imagining bugs crawling on the skin.

References

Ames, S. L., Grenard, J. L., Thush, C., Sussman, S., Wiers, R. W., & Stacy, A. W. (2007). Comparison of indirect assessments of association as predictors of marijuana use among at-risk adolescents. *Experimental and Clinical Psychopharmacology, 15*(2), 204–218.

Azrin, R. D., & Hayes, S. C. (1984). The discrimination of interest within a heterosexual interaction: Training, generalization, and effects on social skills. *Behavior Therapy, 15*, 173–184.

Barnes-Holmes, D., Barnes-Holmes, Y., Stewart, I., & Boles, S. (2010). A sketch of the implicit relational assessment procedure (IRAP) and the relational elaboration and coherence (REC) model. *The Psychological Record, 60*(3), 527–542.

Barnes-Holmes, D., Waldron, D., Barnes-Holmes, Y., & Stewart, I. (2009). Testing the validity of the Implicit Relational Assessment Procedure (IRAP) and the Implicit Association Test (IAT): Measuring attitudes towards Dublin and country life in Ireland. *The Psychological Record, 59*, 389–406.

Barnes-Holmes, Y., McHugh, L., & Barnes-Holmes, D. (2004). Perspective-taking and theory of mind: A relational frame account. *The Behavior Analyst Today, 5*, 15–25.

Bennett-Levy, J., Westbrook, D., Fennell, M., Cooper, M., Rouf, K., & Hackmann, A. (2004). Behavioural experiments: Historical and conceptual underpinnings. In J. Bennett-Levy, G. Butler, M. Fennell, A. Hackmann, M. Mueller, & D. Westbrook (Eds.), *Oxford guide to behavioural experiments in cognitive therapy* (pp. 1–20). Oxford, UK: Oxford University Press.

Bernstein, I. L. (2000). Taste aversion learning. In A. E. Kazdin (Ed.), *Encyclopedia of psychology* (Vol. 8, pp. 11–13). New York: Oxford University Press.

Bushman, B. J., Baumeister, R. F., Thomaes, S., Ryu, E., Begeer, S. & West, S. G. (2009). Looking again, and harder, for a link between low self-esteem and aggression. *Journal of Personality, 77*, 1467–6494.

Carpenter, K. M., Martinez, D., Vadhan, N. P., Barnes-Holmes, D., & Nunes, E.

V. (2012). Measures of attentional bias and relational responding are associated with behavioral treatment outcome for cocaine dependence. *American Journal of Drug and Alcohol Abuse, 38*(2), 146–154.

Cassidy, S., Roche, B., & Hayes, S. C. (2011). A relational frame training intervention to raise Intelligence Quotients: A pilot study. *The Psychological Record, 61*, 173–198.

Catchpole, C. K., & Slater, B. J. B. (1995). *Bird-song: Biological themes and variations.* Cambridge, UK: Cambridge University Press.

Cherner, R. A., & Reissing, E. D. (2013). A psychophysiological investigation of sexual arousal in women with lifelong vaginismus. *Journal of Sexual Medicine, 10*(5), 1291–1303.

Craske, M. G., Kircanski, K., Zelikowsky, M., Mystkowski, J., & Baker, A. (2008). Optimizing inhibitory learning during exposure therapy. *Behaviour Research and Therapy, 46*, 5–27.

Dahl, J. C., Plumb, J. C., Stewart, I., & Lundgren, T. (2009). *The art and science of valuing in psychotherapy: Helping clients discover, explore, and commit to valued action using acceptance and commitment therapy.* Oakland, CA: New Harbinger.

Dawson, D. L., Barnes-Holmes, D., Gresswell, D. M., Hart, A. J., & Gore, N. J. (2009). Assessing the implicit beliefs of sexual offenders using the implicit relational assessment procedure: A first study. *Sexual Abuse: Journal of Research and Treatment, 21*(1), 57–75.

Deacon, T. W. (1998). *The symbolic species: The co-evolution of language and the brain.* New York: Norton.

Devany, J. M., Hayes, S. C., & Nelson, R. O. (1986). Equivalence class formation in language-able and language-disabled children. *Journal of the Experimental Analysis of Behavior, 46*, 243–257.

Dollard, J., & Miller, N. E. (1950). *Personality and psychotherapy: An analysis in terms of learning, thinking, and culture.* New York: McGraw-Hill.

Dougher, M. J., Hamilton, D., Fink, B., & Harrington, J. (2007). Transformation of the discriminative and eliciting functions of generalized relational stimuli. *Journal of the Experimental Analysis of Behavior, 88*(2), 179–197.

Dymond, S., & Barnes, D. (1995). A transformation of self-discrimination response functions in accordance with the arbitrarily applicable relations of sameness, more-than, and less-than. *Journal of the Experimental Analysis of Behavior, 64*, 163–184.

Dymond, S., & Barnes, D. (1996). A transformation of self-discrimination response functions in accordance with the arbitrarily applicable relations of sameness and opposition. *The Psychological Record, 46*(2), 271–300.

Dymond, S., May, R. J., Munnelly, A., & Hoon, A. E. (2010). Evaluating the evidence based for relational frame theory: A citation analysis. *The Behavior Analyst, 33*, 97–117.

Dymond, S., & Roche, B. (Eds.). (2013). *Advances in relational frame theory: Research and application.* Oakland, CA: New Harbinger.

Dymond, S., Roche, B., Forsyth, J. P., Whelan, R., & Rhoden, J. (2007). Transformation of avoidance response functions in accordance with same and opposite relational frames. *Journal of the Experimental Analysis of Behavior, 88*, 249–262.

Ecker, B., Ticic, R., & Hulley, L. (2012). *Unlocking the emotional mind: Eliminating symptoms at their roots using memory reconsolidation.* New York: Routledge.

Foody, M., Barnes-Holmes, Y., Barnes-Holmes, D., & Luciano, C. (2013). An empirical investigation of hierarchical versus distinction relations in a self-based ACT exercise. *International Journal of Psychology and Psychological Therapy, 13,* 373–388.

Foody, M., Barnes-Holmes, Y., Barnes-Holmes, D., Torneke, N., Luciano, C., Stewart, I., et al. (2015). RFT for clinical use: The example of metaphor. *Journal of Contextual Behavioral Science, 3,* 305–313.

Frankl, V. E. (1984). *Man's search for meaning.* New York: Washington Square Press.

Gallagher, M. W., & Resick, P. A. (2012). Mechanisms of change in cognitive processing therapy and prolonged exposure therapy for PTSD: Preliminary evidence for the differential effects of hopelessness and habituation. *Cognitive Therapy and Research, 36*(6), 750–755.

Gawronski, B., & de Houwer, J. (2014). Implicit measures in social and personality psychology. In H. T. Reis & C. M. Judd (Eds.), *Handbook of research methods in social and personality psychology* (pp. 283–310). New York: Cambridge University Press.

Ginsberg, S., & Jablonka, E. (2010). The evolution of associative learning: A factor in the Cambrian explosion. *Journal of Theoretical Biology, 266,* 11–20.

Greenwald, A. G., McGhee, D. E., & Schwartz, J. K. (1998). Measuring individual differences in implicit cognition: The implicit association test. *Journal of Personality and Social Psychology, 74*(6), 1464–1480.

Harris, J. D. (1943). Habituatory response decrement in the intact organism. *Psychology Bulletin, 40,* 385–422.

Hayes, S. C. (1984). Making sense of spirituality. *Behaviorism, 12,* 99–110.

Hayes, S. C. (Ed.). (1989). *Rule-governed behavior: Cognition, contingencies, and instructional control.* New York: Plenum Press.

Hayes, S. C. (2009). *Acceptance and commitment therapy.* Videotape available from the American Psychological Association, Washington, DC.

Hayes, S. C., Barnes-Holmes, D., & Roche, B. (Eds.). (2001). *Relational frame theory: A post-Skinnerian account of human language and cognition.* New York: Plenum Press.

Hayes, S. C., Barnes-Holmes, D., & Wilson, K. G. (2012). Contextual behavioral science: Creating a science more adequate to the challenge of the human condition. *Journal of Contextual Behavioral Science, 1,* 1–16.

Hayes, S. C., Bissett, R., Roget, N., Padilla, M., Kohlenberg, B. S., Fisher, G., et al. (2004). The impact of acceptance and commitment training and multicultural training on the stigmatizing attitudes and professional burnout of substance abuse counselors. *Behavior Therapy, 35,* 821–835.

Hayes, S. C., Brownstein, A. J., Zettle, R. D., Rosenfarb, I., & Korn, Z. (1986). Rule-governed behavior and sensitivity to changing consequences of responding. *Journal of the Experimental Analysis of Behavior, 45,* 237–256.

Hayes, S. C., & Sanford, B. (2014). Cooperation came first: Evolution and human cognition. *Journal of the Experimental Analysis of Behavior, 101,* 112–129.

Hayes, S. C., Strosahl, K., & Wilson, K. G. (1999). *Acceptance and commitment therapy: An experiential approach to behavior change*. New York: Guilford Press.

Hayes, S. C., Strosahl, K., & Wilson, K. G. (2012). *Acceptance and commitment therapy: The process and practice of mindful change* (2nd ed.). New York: Guilford Press.

Hayes, S. C., Villatte, M., Levin, M., & Hildebrandt, M. (2011). Open, aware, and active: Contextual approaches as an emerging trend in the behavioral and cognitive therapies. *Annual Review of Clinical Psychology, 7*, 141–168.

Hesser, H., Westin, V., Hayes, S. C., & Andersson, G. (2009). Clients' in-session acceptance and cognitive defusion behaviors in acceptance-based treatment of tinnitus distress. *Behaviour Research and Therapy, 47*, 523–528.

Hildebrandt, M. J., Fletcher, L. B., & Hayes, S. C. (2007). Climbing anxiety mountain: Generating metaphors in acceptance and commitment therapy. In G. W. Burns (Ed.), *Healing with stories: Your casebook collection for using therapeutic metaphors* (pp. 55–64). Hoboken, NJ: Wiley.

Hollon, S. D., & Beck, A. T. (1979). Cognitive therapy of depression. In P. C. Kendall & S. D. Barlow (Eds.), *Cognitive-behavioral intervention: Theory, research, and procedures* (pp. 153–203). New York: Academic Press.

Hooper, N., Saunders, S., & McHugh, L. (2010). The derived generalization of thought suppression. *Learning and Behavior, 38*(2), 160–168.

Hooper, N., Villatte, M., Neofotistou, E., & McHugh, L. (2010). The effects of mindfulness versus thought suppression on implicit and explicit measures of experiential avoidance. *International Journal of Behavioral Consultation and Therapy, 6*(3), 233–244.

Hughes, S., Barnes-Holmes, D., & Vahey, N. (2012). Holding on to our functional roots when exploring new intellectual islands: A voyage through implicit cognition research. *Journal of Contextual Behavioral Science, 1*, 17–38.

Hussey, I., & Barnes-Holmes, D. (2012). The Implicit Relational Assessment Procedure as a measure of implicit depression and the role of psychological flexibility. *Cognitive and Behavioral Practice, 19*(4), 573–582.

Jackson, M. L., Williams, W. L., Hayes, S. C., Humphreys, T., Gauthier, B., & Westwood, R. (in press). Whatever gets your heart pumping: Using implicit measures to select motivative exercise statements. *Journal of Contextual Behavioral Science.*

Ju, W. C., & Hayes, S. C. (2008). Verbal establishing stimuli: Testing the motivative effect of stimuli in a derived relation with consequences. *The Psychological Record, 58*, 339–363.

Kashdan, T. B., Barrios, V., Forsyth, J. P., & Steger, M. F. (2006). Experiential avoidance as a generalized psychological vulnerability: Comparisons with coping and emotion regulation strategies. *Behaviour Research and Therapy, 9*, 1301–1320.

Kelly, G. A. (1955). *The psychology of personal constructs*. New York: Norton.

Kircanski, K., Lieberman, M. D., & Craske, M. G. (2012). Feelings into words: Contributions of language to exposure therapy. *Psychological Science, 23*, 1086–1091.

Kishita, N., Ohtsuki, T., & Stewart, I. (2013). The Training and Assessment of

Relational Precursors and Abilities (TARPA): A follow-up study with typically developing children. *Journal of Contextual Behavioral Science, 2,* 15–21.

Koerner, K. (2011). *Doing dialectical behavior therapy: A practical guide.* New York: Guilford Press.

Kohlenberg, R. J., & Tsai, M. (1991). *Functional analytic psychotherapy.* New York: Plenum Press.

Kohut, H. (2009). *The analysis of the self: A systematic approach to the psychoanalytic treatment of narcissistic personality disorders.* Chicago: University of Chicago Press. (Original work published 1971)

Levin, M., Hayes, S. C., & Waltz, T. (2010). Creating an implicit measure of cognition more suited to applied research: A test of the Mixed Trial–Implicit Relational Assessment Procedure (MT-IRAP). *International Journal of Behavioral Consultation and Therapy, 6,* 245–262.

Levin, M. E., Luoma, J., Vilardaga, R., Lillis, J., Nobles, R., & Hayes, S. C. (under review). *Examining the role of psychological inflexibility, perspective taking and empathic concern in generalized prejudice.*

Linehan, M. M. (1993). *Cognitive-behavioral treatment of borderline personality disorder.* New York: Guilford Press.

Lipkens, G., & Hayes, S. C. (2009). Producing and recognizing analogical relations. *Journal of the Experimental Analysis of Behavior, 91,* 105–126.

Luciano, C., Ruiz, F. J., Torres, R. M. V., Martín, V. S., Martínez, O. G., & López, J. C. (2011). A relational frame analysis of defusion interactions in acceptance and commitment therapy: A preliminary and quasi-experimental study with at-risk adolescents. *International Journal of Psychology and Psychological Therapy, 11,* 165–182.

Luciano, M. C., Rodríguez Valverde, M., & Gutiérrez Martínez, O. (2004). A proposal for synthesizing verbal contexts in experiential avoidance disorder and acceptance and commitment therapy. *International Journal of Psychology and Psychological Therapy, 4,* 377–394.

Maslow, A. H. (1966). *The psychology of science: A reconnaissance.* New York: Harper & Row.

Masuda, A., Hayes, S. C., Twohig, M. P., Drossel, C., Lillis, J., & Washio, Y. (2009). A parametric study of cognitive defusion and the believability and discomfort of negative self-relevant thoughts. *Behavior Modification, 33,* 250–262.

McCurry, S., & Hayes, S. C. (1992). Clinical and experimental perspectives on metaphorical talk. *Clinical Psychology Review, 12,* 763–785.

McDougall, I., Brown, F. H., & Fleagle, J. G. (2005). Stratigraphic placement and age of modern humans from Kibish, Ethiopia. *Nature, 433,* 733–736.

McHugh, L., Barnes-Holmes, Y., & Barnes-Holmes, D. (2004). Perspective-taking as relational responding: A developmental profile. *The Psychological Record, 54,* 115–144.

McHugh, L., & Stewart, I. (2012). *The self and perspective taking: Contributions and applications from modern behavioral science.* Oakland, CA: New Harbinger.

McMullen, J., Barnes-Holmes, D., Barnes-Holmes, Y., Stewart, I., Luciano, M.

C., & Cochrane, A. (2008). Acceptance versus distraction: Brief instructions, metaphors and exercises in increasing tolerance for self-delivered electric shocks. *Behaviour Research and Therapy, 46*(1), 122–129.

Miller, W. R., & Rollnick, S. (1991). *Motivational interviewing: Preparing people to change addictive behavior.* New York: Guilford Press.

Monestès, J. L., & Villatte, M. (2011). *La thérapie d'acceptation et d'engagement ACT.* Paris: Elsevier Masson.

Monestès, J. L., & Villatte, M. (2015). Humans are the selection criterion in psychological science, not "reality": A reply to Herbert and Padovani. *Journal of Contextual Behavioral Science, 4*, 210–211.

Mowrer, O. H. (1948). Learning theory and the neurotic paradox. *American Journal of Orthopsychiatry, 18*, 571–610.

Mowrer, O. H. (1950). *Learning theory and personality dynamics.* New York: Ronald Press.

Nezu, M., Nezu, C., & D'Zurilla, T. J. (2013). *Problem-solving therapy: A treatment manual.* New York: Springer.

Nichols, J. (1992). *Linguistic diversity in space and time.* Chicago: University of Chicago Press.

Nicholson, E., & Barnes- Holmes, D. (2012). The Implicit Relational Assessment Procedure (IRAP) as a measure of spider fear. *The Psychological Record, 62*(2), 263–277.

Nilsonne, G., Appelgren, A., Axelsson, J., Fredrikson, M., & Lekander, M. (2011). Learning in a simple biological system: A pilot study of classical conditioning of human macrophages *in vitro. Behavioral and Brain Function, 7*, 47.

Nowak, M. A., Tarnita, C. E., & Wilson, O. (2010). The evolution of eusociality. *Nature, 466*, 1057–1062.

O'Hora, D., Barnes-Holmes, D., Roche, B., & Smeets, P. M. (2004). Derived relational networks and control by novel instructions: A possible model of generative verbal responding. *The Psychological Record, 54*, 437–460.

O'Hora, D., Pelaez, M., Barnes-Holmes, D., & Amesty, L. (2005). Derived relational responding and human language: Evidence from the WAIS-III. *The Psychological Record, 55*, 155–174.

O'Hora, D., Roche, B., Barnes-Holmes, D., & Smeets, P. M. (2002). Response latencies to multiple derived stimulus relations: Testing two predictions of relational frame theory. *The Psychological Record, 52*, 51–76.

O'Toole, C., & Barnes-Holmes, D. (2009). Three chronometric indices of relational responding as predictors of performance on a brief intelligence test: The importance of relational flexibility. *The Psychological Record, 59*, 119–132.

O'Toole, C., Barnes-Holmes, D., Murphy, C., O'Connor, J., & Barnes-Holmes, Y. (2009). Relational flexibility and human intelligence: Extending the remit of Skinner's Verbal Behavior. *International Journal of Psychology and Psychological Therapy, 9*(1), 1–17.

Penn, D. C., Holyoak, K. J., & Povinelli, D. J. (2008). Darwin's mistake: Explaining the discontinuity between human and nonhuman minds. *Behavioral and Brain Sciences, 31*, 109–178.

Penton-Voak, I. S., Thomas, J., Gage, S. H., McMurran, M., McDonald, S., & Munafò, M. R. (2013). Increasing recognition of happiness in ambiguous facial expressions reduces anger and aggressive behavior. *Psychological Science, 24*(5), 688–697.

Plassmann, J., O'Doherty, Shiv, B., & Rangel, A. (2007). Marketing actions can modulate neural representations of experienced pleasantness. *Proceedings of the National Academy of Sciences of the USA, 105,* 1050–1054.

Quinones, J., & Hayes, S. C. (2014). Relational coherence in ambiguous and unambiguous relational networks. *Journal of the Experimental Analysis of Behavior, 101,* 76–93.

Ramnero, J., & Törneke, N. (2008).*The ABCs of human behavior: Behavioral principles for the practicing clinician.* Oakland, CA: Context Press/New Harbinger.

Ray, E., & Heyes, C. (2011). Imitation in infancy: The wealth of the stimulus. *Developmental Science, 14,* 1467–1487.

Reese, H. W. (1968). *The perception of stimulus relations: Discrimination learning and transposition.* New York: Academic Press.

Rehfeldt, R. A., & Barnes-Holmes, Y. (2009). *Derived relational responding: Applications for learners with autism and other developmental disabilities.* Oakland, CA: New Harbinger.

Rehfeldt, R. A., Dillen, J. E., Ziomek, M. M., & Kowalchuk, R. K. (2007). Assessing relational learning deficits in perspective-taking in children with high functioning autism spectrum disorder. *The Psychological Record, 57,* 23–47.

Rogers, C. (1951). *Client-centered therapy: Its current practice, implications and theory.* London: Constable.

Rosen, S. (1991). *My voice will go with you: The teaching tales of Milton H. Erickson.* New York: Norton.

Rosenberg, M. (2003). *Non-violent communication: A language of life.* Encinitas, CA: Puddle Dancer Press.

Ruiz, R. J., & Luciano, C. (2015). Common physical properties among relational networks improve analogy aptness. *Journal of the Experimental Analysis of Behavior, 9999,* 1–13.

Sheldon, K. M., Ryan, R. M., Deci, E. L., & Kasser, T. (2004). The independent effects of goal contents and motives on well-being: It's both what you pursue and why you pursue it. *Personality and Social Psychology Bulletin, 30,* 475–486.

Skinner, B. F. (1974). *About behaviorism.* New York: Knopf.

Slattery, B., & Stewart, I. (2014). Hierarchical classification as relational framing. *Journal of the Experimental Analysis of Behavior, 101,* 61–75.

Smith, G. S. (2013). *Exploring the predictive utility of the Implicit Relational Assessment Procedure (IRAP) with respect to performance in organizations.* Unpublished doctoral dissertation, University of Nevada, Reno.

Stewart, I., Barnes-Holmes, D., & Roche, B. (2004). A functional-analytic model of analogy using the relational evaluation procedure. *The Psychological Record, 54,* 531–552.

Stewart, I., Hooper, N., Walsh, P., O'Keefe, R., Joyce, R., & McHugh, L. (2015). Transformation of thought suppression functions via same and opposite relations. *The Psychological Record, 65*(2), 375–399.

Thompson, R. F. (2009). Habituation: A history. *Neurobiology of Learning and Memory, 92*(2), 127–134.

Törneke, N. (2010). *Learning RFT: An introduction to relational frame theory and its clinical applications.* Oakland, CA: New Harbinger.

Troy, A. S., Shallcross, A. J., & Mauss, I. B. (2013). A person-by-situation approach to emotion regulation: Cognitive reappraisal can either help or hurt, depending on the context. *Psychological Science, 24*(12), 2505–2514.

Vilardaga, R., Estévez, A., Levin, M. E., & Hayes, S. C. (2012). Deictic relational responding, empathy and experiential avoidance as predictors of social anhedonia in college students. *The Psychological Record, 62*, 409–432.

Vilardaga, R., & Hayes, S. C. (2010). Acceptance and commitment therapy and the therapeutic relationship stance. *European Psychotherapy, 9*, 117–139.

Villatte, J. L., Villatte, M., & Hayes, S. C. (2012). A naturalistic approach to transcendence: Deictic framing, spirituality, and pro-sociality. In L. McHugh & I. Stewart (Eds.), *The self and perspective-taking: Contributions and applications from modern behavioral science* (pp. 199–216). Oakland, CA: New Harbinger.

Villatte, M., Monestès, J. L., McHugh, L., Freixa i Baqué, E., & Loas, G. (2008). Assessing deictic relational responding in social anhedonia: A functional approach to the development of theory of mind impairments. *International Journal of Behavioral Consultation and Therapy, 4*(4), 360–373.

Villatte, M., Monestès, J. L., McHugh, L., Freixa i Baqué, E., & Loas, G. (2010a). Adopting the perspective of another in belief attribution: Contribution of relational frame theory to the understanding of impairments in schizophrenia. *Journal of Behavior Therapy and Experimental Psychiatry, 41*, 125–134.

Villatte, M., Monestès, J. L., McHugh, L., Freixa i Baqué, E., & Loas, G. (2010b). Assessing perspective taking in schizophrenia using relational frame theory. *The Psychological Record, 60*, 413–424.

Wegner, D. M. (1989). *White bears and other unwanted thoughts: Suppression, obsession, and the psychology of mental control.* New York: Viking/Penguin.

Weil, T. M., Hayes, S. C., & Capurro, P. (2011). Establishing a deictic relational repertoire in young children. *The Psychological Record, 61*, 371–390.

White, M. (2007). *Maps of narrative practice.* New York: Norton.

Wilson, D. S., Hayes, S. C., Biglan, T., & Embry, D. (2014). Evolving the future: Toward a science of intentional change. *Behavioral and Brain Sciences, 34*, 1–22.

Wilson, D. S., & Wilson, E. O. (2007). Rethinking the theoretical foundation of sociobiology. *Quarterly Review of Biology, 82*, 327–348.

Wilson, K. G., & DuFrene, T. (2009). *Mindfulness for two: An acceptance and commitment therapy approach to mindfulness in psychotherapy.* Oakland, CA: New Harbinger.

Zettle, R., Hayes, S. C., Barnes-Homes, D., & Biglan, A. (2016). *Handbook of contextual behavioral science.* Chichester, UK: Wiley-Blackwell.

Index

Note: *f* following a page number indicates a figure; *n* indicates a footnote.

Page numbers in index entries reflect places in the text where concepts and terms are discussed substantively. The index is not meant to be an exhaustive list of all text mentions of terms